DISEASE AND SOCIETY IN PREMODERN ENGLAND

Disease and Society in Premodern England examines the impact of infectious disease in England from the everyday to pandemics in the period c. 500–c. 1600, with the major focus from the eleventh century onward.

Theilmann blends historical research, using a variety of primary sources, with an understanding of disease drawn from current scientific literature to enable a better understanding of how diseases affected society and why they were so difficult to combat in the premodern world. The volume provides a perspective on how society and medicine reacted to "new" diseases, something that remains an issue in the twenty-first century. The "new" diseases of the Late Middle Ages, such as plague, syphilis, and the English Sweat, are viewed as helping to lead to a change in how people viewed disease causation and treatment. In addition to the biology of disease and its relationship with environmental factors, the social, economic, political, religious, and artistic impacts of various diseases are also explored.

With discussions on a variety of diseases including leprosy, tuberculosis, malaria, measles, typhus, influenza, and smallpox, this volume is an essential resource for all students and scholars interested in the history of medicine and disease in premodern England.

John Theilmann is Andrew Helmus Distinguished Professor of History and Politics at Converse University. He has published several articles and book chapters dealing with topics in medieval history and the history of diseases, and a book and several articles in political science dealing with congressional elections.

DISEASE AND SOCIETY IN PREMODERN ENGLAND

John Theilmann

Routledge
Taylor & Francis Group

LONDON AND NEW YORK

Cover credit: Dance of Death. Allegory of universality of the death.
Colored engraving, 14th century © Lanmas/Alamy Stock Photo

First published 2022
by Routledge
2 Park Square, Milton Park, Abingdon, Oxon OX14 4RN

and by Routledge
605 Third Avenue, New York, NY 10158

Routledge is an imprint of the Taylor & Francis Group, an informa business

British Library Cataloguing-in-Publication Data
A catalogue record for this book is available from the British Library

Library of Congress Cataloging-in-Publication Data
A catalog record has been requested for this book

ISBN: 978-1-032-10412-6 (hbk)
ISBN: 978-1-032-10413-3 (pbk)
ISBN: 978-1-003-21521-9 (ebk)

DOI: 10.4324/9781003215219

Typeset in Bembo
by KnowledgeWorks Global Ltd.

CONTENTS

TABLES

ACKNOWLEDGEMENTS

Converse University contributed to this work with a sabbatical leave and a summer research grant. One of the pleasures of teaching at, until recently, a liberal arts college for women has been the chance to engage in research work with superior students who went on to further study in medicine, veterinary medicine, mathematics, public health, epidemiology, and music. Thank you, Frances Cate, Jennifer Jones, Stacy Thrall, Whitney Weeks†, Lindsey Eller, Abigail Sweet, Zoe Kushubar, and Isabel Fangman for stimulating conversation, good ideas, and some laughs along the way. Several aspects of this work have been presented at conferences, most notably the Southern Association for the History of Medicine and Southeastern Medieval Association. Thanks to other attendees for helpful comments and questions. A long lunchtime conversation with Ann Carmichael came at the right time for causing me to rethink some points. I've also engaged in several thought-provoking conversations with Dr. James Thompson

SHORT TITLES

BHM *Bulletin of the History of Medicine*
Creighton, *Epidemics* Charles Creighton, *A History of Epidemics in Britain*, 2 vols., 2d ed. (London: Frank Cass, 1965, 1894)
EconHstRev *Economic History Review*
EETS Early English Text Society
Fracastoro, *Contagion* Girolamo Fracastoro, *De contagion et contagiosis morbis et eorum curatione, libre III*, Wilmer Cave Wright, trans. (New York: G.P. Putnam's Sons, 1930, 1546)
JHM *Journal of the History of Medicine and Allied Sciences*
PNAS *Proceedings of the National Academy of Sciences*
PRHS *Proceedings of the Royal Historical Society*
Riley, *Memorials of London* H.T. Riley, ed. and trans., *Memorials of London and London Life in the XIIIth, XIVth, and XVth* Centuries (London: Longmans, 1868)
Slack, *Impact of Plague* Paul Slack, *The Impact of Plague in Tudor and Stuart England* (Oxford: Clarendon Press, 1985)

INTRODUCTION

Infectious disease has always been part of human life. Dating from the nine-teenth century, society became better able to deal with the threat of disease. Today we are able to control several diseases with preventative measures and treatment and one, smallpox, has been eradicated as a threat to human health. Several commentators writing in the 1970s argued that epidemic disease would soon be a thing of the past; humans only had to fear chronic diseases such as heart disease or cancer. From the perspective of the early twenty-first century with COVID-19, Ebola, or SARS this argument seems to be incredibly naive and misleading. Anyone writing in premodern England (c. 500 to c. 1600) would not have been so optimistic. Chronic disease was a problem, but many people died long before heart disease or cancer would take their toll. Everyday medical problems such as infections or diarrhea were magnified in the pre-antibiotic era and often killed. Violence and accidents also claimed their vic-tims. Epidemic disease, however, could kill large numbers of people, often in a very short period of time.

This study examines the impact of disease on premodern England as well as the measures that society took to try to combat disease. Disease did not occur in a vacuum, and attention will be paid to factors that influenced the severity and overall impact of diseases, most notably, climate change, famine, human action such as the medical response to disease, or population movement. Diseases also had a variety of impacts on premodern society. High mortality rates, especially when concentrated in short periods of time, affected population size and eco-nomic growth and may have contributed to other medical issues. High mortality rates, especially those associated with the Black Death, may well have had a psychological impact that affected society. Even everyday health problems sapped peoples' strength, decreased productivity, and often contributed to high child mortality rates.

DOI: 10.4324/9781003215219-1

The history of disease is not the history of medicine although the two subjects overlap in many ways. The history of medicine examines theories of how diseases are caused and how they are treated. Often it is intellectual history with the focus on learned practitioners and their writings, in part because information about less well-educated practitioners is often scarce. Understanding contemporary medical theory is an important aspect in understanding the impact of diseases in the past. The history of disease goes further as the impact that disease has on people's lives and on society is an important part of its study, as is examining long-term trends that may arise from outbreaks of epidemic disease. Understanding the biology of agents of disease, the progression of disease, and symptoms are also crucial to comprehending the impact of particular diseases. This biological understanding also enables scholars to compare disease outbreaks over time.

Disease and its impact

How people view disease has changed over time. Dating from the late nineteenth century, many medical commentators emphasized the biological reality of each disease, often concentrating on the agent of disease and the symptoms. In this view, usually labeled the ontological approach, disease is seen as a specific entity, and treatment is directed toward controlling the disease rather than treating the patient. The social construction of disease can be seen as a counter to this approach in which diseases are seen as being defined by society at the time based on how a victim reacts to a disease and how society views this reaction. In reality, disease is all this and more. Some diseases are defined by society as when a person's symptoms render them unable to perform daily tasks. Biology is also important as diseases have causes and understanding the causes and the progression of a disease provides a better understanding of how a disease affects individuals and ultimately society. Premodern people assigned causes to diseases and tried to treat the symptoms which were sometimes seen as diseases themselves. One approach to the history of disease would be to simply describe how premodern people tried to explain disease within their worldview, and how disease affected society without any reference to more recent scientific knowledge. Bringing biology into the picture enables comparison of a disease over time as well as yielding a better understanding of how a disease would come to affect society as well as its progression. In sum, understanding disease in the past requires a multi-faceted approach that blends scientific reasoning and historical understanding.

The impact of various diseases has been varied with some causing great loss of life in a short period of time and others causing ongoing problems or death for some individuals. Magnitude is important. A disease such as the plague produced such a profound impact that some commentators almost seemed to lose hope. Commenting on the first outbreak of plague in England in 1348, the chronicler John of Reading spilled out a plaintive cry of pain:

> "And there was those days death without sorrow, marriage without affection, self-imposed penance, want without poverty, and flight without escape....

In the end the plague devoured a multitude of people who left behind them all their worldly riches. Scarcely a tenth of the population survived."[1]

John of Reading's lamentation reflects the overall impact of the plague on society. Glimpsing how diseases affected individuals in premodern England is more difficult, but occasionally something comes to the surface. Henry VIII was still infatuated with Anne Boleyn, his new mistress, in June 1528 when the English Sweat swept across England. Anne was taken sick with the Sweat and retired to her father's country house to recuperate. Henry's heartfelt letter to Anne of 16 June indicates the pain felt by individuals whose beloved were imperiled by disease:

> There came to me in the night the most afflicting news possible. I have to grieve for three causes: first, to hear of my mistress's sickness, whose health I desire as my own, and would willingly bear the half of yours to cure you; secondly because I fear to suffer yet longer that absence which has already given me so much pain.

Henry lamented that his primary physician was absent, but indicated he would send his second physician to tend to Anne who survived the Sweat, but not Henry's desire for a male heir.[2] Even allowing for histrionics on Henry's part, this was a cry from the heart at the illness of a loved one. Sweat outbreaks did not have the impact of the plague, but they still caused loss of life and in this case a genuine fear of loss on Henry's part.

Most of the diseases considered here can be considered to have produced epidemics that affected all or most of England for a time and the First and Second Plague Pandemics affected all of the Western world for considerable periods of time. Even syphilis and leprosy produced so many cases in certain periods that they could almost be considered epidemics. Epidemic and pandemic diseases have a much different impact on societies than what can be labeled as background diseases such as diarrhea. Epidemics and pandemics can help to cause a paradigm shift in society. They do not cause dramatic changes by themselves, but they may reinforce existing trends or interact with other factors, such as war, to produce change over time. Pandemics, in particular, tend to leave a legacy that may take many years to play out, but that can produce changes ranging from how medicine confronts disease, to reinforcing new social trends and even lead to an overall paradigm shift that helps to place society on a new track.

Some of the diseases, such as leprosy, syphilis, influenza, measles, and smallpox are contagious diseases, passed from one person to another. Others, such as plague, typhus, and malaria, are vector-borne diseases with other entities such as fleas, lice, or mosquitos transmitting the disease. Plague is unusual in that bubonic plague is a vector-borne disease, but the pneumonic and septicemic varieties are transmitted from human to human. Diarrheal diseases, too, can be transmitted from human to human and indirectly by vectors. Currently, the means of transmission for the English Sweat which affected England from the late fifteenth to the mid-sixteenth centuries is yet to be understood. Understanding how these diseases are transmitted helps to understand their impact on individuals and ultimately society as a whole.

There are several useful histories of disease available today. Most draw on other secondary works in order to synthesize material over a broad time and space frame. The focus here is more of a case study that enables detailed analysis of specific diseases. England is the primary geographic focus for this study although at times Scotland, Ireland, and the rest of Europe will receive attention in order to complement the English material. Rather than attempting a sweeping description of disease over time, the chronological focus is limited to what is often referred to as premodern England. This focus is derived in part from the availability of source material that becomes more apparent from the eleventh century onward. In order to draw some contrasts between the First and Second Plague Pandemics, the first plague pandemic of the sixth through eighth centuries is examined, but otherwise the focus is largely from 1000 onward. Medicine was beginning to change in the seventeenth century and disease patterns were also changing so the study concludes c. 1600. Examining developments in England in the period from the eleventh through the sixteenth centuries helps to see how English society coped with existing medical problems as well as some new diseases that caused some rethinking of how society should confront disease.

It would be easy to assert that the mortality produced by outbreaks of epidemic disease sapped the strength of society, even leading to an overall fatalistic attitude that accepted the omnipresence of death. Premodern people were certainly aware that death could strike at any moment, but this rarely led them to give up hope. Each disease episode illustrates the resilience of human beings. In spite of the death of loved ones and disabilities produced by disease, people continued to live out their lives. Some diseases, most notably leprosy and syphilis did produce a moralistic response that might blame the victims for their moral failings, but this was not a uniform response. Instead, medical practitioners tried to describe diseases and provide treatments within the limits of existing scientific and medical knowledge.

In order to fully understand the impact of any disease on society, we need to have some knowledge of the biology of the disease. Biological understanding enables us to better describe how epidemic diseases spread, why did they affect some segments of society more than others, as well as the mortality rates of various diseases. Advances in paleobiology and historical epidemiology enable historians to better understand disease in the past. What is needed is consilience, an approach advocated by biologists such as E.O. Wilson and historians such as Michael McCormick that brings together explanations from disciplines such as history and biology. Biological overviews will accompany discussions of all the diseases examined in later chapters.

Everyday diseases such as fevers or diarrheal diseases and inter-personal violence and accidents were part of life and people developed means to try to deal
with these problems. Some diseases such as tuberculosis or malaria had a long
presence in English society and people had developed means of coping with them
as well. Leprosy rose to prominence in the eleventh century but was becoming
less important by the fifteenth century although cases would continue well into
the twenty-first century. Leprosy and tuberculosis are both degenerative diseases
that take some time to kill although kill they will if the patient does not die of
other causes. Leprosy is also of interest because it was the first disease to have
its victims acquire a moral stigma although syphilis would later take on this
stigma as well. Although leprosy cases were numerous in the thirteenth century,
and syphilis in the sixteenth century, neither they nor tuberculosis or malaria
can be labeled epidemic diseases although the number of cases almost seemed
to reach epidemic proportions at times. To be sure, there were regions, such as
marshy areas along rivers, where many people suffered from malaria, but geography helped to confine the disease. The other infectious diseases that afflicted
English society can be considered emerging infectious diseases in the modern
sense. They were new to society or had appeared centuries before and had been
forgotten. They were often highly infectious and produced high mortality rates,
especially for the first outbreaks. Medical practitioners had developed no means
to explain or deal with these diseases and turning for answers to the past was no
help as earlier practitioners did not have to confront these diseases. As they coped
with the "new" diseases, medical practitioners did help to foster medical progress, albeit in halting and not always positive ways. In many cases, these diseases
affected almost all of Europe, not just England.

Going beyond everyday medical issues such as diarrhea or infections and the
longstanding problems arising from malaria, tuberculosis, and leprosy (c. 3),
what diseases affected premodern people in England? Plague earns pride of
place from its geographic spread, longevity, and death toll. The First Plague
Pandemic (c. 4) struck the Byzantine Empire in the fifth century C.E. and
arrived in England in the seventh century. The Second Plague Pandemic
(c. 5–6) arrived in Constantinople in 1347 and had reached England by 1348.
Plague continued to trouble European society until the early eighteenth century although its last major outbreak in England was in 1666. The Third Plague
Pandemic swept across China in the nineteenth century reaching British India
and the United States by the early twentieth century. Its death toll like the
other two pandemics was high, but it did not affect the British Isles directly.
In some ways, plague is the test case against which all other infectious diseases
are evaluated.

The second plague pandemic has justly received a good deal of attention from
scholars and paleobiologists are still trying to tease out some of its secrets. Some
scholars consider the fourteenth-century outbreaks to have led to the Great
Divergence, a time of change for European society that led it into a different
path than most of the rest of the world, although this is a debated point. It is the

disease that other epidemics diseases are compared against, even today, so it will receive a good deal of attention.

Plague was not the only epidemic disease to afflict premodern England. Starting in 1485, a mystery disease, the English Sweat (c. 7) made five appearances and was not seen after 1551. The Sweat did not produce a high mortality rate, but it did generate a good deal of fear. Examining the Sweat helps to provide insight into how people described and reacted to what they considered a new disease.

The English Sweat impacted England and possibly parts of Germany, but another disease that appeared in the late fifteenth century affected all European countries. Generally considered to be part of what is labeled the Columbian Exchange, syphilis (c. 8) seems to have been imported from the Americas in the 1490s and soon spread across Europe. It too was a new disease, although one that people soon came to understand. Syphilis seems to have been quite lethal in its early years but then turned into a degenerative disease that would ultimately kill its victims if they didn't die of something else first. Syphilis, like leprosy, also shows how moralism was applied to diagnosis and treatment.

Three other diseases (c. 9) began to have major impacts on society from the fifteenth century onward. Typhus is a disease that attracts almost no attention today as it is easily preventable. In the past, it was a great killer especially of people packed into less than sanitary conditions such as soldiers and prisoners. While probably present earlier, it began to have a major impact in the sixteenth century. Smallpox would become a great killer by the late seventeenth century, but it appears to have been a childhood disease in the Middle Ages. Developing an understanding of how smallpox evolved from a disease of children to a major killer helps us to understand how infectious diseases evolve and how this evolutionary process affects society.

Much of influenza's origins are shrouded in the mists. It was clearly identified as a distinct disease in the early modern era, but most likely was present long before that. It may have appeared as the various fevers that affected society and some have even suggested that the English Sweat was influenza. Rising population densities from the sixteenth century onward helped to make influenza the major health threat that it potentially remains today. Having some understanding of the earlier history of influenza enables us to understand what is necessary for diseases to evolve from merely troubling medical issues to major health problems.

In order to understand the impact of disease in premodern England, it is important to be aware of what factors affect how infectious diseases affected society and what their impact was likely to be. The first chapter provides an overview of environmental factors that affected the spread of disease, most notably climate change. In addition, some of the basic principles of epidemiology are described as are some basic biological concepts for those readers needing a refresher. The second chapter provides a discussion of how human society reacted to disease with a discussion of medicine in theory and practice as well as sanitation practices and other public health measures. The relationship of famine to disease is touched on in both chapters as environmental factors and human action and inaction affected the impact of dearth. This chapter also contains some discussion of environmental factors such as water quality and the impact of hazardous materials. Taken together, the two chapters help to provide a framework in which to examine various infectious diseases.

The concluding chapter (c. 10) highlights some of the themes that have appeared in the discussion of various diseases. Two notable themes will be an examination of changes in medicine and the public health response brought about by various epidemic diseases. In addition, the relationship of disease and other factors in helping to produce a paradigm shift for society that helped to create the modern world will be examined.

Historians are usually concerned with change over time and that is one of the goals here. The first two chapters and the tenth chapter provide bookends enabling us to see how society's views of disease changed, how society reacted to infectious disease and what broader impacts infectious disease produced, and what lessons people learned from confronting "new" diseases as well as existing medical problems. In all cases, the biological agents of disease and how they affected the progression of the disease will be examined as well as what contemporaries thought caused the disease and what they did to counteract it. Throughout the discussion of various diseases, the relationship of how environmental issues, most notably climate change, interacted with infectious disease. Some potential lessons for us today in confronting emerging infectious diseases can also be drawn from the discussion of the various diseases in the intervening chapters as well as the summary in the final chapter.

Notes

1 James Tait, ed., *Chronica Johannis de Reading et Anonymi Cantaurienis 1346–1367* (Manchester: Manchester University Press, 1914), 109.
2 *Letters and Papers, Foreign and Domestic of the Reign of Henry VIII*, 22 vols (London, 1862–1932), 4: 1921.

1

FINDING THE IMPACT OF DISEASE IN PREMODERN ENGLAND

The impact of infectious diseases continues to link people today with people in the past. People still suffer from infectious diseases, fear them, try to understand them, try to cure them, and attempt to prevent them. People in premodern England were no different. Although we might confront different diseases than our forbearers and possess improved medical technology, we are nonetheless often at the mercy of disease as can be seen with the impact of the novel coronavirus COVID-19. In the past and today, many diseases strike down people one at a time although the overall number of victims may be high, such as those traceable to the two major killers in twenty-first-century American society: cancer and heart disease. Today chronic diseases such as heart disease, cancer, or diabetes are responsible for a large majority of the deaths reported in industrial nations. Medical advances have made the epidemic diseases of the past less of a threat. Child mortality rates tend to be low in industrial nations so that the average life expectancy has increased dramatically from what it was in the Middle Ages. As populations become older, chronic diseases are more likely to be a factor in mortality in industrial nations today.

Although the cumulative impact of diseases affecting single individuals may be great, it is the epidemic diseases that can have a dramatic impact in a short period of time even altering the political and economic development of a region or nation. Today, the specter of the use of infectious disease-causing agents as weapons of terrorism magnifies the fear of some diseases. In the premodern world with a lower ability to respond to any sort of disease, epidemic diseases could be potentially cataclysmic. In both instances, population density plays a factor in the impact of epidemic diseases. Epidemic diseases can spread easily in the closely packed cities of the modern world although they have more difficulty spreading in the largely rural premodern world.

DOI: 10.4324/9781003215219-2

This chapter seeks to lay out the problem of diseases in premodern England by identifying some of the factors that led to the presence of infectious diseases in society and how they affected people. Two sets of factors influence how diseases affect society. There are those factors that society cannot control such as climate or the biology of an agent of disease. Humans can affect how diseases impact society through their actions and knowledge. This chapter provides a brief conceptual model of the two sets of factors and then examines the impact of outside factors. The next chapter will examine how premodern people's actions affected the impact of disease on society. Both sets of factors will be treated more specifically in later chapters that examine particular diseases.

The forces that shaped public health in premodern England

The health of medieval and early modern people was shaped by a variety of forces that came from outside of human society—exogenous factors and those that came from within society—endogenous factors. When we examine their impact, we often find that they interact together to worsen or to improve a situation. This state of interacting factors can be extended to one of the interaction of diseases through the concept of syndemics—the interaction between multiple diseases that can worsen the negative effects of one or more of the diseases.[1]

Exogenous factors (outside forces that people had little control over):

Agent of disease
Disease patterns (also partially an endogenous factor), advent of "new" diseases
Infectivity of diseases present
Climate: temperature, precipitation
Natural events, e.g., volcanoes

Endogenous factors (aspects of diseases that humans could influence):

Government and its intervention in dealing with disease
Diet and nutrition, crop yield (partially exogenous as well)
Medical knowledge
Impact of travel and trade patterns
Population size and growth rate (also affected by these and other factors)
Birth rate, age of menarche

All of these factors interact separately and collectively to influence the state of public health and the impact of infectious disease. Governments can close ports limiting trade which potentially limits the importation of disease. Governments also play a role in enforcing sanitary standards that can make it more difficult for a disease to spread. Crop yields are affected not only by the state of agricultural technology but also by the length of the growing season and the amount of moisture received and when. Large crowded populations make it easier to spread some infectious diseases and are almost essential to spreading diseases to others. Weather varies from year to year producing events such as droughts or especially cold winters that have short-term impacts on human health. Climate can change gradually over time, but events such as major volcanic eruptions can modify weather patterns for a period of time or even help to cause a new climate regime. An infectious disease that newly appears in a region has the potential to be more infective than an already existing one because people possess no innate immunity to the disease. Changes in the virulence of a disease can affect both its morbidity and mortality rates as does population density. Medical knowledge and how society uses this knowledge influence the ability to deal with potential health threats.

Both acute and chronic diseases often interact in ways that can be positive for public health but are more likely to produce additional complications. An often cited positive interaction is the protection that the sickle cell gene affords to those carrying it from malaria infection. Unfortunately, sickle cell anemia is itself a major health problem so the benefit is a mixed one. Negative interactions occur when two or more diseases interact synergistically to produce health issues that may be more deleterious than those produced by individual diseases. For example, AIDS weakens the immune system making the victim subject to more symptoms from diseases such as tuberculosis or some fungal disease that may then accelerate the progress of the HIV infection. Either disease by itself is harmful, but the combination of the two is often deadly.

The biology of infectious disease

Agents of disease are biological entities that serve to infect humans with disease. There are five causative agents of disease: viruses, bacteria, protozoa, fungi, and worms. Almost all epidemic diseases are caused by bacteria or viruses although protozoal diseases such as malaria can reach nearly epidemic proportions, and in parts of Africa, worm-caused diseases such as river blindness or schistosomiasis have occurred in near epidemic numbers. Scientists did not identify bacteria as a disease agent until the late nineteenth century and viruses awaited identification until the mid-twentieth century. Until the agents of disease could be identified clinically, it would be difficult to provide reliable diagnosis and effective treatment for many diseases.

Bacteria would first be identified as a disease agent by Louis Pasteur in 1857. The work of Pasteur and Robert Koch, first with anthrax and then other diseases, opened up a new way of looking at diseases. Based on their work, several other diseases were also diagnosed as being caused by bacteria. A notable example came with the bubonic plague outbreak in Hong Kong in 1894. Both Shibasaburo Kitasato (a student of Koch) and Alexandre Yersin (a student of Pasteur) visited Hong Kong and labored to find the agent responsible for the plague. Yersin received the credit for discovering bacillus that would eventually be named after him, *Yersinia pestis*.

Bacteria the causative agents for several epidemic diseases, such as plague or tuberculosis, are single-celled prokaryotes that can be parasites or free-living. All told less than 40 of about 400 recognized genera of bacteria cause disease in humans. Although too small to be seen with the naked eye, bacteria can be seen with the aid of a microscope. Bacterial cells are held together by a cytoplasmic membrane and many have a rigid cell wall, or capsule, that provides some protection from the outside world but they do not have a nucleus. The bacteria's genetic material (DNA) is contained within a portion of the cell although some species may also have small amounts of DNA (plasmids) outside the nuclear area that can replicate independently from the nucleated chromosomes. Some of these independent chromosomes carry genetic resistance to other substances such as antibodies. Bacteria have the advantage of being able to mutate rapidly enabling them to cope with changing environments. Although bacteria are often agents of disease, they are also an essential part of human life, performing many positive functions within the human body.

Rickettsiae resemble bacteria biochemically (they are both prokaryotes) and they have some cellular structure like bacteria but they resemble viruses in needing a host cell to survive. Rickettsiae generally live in a symbiotic relationship with their insect hosts that are generally blood-sucking in nature such as ticks or fleas. The insect hosts usually transmit the rickettsia to humans through salvia or infected feces deposited at a bite site. Typhus is a rickettsial disease that has essentially vanished from notice today but was important in the past, also Q fever, another rickettsial diseases, is considered a potential biological weapon threat today.

After the discoveries of Pasteur and Koch scientists, and medical practitioners were soon diagnosing bacteria as the causes of almost all diseases. When influenza spread across the globe in 1918–19, scientists looked for the bacterial source of the disease. However, there was another agent of disease, something too small to be glimpsed with a microscope—the virus. It would not be until 1939 that scientists observed viruses using an electron microscope. Several important epidemic diseases such as influenza, smallpox, or - COVID-19 are viral not bacterial.

Viruses are not complete cell, but instead are strands of DNA or RNA and are dependent on other forms of life for their existence. They are found in all animals, plants, protozoa, fungi, and bacteria. Viruses gain entry to a host through a variety of means and once they do so they attach to target cells and begin to replicate. Once they have replicated, the new viral particles need to leave the host cell. In some cases, this is done by the virus encapsulating itself in a lipid (fat) envelope derived from the cell membrane. Another, more destructive approach occurs when the replicated virus causes the cell wall to burst, destroying the cell as the virus spreads. Easily adaptable to environmental change—viruses, especially RNA viruses such as HIV, can mutate very rapidly. Different strains within a host can exchange genetic information between them, creating a new strain. In addition to HIV, several other viruses, such as smallpox, Yellow Fever, influenza, polio, and the emerging hemorrhagic viruses such as Ebola pose health threats to humans.

Protozoa are more complex than either bacteria or viruses as they are single-celled organisms with a nucleus. Some protozoa have elaborate life cycles moving through different hosts at different stages of development, often with growth and reproductive stages in different organs, intermediate hosts, or insect vectors. Their cellular structure enables protozoa to more easily evade a host's immune structure than bacteria or viruses and consequently, they are often more difficult to treat. Examples of protozoal diseases include malaria and *Giardia*, a waterborne intestinal disease.

Fungi are eukaryotic organisms and tend not to be as virulent as the other disease agents. Only a small number of the more than 70,000 fungi are harmful to humans. Most fungal infections, called mycoses, are kept in check by the human immune system. Some, however, can prove highly virulent to those people with a compromised immune system. Many AIDS patients, for example do not die of AIDS but from fungal infections such as cryptococcosis. Other fungal infections such as those resulting from ergot, a fungus that infects grain, especially rye, can cause abortions or wild hallucinations such as those caused by LSD (Lysergic acid diethylamide). On the other hand, the ergot alkaloid ergotamine can be used to treat migraines, and ergonovine can be used to treat vaginal bleeding after childbirth as well as easing childbirth, or in large doses cause an abortion.

Bacteria and viruses evolve rapidly in both less and more deadly directions. In one sense, an extremely deadly virus or bacteria that kills all the hosts that it infects is not displaying a "good" evolutionary approach. Killing a host too readily makes it difficult for a microbe to continue to spread and helps to limit its survival. A bacteria or virus that kills slowly or not at all helps to ensure its survival by guaranteeing the continued presence of a host. Many bacteria or viruses evolve in a more benign direction over time, coming to have a symbiotic relationship with their hosts. Not all bacteria and viruses follow this pattern with some retaining the ability to readily kill their host and some even evolving in a more lethal direction.[2] Indeed, some diseases with origins in the distant past have appeared in several different biovars (biological varieties) with varying degrees of lethality for their hosts.

Another issue to keep in mind when considering infectious diseases is that as an agent of disease evolves over time, it may change so that it can infect new species. There are a variety of zoonotic diseases found in animals that have evolved and have come to infect humans. What might have started out as a disease that co-existed with its original host, became quite deadly when it infected a new host. HIV is the classic case of a virus that has jumped species from monkeys to humans. Moreover, because HIV is an RNA virus, it evolves very quickly, making it difficult to find a means of treating it as the virus quickly develops resistance to whatever drug is used for treatment. The presence of multiple hosts also makes it extremely difficult to eradicate a disease. Even when one host is protected by vaccination, the disease will continue to be present in a different host, presenting an opportunity for re-infection. Smallpox, a disease that has been officially eradicated as the last case occurred in the wild in Somalia in 1977, is an example of a disease with one host—humans. Once vaccinations protected people from the smallpox virus, the disease died out naturally, as there were no other hosts although the virus continues to be preserved in a few highly secure laboratories.

When a disease jumps species or when it is introduced into an area in which it has not been present, what the historian Alfred Crosby called a virgin soil epidemic ensues.[3] In both cases, the newly targeted population has no innate immunity to the new disease. Such an epidemic is likely to produce a much higher death rate than one that strikes an already exposed population that may have some immunity to the disease. With a virgin soil epidemic, because the population has no natural immunity, the disease is likely to infect a large number of people. Such a disease often is highly virulent producing a high mortality rate. A classic case of a virgin soil epidemic is the impact of smallpox on the Native American population when Europeans invaded North and South America. As a population continues to be exposed to a disease, the presence of survivors who possess immunity means that the next outbreak of the disease will often have more difficulty in spreading. If part of the population had immunity to the disease from an earlier outbreak, a new outbreak would burn out as the potential infectable population became exposed to the disease. Smallpox is a good example of this situation as survivors of an outbreak were immune and could not be infected again. Exposure to some diseases, such as plague, confers no lasting immunity so the total population is at risk in a second outbreak.

Scientists have developed an approach for measuring the persistence and spread of infectious diseases in a population. An indication of the contagiousness of an infectious disease is the basic reproduction number (R_0). The potential size of a disease outbreak is related to the magnitude of the R_0 although a variety of other factors also affects the spread of a disease. In order for a disease to continue to spread, it must have an average R_0 of a least one. For example, a person with a disease with an R_0 of two is likely to spread it to two other people assuming that many people are encountered. The same person who is present in a crowded room is likely to spread the disease to even more people. The number of cases grows, often dramatically, as more people are infected. On the other hand, a disease with an R_0 of less than one will be unlikely to spread as infected people often have no one else who is susceptible to come into contact with and the outbreak soon dies out. There are four primary parameters that go into the calculation of an R_0. The first is the duration of the contagious phase of a disease after a person has been infected. A disease with a long contagious phase makes it more likely that an infected person will come into contact with other people to infect. The second parameter is the likelihood of infection per contact between an infected person and a susceptible person, in essence, the number of opportunities an infected person has to spread the disease. An isolated person is likely to come into contact with almost no one, but someone working in a busy market will come into contact with many people. The third factor is the probability that a contact results in a transmission of the disease. The fourth parameter is the susceptibility of the population to the disease. A simplified mathematical model for the spread of disease is $R_0 = (d) \times (o) \times (p) \times (s)$

1. d is the duration of the infective stage of a disease
2. o is the opportunities for contact with susceptible people
3. p is the probability that the pathogen will be transferred from the infected source to a susceptible host.
4. s is the susceptibility of the population

An increase in the size of the susceptible population or in the rate of transmission increases the R_0, while a decrease in the transmission rate or an increase in the mortality rate of the disease will tend to decrease the R_0. If the size of a host population is small, it will be difficult for a disease to reach epidemic proportions as once everyone in the population has contracted the disease, there will no more be susceptibles to infect unless outsiders are introduced and the outbreak dies out. It is possible to find a threshold size for a population necessary to maintain an outbreak by finding the population density necessary to produce an R_0 of one or greater.[4] When a large enough number of a potentially susceptible population has been infected and have gained immunity, the rest of the population may have effective immunity as infected individuals are unlikely to be able to spread the disease. This state is labeled herd immunity and can be produced by creating a large enough number of people who have immunity so as to protect the rest of the population or by vaccination.[5]

The basic reproduction number R_0 is the product of these four factors. There are more sophisticated mathematical treatments, but this simple formula serves our purposes. Urban populations can lead to a higher o value, but in small villages with little contact with the outside, a disease will quickly infect everyone and then die out without spreading. Once outside the few cities in medieval Europe, it was difficult to sustain an epidemic. The evolution of microbes also affect the impact of a disease. Some microbes such as the tuberculosis bacteria seem to have been harmful to humans for a long time. Others have evolved to become harmful or have jumped from one species to another and in doing so, have become harmful to human beings.

Epidemic diseases are often classified into three types depending on how they develop.[6] A type I epidemic has a regular pattern of outbreaks and the disease is endemic, as it never completely disappears from the population and there are always a few cases present between major outbreaks to serve to spark a new outbreak. A type I epidemic requires a large population of susceptibles so that an R_0 of one or greater can be maintained. A type II epidemic displays a regular pattern of the occurrence of cases but the disease pattern is discontinuous with breaks between the infection peaks as the disease is not endemic. Unlike a type I epidemic pattern, the R_0 for the disease is less than one. Type III epidemics occur in communities with small populations. There are occasional outbreaks of the disease but often with long periods of time with no cases of the disease.

Vaccinations can reduce the size of a susceptible population and gradually turn a type I epidemic into a type II and then type III epidemic as countries such as the United States have done with measles and mumps. However, if a disease can maintain itself in a few "hot" spots, it can reappear as a new epidemic. The calculation of an R_0 and the population size necessary to maintain an outbreak is important when applied to premodern England which had almost no large cities and only a few towns of 10,000 or more people so that it was difficult to sustain an epidemic.

This classification scheme is related to the ease in transmission of disease over space. Some agents of disease are fragile and cannot exist long outside a host while others are hardy and can live, or go dormant, for long periods of time outside a host. The latter parasites are easily transmitted from place to place making it possible for the microbe to reach new susceptible populations. Today, many diseases can be easily transmitted from one continent to another in the time it takes for an airplane to fly from say Nairobi to Chicago. In the Middle Ages, some diseases infected a community and once everyone had been infected the disease died out. Trade or pilgrimage routes, however, made it possible for hardier microbes to move from place to place finding new populations to infect. A disease might start as a regional or even national epidemic and the epidemic would expand along trade routes to another country. In the meantime, the disease usually died out in the first country so what existed was a rolling series of epidemics rather than a pandemic. In the twenty-first century, it is possible for several diseases to become pandemics, infecting several continents at once rather than the local, regional, or national epidemics of the past. Currently, the world is experiencing a seventh cholera pandemic, the fear of pandemic influenza persists, and the COVID-19 pandemic shows how it is possible for a disease to impact almost all parts of the world.

It is possible to model the development of an epidemic once basic demographic information is combined with the R_0 of the disease. The basic model used to describe the progress of an infectious disease is the SIR model, where the susceptible population is labeled S, the infected population is labeled I, and the removed (recovered or dead) is labeled R.[7] Sometimes, another term (E) is inserted after S to capture the exposure period. The SIR model is a compartmental model in which different parts of the population are neatly categorized. The model is based on several assumptions such as the total population is initially susceptible, that recovery means permanent immunity, and the latent period between exposure and infection is so short that it can be ignored. As time passes, it is possible to track the progress of a disease from an uninfected population to one in which the epidemic is over. The SIR model has served epidemiologists well because of its simplicity. Because the SIR model does not take into account all real-world circumstances, it has been expanded to include geography, external factors such as migration, or governmental intervention (quarantine). In some cases, epidemiologists have developed stochastic models with parameters that are continually changing in response to changing situations.

The computations involving R_0 and the SIR model enable epidemiologists to predict the course of an epidemic with some degree of accuracy. In many cases, with a large enough population, this produces a logistic growth curve model derived from a basic differential equation representing the rate of the spread of the disease. Logistic growth curve models have three phases. The first phase is a slow growth phase with a few but a growing number of cases. It is easiest to halt a potential epidemic during this stage. The second stage is one of explosive growth, in which much of a susceptible population becomes infected. The third, or burnout, stage is reached when the target population has been completely infected or is protected through vaccination. The predicted course of an epidemic requires a good deal of information that would be difficult if not impossible to achieve for a premodern epidemic. Using a modern prediction, however, it is possible to gain an appreciation for how an epidemic developed in the past as well as its potential impact. For example, it is possible to predict how an infectious disease might affect a medieval village and test the prediction against what information is available and in doing so fill in some potential gaps in our information. [8]

Three terms, outbreak, epidemic, and pandemic, are used to describe the impact of an infectious disease. The three terms are not overly precise but they give an indication of the geographic spread of a disease, how many people fell ill, and how many died. Simply put an outbreak is one of limited geographic size and number of people involved, say a monastic community or small village. An epidemic is when a disease infects a large number of people over a large area such as a province or nation. Finally, a pandemic is transnational and covers one or more continents with a very large number of people (often in the millions) involved. Especially if the disease is one with a high case fatality rate, a pandemic is extremely destructive and may stress the normal bonds of society. A good example is how COVID-19 spread from China across every continent, save Antarctica, and with hundreds of millions of cases recorded worldwide.

An understanding of how infectious diseases spread enables us to have a better understanding of the impact of the diseases on premodern society that we will encounter in later chapters. Many of the diseases examined in later chapters are the same as modern diseases. Even if they are not, the basic principles of biology and epidemiology will help to better understand how they were able to affect premodern England. A strictly biomedical approach to disease tends to concentrate on the agents of the disease and how they are transmitted. As indicated above, a variety of factors affect the transmission of a disease pathogen. The basic reproductive number captures some of this relationship, but generally leaves environmental factors unexamined and social and political factors under-examined. In sum, a more broad-based approach to understanding disease in the past is necessary especially if we want to understand the impact of a disease on society.[9] Such an approach involves biologists, archaeologists and other paleo-scientists, as well as historians. The next chapter will examine how human impacts affect the role of infectious diseases in society.

Climate and disease

Climate is another external factor that influenced the transmission of diseases and how they affected the human population in the premodern era through an impact on food supply, and the ease of movement of the human and disease host populations. The relationship of climate, famine, and disease is complex and must be treated with care as Timothy Newfield points out regarding the Early Middle Ages.[10] The climate, or more properly weather for limited time frames, can vary from year to year and lead to crop failures and even an outbreak of a disease such as malaria in an especially wet year.[11] Climate change over a few centuries is sometimes hard to detect but over time it can begin to have an almost imperceptible on human health and the prevalence of certain types of disease.

Understanding climatic and environmental change in the past is a challenging topic. Nonetheless, some scholars, such as Bruce Campbell, indicate that the relationships between society, the economy, and the environment must be examined together in order to gain an accurate picture of the past.[12] Researchers need to draw on a variety of records in order to achieve an accurate picture. The usually written records of the historian have much to tell us, but also ignore or obscure a lot. Archaeologists and historians have often engaged in complementary work such as the excavations of the London plague cemeteries. Science too can provide useful information drawing on dendrochronology and climatic research. Some scholars advocate a disciplinary consilience that blends the humanities and sciences.[13] The term consilience was introduced by the biologist E.O. Wilson in a book of the same name as he advocated that the sciences and humanities come together as both sets of disciplines have much to offer the other. Care must be taken to avoid misunderstandings arising from how various disciplines use language, treat their sources, and approach their research topics.[14] In spite of possible pitfalls, disciplinary collaboration has much to offer in treating environmental issues and the history of disease.

The impact of climate in the past took many forms such as limited mobility through adverse weather conditions and various heat and cold-related health problems. Frostbite results from exposure to cold temperatures for too long a period. Sunstroke and heat exhaustion were unlikely to affect most people in northern Europe, but their impact can be severe even leading to death. Probably the most important relationship is that of climate and nutrition. Weather can both positively and adversely affect the growing season as well as have an impact on livestock. Unusually "bad" years could lead to severely restricted food production that could lead to malnutrition or even famine. A series of poor harvests could produce a famine. One tendency is to make the correlation, bad weather = bad harvest = crisis.[15] When the next step of correlating malnutrition and famine with disease is made, the relationship between climate and disease is clearly established. However, a variety of other factors influence whether a food shortage turns into a famine and how poor diet affects health. Taking a reductionist approach that indicates correlation, indicates causation, is a research flaw that all students in statistics classes are warned against, and it is easy to fall into this trap when assessing the relationship between climate and food shortages.[16] In examining the relationship between climate and past society, it is also important to avoid relying on outdated data or reading more into a data set than is prudent.[17] There is a relationship between poor nutrition and disease, and a relationship between climate and nutrition that exists, but both are complex. A brief overview of premodern climate and factors that influenced it follows, but specific relationships of climate, nutrition, and individual diseases will be detailed in later chapters.

Determining the climate of the past has proven to be a challenging task. Overall it has been possible to establish some broad climate signatures over time. The earth's climate has been much warmer than it is today such as the Paleocene-Eocene Thermal Maximum, some 55 million years ago when palm trees and camels could be found in the Arctic because the planet was ice-free. The earth has also undergone several ice ages, the most recent ending some 11,000 years ago with the transition to the Holocene era of relatively mild climate. Proxy measures of climate in the past include documentary sources such as chronicles and records of famines or dearth and may indicate some of the human impact deriving from climate change, but these records before 1000 are not always accurate or speak in generalities. Tree ring data provide much older series but coverage is spotty with better records for some parts of the globe than others. Ice core data from boreholes in Antarctica and Greenland enable an extension of knowledge about the climate several thousand years into the past in dealing with some types of pollution and the chemical content of the atmosphere. Ice core and tree ring data provide an accurate reading of past climates, but unfortunately, these sources tell us little about the impact on human societies in the past. Today proxy climate records extend back to 0 CE with increasing numbers of data series as we move forward in time.[18] Ice core data supplement and expand these records by providing chemical records such as sulfur from the atmosphere that may have been generated by volcanic activity.

The periodization of climate is not a smooth or even process. Colder periods may enjoy a year with warmer temperatures and warm periods still had cold and wet years. Climate has not changed uniformly around the globe with climate change starting earlier or ending later in some regions or even not occurring at all in some places. Nonetheless, there is some agreement as to a rough periodization of climate in Europe from the time of the Roman Empire onward:

Roman Climate Optimum ca. 200 BCE–400 CE
Roman Transitional Period ca. 150 CE–450 CE
Late Antique Little Ice Age ca. 450–800
Medieval Climate Anomaly ca. 800–1300
Little Ice Age ca. 1300–1850

All of these periods are approximate, but they give some idea of the progression from warmer to colder and back again. Unlike climate in the pre-Holocene era, the temperature ranges of these periods did not differ a great deal as there were no full-scale ice ages.

European climate during the Roman Climate Optimum and the Medieval Climate Anomaly (MCA) was slightly warmer than that of the first half of the twentieth century (probably 0.4° C warmer than 1961–1990 temperatures). The MCA was once known as the Medieval Warm Era, but recent research has indicated that this did not seem to be a global phenomenon and its warmth may have been exaggerated.[19] In England, there seem to have been three notable warm periods (1010–1040, 1070–1105, and 1155–1190), but there were also some notable cold years such as 1205, 1282, 1310, and 1408, during which the Thames at London was reported to be frozen over during the winter.[20] Temperatures seemed to rebound a bit in the late fourteenth century from a slightly lower trend in mid-century.[21] From the fourteenth century onward until the early eighteenth century, temperatures trended downward, reaching troughs in the late sixteenth and seventeenth centuries, producing what is referred to as the Little Ice Age with temperatures approximately 1° C lower in the troughs than during the late twentieth century. Even during the Little Ice Age, temperatures were not uniformly low with warmer than average temperatures in 1434, 1453, 1504, 1565, 1587, and 1601.[22]

The past climate history of the globe has been one of the gradual cycles of change as well as sudden changes. A change in the climate regime could be precipitated and maintained by events such as volcanic eruptions or sunspots. A few sharply colder or warmer years could affect the flow of ocean currents that influenced the climate of Western Europe known as the North Atlantic Oscillation. The ocean currents of the Atlantic have changed course over time, bringing colder and wetter winters to northern Europe as well as warmer summers. The Medieval Climate Anomaly seems to have been dominated by North Atlantic currents that brought warmer water farther north and closer to the European continent than in preceding years.[23] Why the North Atlantic currents change path is not fully understood, but it appears that low solar activity can force a change to the lower index state of the North Atlantic Oscillation.[24]

Sunspots and eclipses can have a profound impact on how people perceive their world, and sunspots in particular, are often recorded in the records of the past. Probably the most notorious period of low solar activity is the Maunder Minimum in the seventeenth century. The Maunder Minimum led to reduced growing seasons in an already colder than usual period, helping to produce malnutrition and famine, and has been credited as part of the causation for what is known as the Crisis of the Seventeenth Century.[25] During the Middle Ages, there were three other periods of decreased solar activity. At present little is known about the Oort Minimum of 1010–1060 and the Wolf Minimum of 1280–1350. The Oort Minimum may be related to a somewhat colder period during the MCA. The Wolf Minimum came at a time of increased volcanic activity and the combination of the two may have helped precipitate the early stages of the Little Ice Age. During the critical years of the Wolf Minimum in the 1310s, Northern Europe faced the Great Famine that was caused in part by several cold, wet years. The impact of the Spörer Minimum (1460–1550) helped to reinforce the climate changes that were occurring and that led to the Little Ice Age.[26] Additional reinforcement for the colder climate regime may have also occurred during the 1430s. Winters during the decade were wetter than usual although summer temperatures seemed to be warm. The situation of the 1430s appears to have been one caused by the chance occurrence of various factors rather than external forcing.[27]

The impact of volcanic eruptions can be measured with a combination of ice core data and various sources such as written records, tree ring data, speleothems (stalactites or stalagmites). Ice core records from Antarctica and Greenland reveal the chemical composition of an eruption, most notably sulfates, which served to block some solar radiation, and the amount of particulate matter. When used with other sources, ice cores and tree ring data help to reveal the magnitude of an eruption, the amount of solar radiation blocked, and often its location. The impact of an eruption is also dependent on location. The rain of particulate matter from a nearby volcano is more severe than one from the other side of the world. With large eruptions, particulate matter is ejected high into the atmosphere to circle the globe over the next one or more years, producing phenomena such as dust clouds and intensely red sunsets. Tropical eruptions during the Middle Ages tended to produce sulfur aerosols that affect solar radiation more than the aerosols from northern hemisphere volcanoes.[28] Fortunately for northern Europe, Icelandic volcanoes were relatively inactive during the period with the largest eruptions occurring in the tropics

The science of volcanology made great strides in the late twentieth century, but even today volcanic eruptions and the amount of their discharge are not entirely predictable. The ability to predict the occurrence of volcanic eruptions is important because many population centers are near potentially active volcanoes. In the past, volcanoes profoundly altered the landscape and climate of the planet. Fortunately for us, the super volcanoes that erupted millions of years ago are no longer a problem. The eruption on the Indonesian island of Tambora in 1815 did have a multi-year climatic impact, producing the year without summer and the next year in which snow fell in eleven of twelve months in New England. The last volcano that even approached magnitude of the great volcanoes of the past was Toba in the Indonesian archipelago that erupted some 74,000 years ago. While estimates of Toba's impact on the human population have been disputed, it had a global environmental impact and it seems to have created a population bottleneck that had a potentially drastic impact on humans.[29] Fortunately, for people in medieval Europe, no Toba level eruptions took place. Unfortunately, some medieval eruptions still had deleterious impacts on the climate, contributing to short and long-term cooling.

Medieval chroniclers in northern Europe were unaware of volcanic eruptions that left ice core signatures beyond any that occurred in Iceland, but they often reported weather impacts on society. Notice of shorter growing seasons, colder and wetter winters, and the resulting food shortages often appear in the chronicle record. For example, Matthew Paris, writing at the monastery of St. Albans near London indicated that the summer of 1258 was hot and dry but that autumn rains caused the crops to rot in the fields as well as leading to a food shortage and distress. He also notes famine near London in May and later in the summer in 1258. It might be possible to assume the famines were weather-related, but he does not provide enough details to reach a definitive conclusion.[30] Not all chroniclers were as meticulous as Matthew Paris in noting weather events, but notices of abnormally cold winters, hot summers, and spoiled harvests often appear. Also, written accounts and some artistic representations noted that the sun turned dark almost blue in color or dry fogs that colored the sky a dark red that arose from particulate matter in the atmosphere coming from a large volcanic eruption.[31] These accounts often appear one to two years after the eruption occurred (based on ice core dating). Written accounts in conjunction with tree ring data help to provide confirmation for ice core dating of volcanic eruptions in the Middle Ages.

Climate scientists, historians, and archaeologists have been able to pinpoint several volcanic eruptions large enough to have an impact on the climate of medieval Europe. In some cases, the impact lasted only a year or two. In other cases, especially when the eruption occurred during a period in which the North Atlantic Oscillation had moved the warmer ocean currents away from Europe, the combination of the two factors helped to precipitate a changing climate.

The Late Antique Little Ice Age lasted from about 536 to about 800 and appears to have produced colder and wetter winters and summers and shortened growing seasons as well as having public health impacts such as increased incidence of disease. It encompassed much of northern Europe including England. Examination of Greenland and Antarctic ice cores indicate a near-equatorial and large explosive eruption producing an atmospheric dust veil around 536.[32] The short-term dust cloud of about a year seems to have produced little immediate political or social impact in the Mediterranean region although it was well described.[33] The 536 dust cloud was supplemented by further tropical eruptions over the next few years and most likely a forcing of the North Atlantic Oscillation that helped to sustain the trend toward lower temperatures.[34] The 536 eruption may have caused a temperature decrease of 1.5° to 2.5° C that when combined with the effects of later eruptions produced the coldest decade in the last 2300 years, leading some scholars to call 536 the worst year to be alive.[35] Although care must be taken in interpreting the impact of the Antique Little Ice Age, malnutrition and even famine seem to have occurred quite often during this period. Climate alone was not the cause as transportation difficulties, lack of political capacity and political disorder also played a role. While the climate appears to have warmed after 800, there continued to be cold spells well into the tenth century in parts of Europe. Charlemagne and his successors faced six cold years from 763 through 940. The resulting crop failures negatively affected human life, and in conjunction with animal murrains, also led to horse, cattle, and oxen loss.[36] Dearth on the continent was not necessarily dearth in England, but the suspicion remains that there were several hard years for the English people during this period.

Gradually the weather improved and so by 1000 and likely earlier, northern Europe was enjoying the Medieval Climate Anomaly. Growing seasons expanded allowing better crop yields. Population may have grown slightly, but there were still too many factors such as high child mortality rates and the threat of Viking invaders to enable a large expansion of the English population. At least there were no large-scale epidemics to trouble people.

The good times did not last. Starting in the latter part of the thirteenth century, ice caps began to grow in Iceland and Arctic Canada coming from colder summers and sea ice feedback arising from a new pattern in the North Atlantic Oscillation and a general colder and wetter climate. Volcanic eruptions may have served as the trigger for this climatic shift, but other factors such as a decrease in solar radiation also played a part.[37] The Little Ice Age had begun although contemporaries would not have made the connection. The Little Ice Age was not always uniformly cold and the coldest temperatures did not occur until the seventeenth century.

A decrease in solar activity, the Wolf Minimum, started about 1280, but volcanic activity was already beginning to have a negative impact on Europe. The volcanic eruption of Samalas on Lombok Island in Indonesia in 1257 produced what was probably the largest volcanic sulfur release in the last 7000 years, much greater than that of Tambora in 1815.[38] People in northern Europe experienced the coldest summers in the last millennium in 1258 and 1259 although North America experienced warmer summers than usual, probably influenced by a positive phase of the El Nino-Southern Oscillation.[39] The impact of the Samalas sulfate cloud was short-lived but did produce heavy summer and autumn rains in 1258 as well as a cold winter. Crop failures seem to have been common across England with a dramatic increase in food prices.[40] The decreased crop yields were accompanied by a sheep murrain further adding to the trials of the English people with a famine. In addition, the chronicler Matthew Paris reported a "great pestilence" that struck London in 1258.[41] The famine of 1258 appears to have come from poor harvests in 1256 and 1257, caused by floods. The drop in temperature in 1258 caused by the Samalas eruption of 1257 reinforced an already developing crisis. Bruce Campbell's careful reading of the sources and the timing of the famine illustrates the necessity to combine climate data with material from other sources.[42] Details are sketchy with some victims dying quickly while others exhibited listlessness and chills over several months. The Samalas eruption did not lead to the onset of the Little Ice Age by itself, but when coupled with other factors such as changing ocean currents, northern ice caps were expanding by 1300, a sign that a new and colder climate regime was beginning.[43] Thereafter the LIA received several additional stimuli that continued to propel the colder and wetter temperatures.

Both a changed North Atlantic Oscillation and volcanic activity reinforced the downward pressure on temperature in the fifteenth century. Some of the colder weather such as the colder winters of the 1430s seem to have been unrelated to solar activity or volcanic action but did have societal impacts at least in northwestern Europe.[44] Dating from mid-century, the Spörer Minimum influenced the North Atlantic Oscillation so as to withdraw a warming current from the south from northern Europe. In 1458, the tropical volcano Kuwae erupted, producing a sulfur discharge greater than that of Tambora.[45] By the end of the fifteenth century, the LIA was well underway although the coldest temperatures would come later.

Because climate changed gradually, people were able to adapt so that the climate change by itself had little direct impact on human health. Changes in climate did, however, affect which disease agents were present as well as leading to food shortages that adversely affected people's health. The chapter dealing with the second plague pandemic considers the possibility of climatic factors in initiating the initial spread of the disease. One of the issues related to global warming today is the spread of certain disease agents such as malaria beyond the tropics to more temperate climates as temperatures warm. One study indicates that warmer temperatures and increased rainfall in the western United States influenced by changes in the Pacific Decadal Oscillation helped to enhance the habitat for small mammals that serve as hosts for plague-carrying fleas. The relationship between climate change and the onset of the plague in the fourteenth century will be examined in Chapter 5, but there is an overall consensus that climate change in Asia played a role in the onset of the plague.[46] Climatic changes also could lengthen or shorten the growing season or lead to higher or lower amounts of rainfall. Overall, the gradual warming of the English climate helped to lengthen the growing season and made growing new plants possible, such as wine grapes. The cooling effect would not be felt during the Middle Ages but led to a few years with very short growing seasons in the seventeenth century.

In addition to long-term climate changes, short-term climatic fluctuations, or what might be called weather, also had an impact on English society. Because it was difficult to move large amounts of food from one place to another, too much or too little rainfall could produce localized famines, or even animal disease. A series of cold and wet years from 1316 to 1318 produced shortened growing seasons and localized flooding that led to widespread malnutrition and even starvation. Climate fluctuations were thus related to the ever-present possibility of famine. Examination of the *Anglo-Saxon Chronicle* and other sources indicates that several major famines troubled England from the fifth century to the end of the eleventh century plus a host of smaller events, many of which were caused by cold, rain, or drought (too much and not enough rain led to problems).[47] Famine on this scale led to at least a few deaths from starvation as well as weakening the resistance of the population, making it somewhat more susceptible to disease. On most occasions, famine was not a major killer but may have weakened the immune system of some people making them susceptible to disease.

Today, humans are in the process of changing the global climate, but in the past, they had little impact on climate although land clearing could modestly affect the climate of a relatively small area. The rotational axis of the earth has changed gradually over time and has helped to produce some of the major changes of the past. The oscillation of ocean currents also affects climate on a year-to-year basis. Two, more short-term impacts that are less predictable are solar activity and volcanic eruptions. Both of these affect the amount of sunlight received, an important determinant of the growing season. The impact of weather and climate in affecting the disease regime of premodern English people is difficult to measure accurately but provided an environmental background that influenced the impact of disease.

Conclusion

This chapter has examined some of the biological and environmental factors that can affect the onset of disease as well as its severity. These exogenous factors were beyond the control of people in premodern England. They tried to adapt to colder or hotter years, but they had no influence over the climate. Extreme climate events had the potential to create food shortages leading to malnutrition. Government, landowners, and individuals did have some influence over the threat of dietary deficiency. Relief efforts such as opening granaries could be organized in a bad year. Conversely, profiteering or withholding food supplies could turn a food shortage into a famine. Trying new crops, improving agricultural techniques, and putting more land into cultivation had a positive impact on food supplies, helping to reduce the likelihood of malnutrition. Nutrition was influenced by outside factors but also by society itself.

In addition to impacting nutritional standards, climate also had the potential to influence which diseases were present and how widespread they became. Climatic change, either short-term events or long-term trends, also made it possible for new or existing diseases to spread more readily. The course of measles, malaria, and plague, for example, are affected by climatic change.

Society could try to limit the spread of infectious disease, curtail its impact, and even prevent it with such tools as sanitation standards. Medieval medical men did not understand how diseases spread and how people became infected although they did advance some explanations. Bacteria and viruses did not care about these explanations; they continued to evolve and survive. Understanding these agents of disease and how society reacted to them, as discussed in later chapters, will help lead to greater comprehension of the impact of disease on premodern England. Premodern people had no real way to ward off infectious disease so it remained an exogenous factor that affected the lives of contemporaries. Medical practitioners and even individuals tried to devise means of coping with infectious disease, and we'll turn to some of these in later chapters. The next chapter will deal with how humans affected medieval public health in positive and negative ways.

Notes

1 Merrill Singer and Scott Clair, "Syndemies and Public Health: Reconceptualizing Disease in Bio-Social Context," *Medical Anthropology Quarterly*, new ser. 17 (2003), 423–41. Ron Barrett and George J. Armelagos, *An Unnatural History of Emerging Infections* (Oxford: Oxford University Press, 2013), 10–11, 38, 68–9.
2 A good discussion of the evolutionary relationship of humans and microbes is Paul Ewald, *Evolution of Infectious Disease*. (New York, 1994).
3 Alfred W. Crosby, "Virgin Soil Epidemics as a Factor in the Aboriginal Depopulation in America," *William and Mary Quarterly*, 33 (1976), 289–99.
4 The actual calculation of an R_0 is more complex than is evident here. J.P. Heesterbeek and K. Dietz, "The Concept of R_0 in Epidemic Theory," *Statistica Neerlandica*, 50 (1996), 89–110. Paul Delamater, Erica J. Street, Timothy F. Leslie, Y. Tony Yang, Kathryn H. Jacobsen, "Complexity of the Basic Reproduction Number (R_0)," *Emerging Infectious Diseases*, 25 (2019), 1–4. A more simplified approach, but one that also shows how the concept of contagion can explain other issues such as financial panics or social movements is Adam Kucharski, *The Rules of Contagion* (New York: Basic Books, 2020).
5 For a review of the concept of herd immunity see Paul E.M. Fine, "Herd Immunity: History, Theory, Practice," *Epidemiologic Reviews*, 15 (1993), 265–302, which is updated in Paul Fine, Ken Eames, David L. Heymann, "'Herd Immunity': A Rough Guide," *Clinical Infectious Diseases*, 52 (2011), 911–16.
6 Much of the discussion in this section relies on the discussion in Irwin W. Sherman, *The Power of Plagues* (Washington DC: ASM Press, 2006), 15–18.
7 An excellent brief introduction is Juliana Tolles and ThaiBinh Luong, "Modelling Epidemics with Compartmental Models," *JAMA*, May 27, 2020. An approach that emphasizes the role of geography is Lisa Sattenspiel, *The Geographic Spread of Infectious Diseases* (Princeton: Princeton University Press, 2009). More sophisticated approaches are detailed in Emilia Vynnycky and Richard G. White, *An Introduction to Infectious Disease Modeling* (Oxford: Oxford University Press, 2010). A sophisticated, broad-based approach is Odo Diekmann, Hans Heesterbeek, Tom Britton, *Mathematical Tools for Understanding Infectious Disease Dynamics* (Princeton: Princeton University Press, 2013). A comprehensive approach to analyzing infectious diseases and their impacts is Roy M. Anderson and Robert M. May, *Infectious Diseases of Humans* (Oxford: Oxford University Press, 1991).
8 See, for example, Stacy Thrall and John Theilmann, "Modeling the Black Death," paper presented at the meeting of the Southeastern Medieval Association, 2007.
9 The call for a multi-disciplinary approach to understanding emerging infectious diseases can also be applied with more urgency to understanding disease in the past. Margot W. Parkes, Leslie Bienen, Jamie Breilh, Lee-Nah Hsu, Marian McDonald, et al., "All Hands on Deck: Transdisciplinary Approaches to Emerging Infectious Diseases," *EcoHealth*, 2 (2005), 258–72.
10 Timothy P. Newfield, "Mysterious and Mortiferous Clouds: the Climate Cooling and the Disease Burden of Late Antiquity," *Late Antique Archaeology*, 12 (2016), 89–115. Newfields's points carry weight for the relationship of climate and disease through the Middle Ages and into the sixteenth century.
11 A useful summary of the impact of extreme weather events is Paul R. Epstein, "Detecting the Infectious Disease Consequences of Climatic Change and Extreme Weather Events," in Pim Martens and Anthony J. McMichael, (eds.), *Environmental Change, Climate and Health* (Cambridge: Cambridge University Press, 2002), 172–96.
12 Bruce M.S. Campbell, "Nature as Historical Protagonist: Environment and Society in Pre-Industrial England," *EconHistRev*, 63 (2010), 281–314.
13 Adam Izdebski, Karin Holmgren, Erika Weiberg, Sharon R. Stocker, Ulf Buentgen et al., "Realising Consilience: How Better Communication between Archaeologists, Historians and Natural Scientists Can Transform the Study of Past Climate Change in the Mediterranean," *Quaternary Science Reviews*, 136 (2016), 5–22. Timothy P. Newfield

and Inga Labuhn, "Realizing Consilience: Studies of Pre-Industrial Climate and Pre-Laboratory Disease," *Journal of Interdisciplinary History*, 58 (2017), 211–40. Sverker Sörlin and Melissa Lane, "Historicizing Climate Change—Engaging New Approaches to Climate and History," *Climatic Change*, 151 (2018), 1–13. John Haldon, Lee Mordechai, Timothy P. Newfield, Arlen F. Chase, Adam Izdebski et al., "History Meets Palaeoscience: Consilience and Collaboration in Studying past Societal Reponses to Environmental Change," *PNAS*, 115 (2018), 3210–3218. Michael McCormick, "Climates of History, Histories of Climate: From History to Archaeoscience," *Journal of Interdisciplinary History*, 50 (2019), 3–30. E.O. Wilson coined the term in *Consilience: The Unity of Knowledge* (New York: Alfred A. Knopf, 1998).

14 Although advocating disciplinary collaboration Heather Sangster, Cerys Jones, and Neil Macdonald warn of some pitfalls to be found along the way: "The Co-Evolution of Historical Source Materials in the Geophysical, Hydrological and Meteorological Sciences: Learning from the Past and Moving Forward," *Progress in Physical Geography*, 42 (2018), 61–82. They and some of the authors in the previous note indicate that team approaches that combine scholars from multiple disciplines may be productive. A more negative approach that warns of the danger of climatic determinism, especially in relating climate change and the evolution of societies and that argues some modern scholars are falling into the discredited approach of such twentieth century scholars as William Diller Matthews and Ellsworth Huntington is David N. Livingstone, "Changing Climate, Human Evolution, and the Revival of Environmental Determinism," *BHM*, 86 (2012), 564–95.

15 D.D. Zhang, P. Brecke, H.F. Lee, H. Yuan-Qing, J. Zhang, "Global Climate Change, War, and Population Decline in Recent Human History," *PNAS*, 104 (2007), 19214–19.

16 Two scholars who warn against climate reductionism are Mike Hulme, "Reducing the Future to Climate: A Story of Climate Determinism and Reductionism," *Osiris*, 26 (2011), 245–66, and Philip Slavin, "Climates and Famines: A Historical Reassessment," *Wiley Interdisciplinary Reviews*, 7 (2016), 433–47.

17 A discussion of some of the pitfalls in interpreting the impact of climate on different aspects of society see Fredrik Charpentier Ljungvist, Andre Seim, and Heli Hubtamaa, "Climate and Society in European History: *Wiley Interdisciplinary Reviews: Climate Change*, 12 (2021), e691, and B.J. Van Bavel, D.R. Curtis, M.J. Hannaford, M. Moatsos, J. Rosen, and T. Soens, "Climate and Society in Long-Term Perspective: Opportunities and Pitfalls in the Use of Historical Datasets," *Wiley Interdisciplinary Reviews: Climate Change*, 10 (2015), e611.

18 Michael E. Mann, Zhihua Zhang, Malcolm K. Hughes, Raymond S. Bradley, Sonya K. Miller, et al., "Proxy-Based Reconstructions of Hemispheric and Global Surface Temperature Variations over the Past Two Millennia," *PNAS*, 105:36 (2008), 13252–57. The authors utilized 1,209 proxy series for this study with 25 extending back to 0 CE, 36 back to 500 CE, 59 back to 1000, 177 back to 1400 and 460 back to 1600.

19 The changing perspective that led the term Medieval Climate Anomaly to replace the term Medieval Warm Era is examined with numerous references in Henry F. Diaz, Ricardo Trigo, Malcolm K. Hughes, Michael E. Mann, Elana Xoplaki et al., "Spatial and Temporal Characteristics of Climate in Medieval Times Revisited," *Bulletin of the American Meteorological Society*, 92 (2011), 1487–1500.

20 Thomas J. Crowley and Thomas S. Lowery, "How Warm was the Medieval Warm Period," *Ambio: A Journal of the Human Environment*, 29 (2000), 51–54. A. Oglive and G. Farmer, "Documenting the Medieval Climate," in Mike Hulme and E. Barrow (eds.), *Climates of the British Isles* (London: Routledge, 1997), 84–111.

21 Oglive and Farmer, "Documenting Medieval Climate," Mann et al., Proxy-Based Reconstructions of Hemispheric and Global Surface Temperature Variations," Michael E. Mann, Zhihua Zang, Scott Rutherford, Raymond S. Bradley, Malcolm K. Hughes, et al., "Global Signatures and Dynamical Origins of the Little Ice Age and Medieval Climate Anomaly," *Science*, 326 (2009), 1256–60.

22 K.R. Briffa, T.J. Osborn, F.H. Schweingruber, "Large-Scale Temperature Inferences from Tree Rings: A Review," *Global and Planetary Change*, 40 (2004), 11–26.

23 Valérie Trouet, Jan Esper, Nicholas E. Graham, Andy Baker, James D. Scourse, and David C. Frank, "Persistent Positive North Atlantic Oscillation Mode Dominated the Medieval Climate Anomaly," *Science*, 324 (2009), 78–80.

24 Drew T. Shindell, Gavin A. Schmidt, Michael E. Mann, David Rind, and Anne Waple, "Solar Forcing of Regional Climate Change during the Maunder Minimum," *Science*, 294 (2001), 2149–52.

25 John A. Eddy, "The 'Maunder Minimum': Sunspots and Climate in the Reign of Louis XIV," in Geoffrey Parker and L. M. Smith (eds.), *The General Crisis of the Seventeenth Century* (London: Routledge, 1978), 264–97. Geoffrey Parker examines the role of climate change along with other factors in his history of the crisis of the seventeenth century. *Global Crisis* (New Haven: Yale University Press, 2013).

26 Giford H. Miller, Áslaug Geirsdóttir, Yafang Zhong, Darren J. Larsen, Bette L. Otto-Bliesner, et al., "Abrupt Onset of the Little Ice Age Triggered by Volcanism and Sustained by Sea-Ice/Ocean Feedbacks," *Geophysical Research Letters* 39 (2012), L02708.

27 Chantal Camenisch, Kathrin M. Keller, Melanie Salvisberg, Benjamin Amann, S. Brázdil, et al., "The 1430s: A Cold Period of Extraordinary Internal Climate Variability during the Early Spörer Minimum with Social and Economic Impacts in North-Western and Central Europe," *Climate of the Past*, 12 (2016), 2107.

28 M. Sigl, M. Winstrup, J.R. McConnell, K.C. Welten, G. Plunkett, et al., "Timing and Climate Forcing of Volcanic Eruptions for the Past 2,500 Years, *Nature* 523 (2015), 543–49.

29 The debate over the impact of the Toba eruption illustrates the difficulty of finding a clear connection between volcanic activity and human life. Michael R. Rampino and Stephen Self, "Climate-Volcanism Feedback and the Toba Eruption of ~ 74,000 Years Ago," *Quaternary Research*, 40 (1993), 269–80. Clive Oppenheimer, "Limited Global Change Due to the Largest Known Quaternary Eruption, Toba ≈ 74 kyr BP?" *Quaternary Science Research*, 21 (2002), 1593–1609. F.J. Gathorne-Hardy and W.E.H. Harcourt-Smith, "The Super-Eruption of Toba, Did it Cause a Human Bottleneck," *Journal of Human Evolution*, 45 (2003), 227–30. Martin A.J. Williams, Stanley H. Ambrose, Sander Van Der Kaars, Carsten Ruehlemann, et al., "Environmental Impact of the 73 ka Super-Eruption in South Asia," *Palaeogeography, Palaeoclimatology, Palaeoecology*, 284 (2009), 295–314. Donald R. Prothero, *When Humans Nearly Vanished* (Washington DC: Smithsonian Books, 2018).

30 Matthew Paris, *Chronica Majora*, H.R. Luard, (ed.), 7 vols. (Rolls Series, 1872–83), 5: 706, 710–11, 693, 701–02.

31 Care needs to be taken to not over-emphasize terrestrial phenomena such as blue suns as illustrating the impact of volcanic eruptions although they can be indicative of some sort of event. Martin Bauch, "The day the Sun Turned Blue: A Volcanic Eruption in the Early 1460s and its Possible Climatic Impact—Natural Disaster Perceived Globally in the Late Middle Ages," in Gerrit Jasper Schenk, (ed.) *Historical Disaster Experiences: Toward a Comparative and Transcultural History of Disasters across Asia and Europe* (Cham, Switzerland: Springer, 2017), 107–38.

32 Richard B. Strothers and M.R. Rampino, "Volcanic Eruptions in the Mediterranean before A.D. 630 from Written and Archaeological Sources," *Journal of Geophysical Research*, 88 (1983), 6357–71. Richard B. Strothers, "The Mystery Cloud of A.D. 536," *Nature*, 307 (1984), 344–5; L.B. Larsen, B.M. Vinther, K.R. Briffa, T.M. Melvin, W.B. Clausen, et al., "New Ice Core Evidence for a Volcanic Cause of the A.D. 536 Dust Veil," *Geophysical Research Letters*, 35 (2008), L04708. Matthew Toohey, Kirstin Krüger, Michael Sigl, Frode Stordal, Henrik Svensen, "Climatic and Societal Impacts of a Volcanic Double Event at the Dawn of the Middle Ages," *Climatic Change*, 136 (2016), 401–12.

33 Antti Arjava, "The Mystery Cloud of 536 CE in the Mediterranean Sources," *Dumbarton Oaks Papers*, 59 (2005), 73–94. Relying on contemporary narrative sources Arjava casts a very narrow net that embraces only immediate political and social events and that ignores any potential long term climatic impacts that would ultimately have an impact on society.

34 Ulf Büntgen, Vladimir Mygian, Fredik Charpentier, Michael McCormick, Nicola Di Cosmo, et al., "Cooling and Societal Change during the Late Antique Little Ice Age from 536 to around 660 A.D," *Nature Geoscience*, 9 (2016), 231. Sigl, et al., "Timing and Climate Forcing of Volcanic Eruptions for the Past 2,500 Years,"

35 Ann Gibbons, "Eruption Made 536 'The Worst Year to be Alive,'" *Science*, 362 (2018), 733–34; Robert A. Dull, John R. Southon, Steffen Kutterolf, Kevin J. Anchukaitis, et al., "Radiocarbon and Geologic Evidence Revel Ilopango Volcano as Source of the Colossal 'Mystery' Eruption of 539–40 CE," *Quaternary Science Reviews*, 222 (2019), 105856.

36 Michael McCormick, Paul Edward Dutton, and Paul A. Mayewski, "Volcanoes and Climate Forcing of Carolingian Europe, A.D. 750–950," *Speculum*, 82 (2007), 865–95. Carroll Gillmor, "The 791 Equine Epidemic and Its Impact on Charlemagne's Army," *Journal of Medieval Military History*, 3 (2005), 23–45. Timothy Newfield, "A Great Carolingian Panzootic: The Probable Extent, Diagnosis and Impact of an Early Ninth-Century Cattle Pestilence," *Argos*. 46 (2012), 200–10. Newfield, "Domesticates, Disease and Climate in Early Post-Classical Europe: The Cattle Plague of c. 940 and its Environmental Context," *Post-Classical Archaeologies*, 5 (2013), 95–126. Irish chronicles also reveal volcanic forcing of cold weather, with several of the events coinciding with the continental cold years. Francis Ludlow, Alexander R. Stine, Paul Leahy, Enda Murphy, Paul A. Mayewski, et al., "Medieval Irish Chronicles Reveal Persistent Volcanic Forcing of Severe Winter Cold Events, 431–1649 CE," *Environmental Research Letters*, 8 (2013), 024035.

37 Joanna Slawinska and Alan Robock, "Impact of Volcanic Eruptions on Decadal to Centennial Fluctuations of Arctic Sea Ice Extent during the Last Millennium and on Initiation of the Little Ice Age," *Journal of Climate* 31 (2018), 2145–67.

38 Richard B. Stothers, "Climatic and Demographic Consequences of the Massive Volcanic Eruption of 1258," *Climatic Change*, 45 (2000), 361–74. Clive Oppenheimer, "Ice Core and Paleoclimatic Evidence for the Timing and Nature of the Great Mid-13th Century Volcanic Eruption," *International Journal of Climatology*, 23 (2003), 417–26. Frank Lavigne, Jean-Phillippe Degeal, Jean-Christophe Komorowski, Sébastien Guillet, Vincent Robert, et al., "Source of the Great A.D. 1257 Mystery Eruption Unveiled, Samalas Volcano, Rinjani Volcanic Complex, Indonesia," *PNAS*, 110 (2013), 16742–47. David C. Wade, Céline M. Vidal, N. Luke Abraham, Sandip Dhomse, Paul R. Griffiths, "Reconciling the Climate and Ozone Response to the 1257 CE Mount Samalas Eruption," *PNAS*, 117 (2020), 26651–59.

39 Sébastien, Guillet, Christophe Corona, Markus Stoffel, Myriam Khodri, Frank Lavigne, et al., "Climate Response to the Samalas Volcanic Eruption in 1257 Revealed by Proxy Records," *Nature Geoscience*, 10 (2017), 123–27.

40 Stothers, "Climatic and Demographic Consequences of the Massive Volcanic Eruption of 1258."

41 Matthew Paris, *Chronica Majora*, 5: 710–11, 674, 701–02, 690.

42 Bruce M.S. Campbell, "Global Climate, the 1257 Mega-Eruption of Samalas Volcano, Indonesia, and the English Food Crisis of 1258," *TRHS*, 27 (2017), 87–121.

43 Miller, et al., "Abrupt Onset of the Little Ice Age Triggered by Volcanism and Sustained by Sea-Ice/Ocean Feedbacks."

44 Camenisch, et al., "The 1430s: A Cold Period of Extraordinary Internal Climate Variability during the Spörer Minimum with Social and Economic Impacts in North-Western and Central Europe."

45 Chachao Gao, Alan Robock, Stephen Self, Jeffrey B. Wittier, Jørgen P. Steffenson, et al., "The 1452 or 1453 AD Kuwae Eruption Signal Derived from Multiple Ice Core Records: Greatest Volcanic Sulfate Event of the Past 700 Years," *Journal of Geophysical Research: Atmospheres*, 111 (2006), D12. J.B. Witter, Stephen Self, "The Kuwae (Vanuatu) Eruption of AD 1452: Potential Magnitude and Volatile Release," *Bulletin of Volcanology*, 69 (2007), 301–18. Christopher Plummer, Mark A.J. Curran, T.D. Van Ommen, Sune O. Rasmussen, Andrew D. Moy, et al., "An Independent Dated 2000-yr Record from Law Dome East Antarctica, including a New Perspective on the 1450s CE Eruption of Kuwae, Vanuatu, *Climate of the Past*, 8 (2012), 1929–1940. Dating of volcanic eruptions is difficult and recent research puts the eruption in 1458 not 1452 as first indicated. Sigl, et al, "Timing and Climate Forcing of Volcanic Eruptions for the Past 2,500 Years."

46 J.N. Mills, J.L. Gage, A.S. Khan, "Potential Influence of Climate Change on Vector-borne and Zoonotic Diseases: A Review and Proposed Research Plan," *Environmental Health Perspectives*, 118 (2010: 1507–1514. Nils Chr. Stenseth, Noelle I. Samia, Hildegunn Viljugrein, Kyrre Linné Kausrud, K.L. Begon, et al., "Plague Dynamics Are Driven by Climate Variation," *PNAS*, 103 (2006), 13110–13115.

47 Ann Hagen, *Anglo-Saxon Food and Drink* (Hockwold Cum Wilton: Anglo-Saxon Books, 2006), 438–44.

2

HUMAN IMPACTS ON HEALTH IN PREMODERN ENGLAND

Life expectancy was short in premodern England, often less than 40 years. Even though people in the past did not have to contend with many of the problems of modern society such as chemical pollution or some modern diseases such as cholera or Ebola, good health was at a premium. Childhood was a particularly dangerous time although children who lived to their tenth birthday had a better chance of survival to old age, which came earlier than today even though there were people who lived into their 70s and 80s.

Threats to health and life itself were commonplace. Medical knowledge was limited and there were no antibiotics or other drugs that we take for granted today so that fevers or wounds could easily lead to death. Poor diet also complicated the pursuit of good health for many people; especially in the early Middle Ages famine or at least malnutrition often stalked the land. Obesity was rarely a problem for medieval people but complications arising from malnutrition made people susceptible to disease and recovery from some ailments more difficult. In some places, violence from family, neighbors, or outsiders also threatened the survival of people. Accidents too threatened the lives of people, especially children. Even when an accident did not kill, the quality of life might be severely diminished if a person was permanently crippled.

The first chapter introduced a conceptual relationship of the factors that influenced health in the past. It also examined exogenous factors that affected the health of the people. This chapter turns to endogenous factors affecting health, those factors that society had some means to control, in essence, human action that had a positive or negative impact on the health of the population. Medical practitioners, diet, settlement patterns, and population size, and sanitation all had impacts on the health of the population especially the threat of infectious disease.

DOI: 10.4324/9781003215219-3

Medicine and medical care in premodern England

Today people in economically advanced countries turn to medical profession-als when they face health issues. In premodern Europe, this was not always an option as professionally trained medical practitioners were rare. Medical care was available from five overlapping sources in the Middle Ages. Educated at universities from the twelfth century onward, physicians were at the top of the pyramid, followed by surgeons who may have had some university training and often underwent a period of apprenticeship. Apothecaries came to play a role in late medieval medicine as they were responsible for preparing compounds prescribed by physicians. Some also engaged in medical practice, something that physicians tried to restrict. The largest and least well-described category included the empirics who were the medical practitioners that most people had contact with. This category included midwives, bone setters, practitioners of herb lore, and increasingly by the fifteenth century educated people who had read some of the medical literature of the day. Some of these practitioners also utilized magical practices, such as gathering herbs by the light of the moon while reciting a Bible verse, but physicians, too, were influenced by astrology. When all else failed, people sought divine intervention by asking the saints to intervene with God on their behalf. These five categories were not mutually exclusive and a person might make use of any of them on different occasions or simultaneously. Sadly, there was also a sixth category, the out and out quack, a person with little medical knowledge and few scruples who took advantage of others for profit.

Intellectual medical knowledge in the medieval West was a product of the Greek world.[1] Scholars consider Hippocrates of Kos—the father of physi-cians, although few works ascribed to him were available to medieval scholars. Hippocrates who lived from approximately 475 BCE to 370 BCE has had more than 60 works ascribed to him. They seem to have been written over a two-hundred-year period and it is even possible that he was the author of none of them. More directly, Galen, the second-century Greek physician who practiced for a time in Rome, was seen as the authority from which medical knowledge flowed in the Middle Ages. Galen's work was available in Greek in the early Middle Ages but gradually vanished from view as knowledge of Greek waned. By the eleventh century, Galen's work was once again becoming available, first through translations and commentaries by Arab physicians and then as transla-tions from Greek to Latin. Galen's work, particularly his *Aphorisms*, became the foundation of university medical education throughout the high and late Middle Ages. Starting in the thirteenth century, especially in Italian medical schools, Aristotle's works also influenced medical education.[2]

Galen described a medical regime predicated on maintaining a balance within the body. He indicated that the naturals (e.g., age, sex, or climate) influenced health but that people had no control over them. The six non-naturals, which he described in his *Ars Medica* (*The Medical Art*), however, could be manipu-lated in order to bring the humors back into balance and return a sick person to good health. The non-naturals were: air, food and drink, sleep and waking, movement and rest, retention and evacuation which included sexual activity, and the passions of the soul or the emotions. Premodern physicians were aware of the six categories and their roles in the provision of good health. Unlike Hippocrates, Galen thought that the non-naturals could be controlled so that a skilled physician could enable his patients to regain good health by making changes in their lives such as changing their diet or receiving a purgative or engaging in less sexual activity.

The humor theory of disease, which was derived from the concept of the non-naturals and incorporated human temperament, dated from the ancient world and continued to be accepted well into the seventeenth century by many people. Because of its association with Galen, medical men regarded humor theory as the authoritative approach to describing the cause of disease particularly with the reinforcement provided by Avicena's *Canon of Medicine* (1095). Andreas Vesalius first challenged humor theory in the mid-sixteenth century although its impact lingered well beyond his initial attack. Even today, we still use the terminology of the humors in a descriptive sense even if not for medical diagnosis. The humors were part of a descriptive structure that related temperament, humors, disposition, and the elements of the natural world:

Element	Humor	Qualities	Temperament
Fire	yellow bile	warm and dry	choleric
Water	phlegm	cold and wet	phlegmatic
Earth	black bile	cold and dry	melancholic
Air	blood	warm and wet	sanguine

Too much of any one element caused the humors to go out of balance producing a medical problem so that an excess of say black bile originating from the spleen's failure to absorb black bile produced a melancholic temperament. A melancholic temperament, if left unchecked, led to an unhealthy pallor, cowardice, and guile, and eventually severe medical problems.[3] In this case, the physician needed to reduce the excess of black bile, a task carried out by purging the afflicted person. Excesses of other humors required the same sort of treatment such as bleeding the patient or dietary prescriptions. Dietary remedies, at least, generally did not harm patients and an improved diet might have been helpful in many cases. Purging and bloodletting could be potentially disastrous for a patient already weakened by disease.

Humor theory was the dominant approach to medicine among educated practitioners although it also trickled down to other practitioners. It was based on the premise that God was the prime mover, but that the relationship of the humors explained everyday problems. The explanatory power of humor theory was reinforced by the natural world as it was believed that natural occurrences such as comets or the conjunction of certain planets could lead to an imbalance in the humors.

"Bad" air influences the balance of the humors in the Galenic approach. It could lead to extrinsic putrid effluvia that produced disease. Galen had emphasized that bad air was one of the most dangerous things that people could encounter and this became a driving force behind miasma theory.[4] Miasmas might come from volcanic eruptions or rotting vegetation, but human action or inaction often produced the miasma that people thought led to disease. In May 1354, the Prior of the Hospital of St. John petitioned the King concerning the butchering waste being deposited in the Fleet River near the Fleet Prison. The London authorities had ignored the matter so King Edward III ordered in no uncertain terms that action be taken to clean up the mess because "the stench arising (from the waste) was so bad as to be injurious to the health of the free prison of the Flete and the neighborhood."[5] Butchering waste produced an unpleasant stench often regarded as a source of disease, but it was not alone in being a public health threat. Today we know that the stench from human and animal wastes does not kill although chemical odors can be harmful. The stench from butchering or dung, however, is a sign that a biological hazard may exist. Human and animal waste can be hosts for bacteria and parasites such as for diarrhea, dysentery, and typhoid among other problems. Dealing with waste issues in the context of miasma theory did help to promote a healthier environment.

The stench emanating from piles of human and animal dung was something that almost everyone reacted to negatively as anything that smelled (and looked) that bad had to be harmful to public health. The negative impact of "bad" air also received intellectual endorsement. Writing in the thirteenth century, and echoing the Arab physician Avicenna's *Canon,* Bartholomew Anglicus noted, "if the vapor is malicious, stinking and corrupt, it corrupted the spirit that is called *animalis* and often brings pestilence."[6] This continued to be the driving force behind trying to ensure healthy air. In his work written for a popular audience in the mid-sixteenth century, Andrew Boorde noted that "there is nothing, except poison, that does putrefy the blood of man, and also does mortify the spirits of man as does a corrupt and contagious air" and then went on to list the agents responsible for impure air.[7] Pestilence was a generic term used to refer to any disease, not just the plague. Nonetheless, contemporaries seemed to have made a connection between "bad" air and the plague as E.L. Sabine indicated that the number of entries in the London Letter Books dealing with stenches was 16 in the period from 1300 to 1350 but rose to 64 in the next 50 years as the plague took hold in England.[8] Although there could be many reasons for this change, a connection between the plague and "bad" air cannot be neglected.

Medical practitioners before the rise of universities were self-educated from reading texts, serving as apprentices, and their own observations. Most physicians and surgeons before 1000 were monks as some monasteries remained repositories of ancient knowledge. Some scholars have criticized the texts that they wrote for being bizarre mixtures of old texts, folklore, magic, and some observations. However, more nuanced views indicate a coherence and logic to their works.[9] In addition to monastic education, early medieval medical practitioners drew on extensive collections of herbal remedies, most notably Bald's *Leechbook* and the *Lacnunga*. Some of the herbal remedies appear to be plausible, but recent laboratory testing often has shown them valueless.[10] Even if ineffective in a chemical sense, the remedies may well have had value because of the placebo effect they created.

University medical education occurred first in southern European universities such as Salerno, Bologna, and Montpelier. By the late Middle Ages, the universities at Padua and Paris had surpassed the first medical schools in influence. Oxford and Cambridge awarded medical degrees, but they were few in number in the Middle Ages as both universities concentrated their efforts on theology.[11] University-trained medical practitioners first followed a course in the Arts and then delved deeper into the works of Galen and Aristotle. Their education was theoretically based with little empirical practice.[12] It revolved around the necessity to maintain the body in equilibrium by keeping the four humors in balance.

Doctors saw diet as the primary means of achieving humoral balance although physical remedies such as purging and bleeding were also used. Physicians also indicated behavioral norms as necessary for keeping the humors in balance so, for example, they indicated that too much sexual activity was harmful. Medieval physicians' diagnostic tools included observation of patients and their complexions and especially uroscopy, the examination of a patient's urine. The physician then prepared a diagnosis as well as a treatment regime that took into account environmental factors as part of the process of returning the patient's humors to a balanced state. This approach regarded each individual case as unique, which required the physician to construct a treatment regime specific to the patient. As such, physicians treated patients rather than curing diseases.

Physicians were the aristocrats of the medieval medical universe. Physicians might write treatises in Latin available to the literate, but they tended to render their services in noble and royal courts and religious establishments as many were in holy orders. Their services were intended to maintain the whole body in equilibrium but were less helpful in cases such as wounds or accidents. Infectious diseases were largely beyond their ability although the possibility exists that some of their prescriptions were helpful, and treatment of any sort can produce a placebo effect that may have been helpful.

Surgeons came to perform the physical side of medieval medical practice. Some were university educated, most were not. In some cases, such as Guy de Chaulaic, who received medical training at the universities of Paris and Bologna and who was the chief papal medical adviser at the time of the plague in the mid-fourteenth century, a surgeon reached the apex of the medical profession. Working with a surgeon as an apprentice was the most common route to becoming a surgeon. Surgeons' skills varied. Some connected with the barbers' guild were little more than tooth-drawers and bone setters. Barber-surgeons were more common than surgeons and tended to have a lower skill level than practitioners who were strictly surgeons. Other practitioners had more sophisticated skill sets that could involve surgery for fistulas, draining abscess, treating wounds, including cauterization to prevent infection and even primitive brain surgery—trephining. The work of sophisticated surgeons was available to only a few but almost anyone could have access to a tooth-drawer or bone setter. Surgery had evolved by the fourteenth century and people came to see surgeons as distinct from physicians because of their education differences and surgeons' emphasis on physical, not dietary remedies. Michael McVaugh argues that this situation may not have been to the advantage of surgeons, as they increasingly needed to defend their turf from encroachment by various sorts of empirics.[13]

Surgeons had the organizational advantage over physicians, in part because of their larger numbers and in part because of their quasi-guild status. It seems that the Fellowship of Surgeons was first formed in 1368 although the Fellowship was never incorporated as a guild.[14] While somewhat suspicious of the motivations of each other, both physicians and surgeons saw they had a common enemy in empirics and surgeons wanted to emphasize their superiority to barber-surgeons. The result was a petition to the London Common Council in May 1423 for a joint college of physicians and surgeons.[15] The petitioners included distinguished physicians such as Gilbert Kymer, who went on to serve as physician to Henry VI, and the two masters of the craft of surgery, Thomas Morstede and John Hawe with Kymer serving as its first rector. The College had high-sounding goals, but neither surgeons nor especially physicians had any real interest in seeing it work and it soon died. The Fellowship of Surgeons continued to be somewhat of a regulatory body in London although not in the provinces. The physicians finally organized and received a royal charter as the College of Physicians of London in 1518. These various professional groups had the professed goal of providing better medical care, but they often worked to limit medical practice by barber-surgeons and other empirics and concentrated their attention in London.

Because physicians relied on various prescriptions to help return the humors to balance, an important adjunct to their work was the apothecary. Apothecaries mixed prescriptions including theriac—the widely recognized cure-all. By the fifteenth century, some advocates said that theriac could cure dropsy, induce sleep, remove a dead child from a mother's womb, cure fevers and heart trouble, heal wounds, and counteract poison among other cures.[16] Theraic, or treacle as it was sometimes known, could be quite expensive depending on the ingredients, such as gold dust, leading some commentators to be critical of what they saw as collusive practices between physicians and apothecaries to rob patients. In addition to compounding medicines, some apothecaries seemed to have also engaged in an illicit practice of medicine on occasion.

Neither physicians nor surgeons were numerous in the premodern world although their numbers increased over time. Both groups tried to defend their status against each other and especially against the far more numerous empirics, whose numbers included all sorts of practitioners from the learned to local cunning men and women who provided herbal cures and at times some physical remedies. Barber-surgeons, who combined barbering with minor surgery, were the most organized achieving a royal charter in 1462 that granted them a medical role within a typical guild structure.[17] The Barber–Surgeons were better organized and more numerous than the surgeons. The surgeons recognized the situation and agreed to merge with the barbers as the Company of Barbers and Surgeons in 1540 although the surgeons broke away in 1745 to found the Royal College of Surgeons. Unfortunately, we know very little about empirics, the largest segment of medical practitioners. Some appear to have been self-educated laymen such as John Crophill, a fifteenth-century rural practitioner who derived his learning from reading vernacular medical texts and the application of common sense and was a fulltime practitioner.[18] Empirics might devote their full attention to the practice of medicine, as did Crophill, but many others occasionally provided an herbal remedy or provided a poultice. Herb lore had been a staple of Anglo-Saxon medicine and continued to be handed down in various families. Physicians had long incorporated herbal remedies into their medicine, but William Bullein, a sixteenth-century physician, was contemptuous of folk knowledge, indicating that the herbal knowledge of practitioners he labeled as herb women was scant in comparison to the superior knowledge of herbal medicine that came from the literate tradition.[19] He was critical of herbalists for not recognizing the medical power of dandelions in this passage. In essence, literate practitioners incorporated earlier herbal traditions and gave them new authority by presenting them in written form even though they denigrated folk practitioners at the same time.

Only occasionally did folk medical practice surface in such a way that merited description. People turned to folk practitioners and may have received relief or not, but little written record of the transaction was likely to be compiled. One important exception to this lack of information, at least for the late Middle Ages, was when something went wrong and a malpractice suit was lodged by the afflicted victim. As Madeleine Pelner Cosman and Sara Butler have indicated, court records can give us a greater understanding of medieval medical practice.[20] On 24 February 1354, a group of surgeons were sworn before the mayor, aldermen, and sheriffs of London to give testimony whether the attempted cure of "a certain enormous and horrible hurt on the right side of the jaw" of Thomas de Shene was possible. John le Spicer (a spice seller, not a surgeon) of Cornhill had promised Thomas that he was expert in the trade of medicine and promised to cure him but instead failed and the injury became incurable.[21] Good health was important to people and general medical practitioners such as John le Spicer promised a cure in return for payment. We don't know what remedy Spicer tried, but it clearly was unsuccessful.

Unfortunately, healers such as Spicer were more common than not, and in 1377, the London authorities committed Richard Cheyndut to prison for failing to cure a sore on the left leg of John del Hull and leaving him in danger of losing the leg.[22] As was the case with Spicer, the authorities admonished Cheyndut for not consulting with better-educated medical practitioners. At least neither Cheyndut nor Spicer had claimed to be physicians, they had simply claimed to have the ability to heal. Roger Clerk, on the other hand, claimed to be a physician, in 1382, when he promised Roger atte Hacche that he could cure his wife Joanna who was lying ill with bodily infirmities, indicating "that he was experienced and skilled in the art of medicine," implying that he was a physician or at least a surgeon. Roger atte Hache provided 12p as partial payment and Roger Clerk set to work. He gave Hache an old parchment wrapped in a cloth of gold, indicating it would cure Joanna's fever and other ailments when it was put around her neck. Nothing happened. Rightly affronted, Roger atteHache sued in the Mayor's court. Perhaps unwisely, Roger Clerk appeared in court and produced the parchment on which he said was written the charm *Anima Christi, sanctifica me; corpus Christi, salve me, in isanguis Christi, nebria me; cum bonus Christus tu, lava me* or "Soul of Christ, sanctify me; body of Christ, save me; blood of Christ, drench me; as thou art good Christ, baptize me." The Mayor and Aldermen were singularly unimpressed and pointed out that nothing was written on the parchment and told Roger that "a straw beneath his foot would be just as much avail for fevers, as this said charm of his was."[23] The court judged the illiterate Roger Clerk to be neither a physician nor a surgeon but it took some pity on him for he was neither fined nor imprisoned. Instead, Roger was to be paraded through the middle of the city on a horse with trumpets and pipes playing and the parchment and a whetstone for his lies and a urinal hung on him before and after. Public humiliation often was used as a punishment, and in this case, we might suppose that it put an end to Roger Clerk's medical career. With Roger Clerk, we have arrived at our sixth category of medical practitioner, the out and out quack. Spicer and Cheyndut may have some good intentions, but Roger Clerk was an outright fraud who tried to prey on the fearful and gullible.

Many empirics, especially village practitioners, often engaged in some sort of magical practice such as gathering herbs by the light of a full moon. Others used healing charms as Roger Clerk tried to do. Galenic medicine had been opposed to magical practice but gradually astrology crept in and some physicians described the causation for various natural events such as epidemics as coming from a conjunction of the planets.

This conjunction of astrology and medical snobbism can be seen in one final malpractice case. In September 1424, William Forest brought suit in the Mayor's court against three surgeons, John Hawe, John Dalton, and Simon Rolf, for incorrectly treating a wound in the muscles of his right thumb. Their treatment proved a failure and they cauterized the wound to prevent further bleeding, maiming his hand. The court appointed a distinguished group of physicians and surgeons including John Morstede, surgeon and one of the founders of the College of Physicians and Surgeons, and Gilbert Kymer, physician and another founder of the College to examine the evidence. We have met Kymer and Hawe before as petitioners to the Common Council in 1423. The investigators found that Forest had been first injured when "the moon being consumed in a bloody sign, to wit, Aquarius, under a very malevolent constellation," and that "on 9 Feb., the moon being in the sign of the Gemini, a great effusion of blood took place." The three surgeons staunched the flow of blood "which broke out six several times in a dangerous fashion, and that on the seventh occasion, the wounded man preferring a mutilated hand rather than death, the said John Hawe (one of the three surgeons), with the consent of the patient, and for lack of other remedy, finally staunched the blood by cautery, as was proper, and thus saved his life." On 9 June 1424, the panel of specialists found that the three surgeons had acted correctly and absolved them from all charges, ordering Forest to remain silent about the matter. They went on to say "that any defect, mutilation or disfigurement of the hand was due either to the constellation aforesaid or some defect of the patient or the original nature of the wound."[24]

There are three underlying factors in the Forest malpractice case that help to illustrate aspects of late medieval medicine. First, the implied, and in some cases actual contract in, which the physician or surgeon agreed to cure the patient before starting treatment leading Forest to think that he had legal recourse for breach of contract. Even when surgeons did their best, as the three seemingly tried to do, the failure to provide the promised cure could lead the aggrieved patient to take action. This contractual relationship led some physicians and surgeons to be reluctant to treat patients whose prognosis was not good. Second, the role of astrology in determining human affairs, as an unfortunate conjunction of the planets helped to create Forest's problem. Knowledge of astrology had come to be part of physicians' and surgeons' tool kits and the implication, in this case, was that Forest was lucky to have survived. Third, the power of position in influencing legal outcomes as Simon Rolf served as master of the Craft of Surgeons in 1415 and John Hawe served as its master in 1423. One interpretation of the events could be that professional distinction granted little protection from malpractice suits and that was the case here. A suspicion arises that distinction, however, also shaped the verdict as the investigating panel and the accused served together in leadership positions in the London medical community. Astrology may have been seen as contributing factor for Forest's problem, but it could also have been a convenient means to exculpate the three leading surgeons.

Overall, medical practitioners did not enjoy a high reputation in medieval England. Their ability to heal was often lacking and many people saw them as grasping and money-hungry. In *Piers Plowman,* William Langland put it eloquently: "For these doctors are mostly murderers, God help them! – their medicines kill thousands before their time."[25] Another anonymous fourteenth-century author put it more bluntly:... "these physicians that help men die."[26] John Mirfield, a late fourteenth century cleric and author of an advice book for medical men, indicated that a physician should cure even the poorest man with no thought to payment although he should be able to expect payment when such was possible.[27] Mirfield seems to have recognized the inability of doctors to cure all ailments for he also indicated that physicians and surgeons should refuse to undertake hopeless cases for fear of damaging their reputations.[28] The thirteenth-century physician Lanfranc of Milan advocated that the wealthy should help to pay for treatment for the poor although the fourteenth-century surgeon John Arderne may have been more typical in indicating that the practitioner should put the patient's welfare first, but he should always be sure to know that he would be paid.[29] The perceived avarice of physicians as well as their inability to heal seems to be a thread that ran through much of popular literature including Chaucer and Langland and still was apparent in the fifteenth century. In offering advice to her son John for his upcoming visit to London, Agnes Paston urged him to avoid physicians during his visit.[30] No wonder that Agnes Paston advised her son to avoid physicians. Try as they might, there were many ailments that were beyond the ability of medical practitioners to heal. Even though their knowledge was improving in the sixteenth and seventeenth centuries, it would take the work of physicians such as William Harvey who identified the circulatory system before meaningful advances in medical treatment could be made.[31]

Not all people in medieval and early modern England came in contact with any of the practitioners noted above. Some people were their own medical practitioners with more educated people turning to medical self-help books and other people relying on herb lore. There were even a few female physicians as was the case with two sisters and their brother who practiced in Herefordshire in the thirteenth century.[32] Midwives played an important role in childbirth and some also provided other forms of medical assistance although, as Monica Greene has shown, the medical establishment moved overtime to limit the role of women in medicine even in childbirth.[33]

Many people afflicted with medical issues also availed themselves of saintly medicine instead of turning to medical practitioners or in addition to more conventional forms of medicine. People called on the saints to intercede with God for almost any sort of issue from the apparent death of a child from drowning, to wounds, and fevers, to long-term crippling or lost animals. Saintly medicine was both an immediate resort in times of emergency and a last resort for those for whom conventional medical practice had failed. In some cases, such as leprosy, a period of remission enabled a saint to receive credit for a cure even though the problem reappeared. In other cases, natural healing of a crippling event or the eventual revival of a child who had fallen into a well enabled people to credit the saints with a cure.

Given the inability of medical practitioners (and their unavailability) to deal with many ailments, saintly medicine offered a clear alternative, one that people turned to for almost any sort of problem.[34] A study of the miracles of 11 English saints and would-be saints from the eleventh to the early sixteenth century found that slightly over fifteen percent (261) of the 1695 miracles were reputed returns from the dead as people turned to the saints in emergencies when no other help was available. The largest category of miracles was that of the cure of crippling and continuing ailments at 21.6% (366). Smoky interiors and other problems often led to blindness and the third-largest category (11.2% [189]) was that of blindness. Miracles involving adults outnumbered those involving children at a nearly three to one ratio with one exception. Children outnumbered adults at a nearly two to one ratio in recovery from death miracles as parents turned to the saints in various emergencies such as drowning. Many of the miracles touched everyday problems such as wounds, broken bones, or insanity, not infectious disease although 39 of the miracles were reputed cures of leprosy, a disease subject to remission in its early stage.[35] Even when the medicine of the saints might not have provided a cure, saintly medicine did provide a placebo effect that led people to think their condition was improving.

The various sorts of healers described above could be quite effective in dealing with everyday problems afflicting society. Infection was the great problem as once a wound became infected or a fever failed to abate, there was little that practitioners of any sort could do. As later chapters will indicate, infectious and especially epidemic diseases presented special problems for all medical practitioners. New diseases, especially infectious diseases proved to be problematic. Physicians based their work on the Galenic corpus which described diseases in detail. They had to find some way to incorporate a new disease into this body of work in order to describe it and find a remedy.

Medicine was reactive for the most part as practitioners dealt with problems as they appeared but there were efforts to be proactive in providing good health. The number of vernacular texts dealing with health and hygiene expanded during the Late Middle Ages and the trend would continue in the sixteenth century with works such as Boorde's *Dietary of Health*.[36] Sanitation and the provision of clean water and food were areas of society in which individuals and governments, both local and national, tried to prevent health problems from occurring.

Doctors tried to prevent medical problems with remedies such as dietary remedies that were intended to keep the humors in balance. Practitioners often modified a patient's diet in order to bring the humors back into balance. This remedy, however, was predicated on people having enough to eat. When we consider diet in the medieval and early modern periods, we need to examine what people ate and if they had enough to eat so we now turn to food and its provision as another way in which individuals and society affected health.

Diet, good health, and illness

Although modern dieticians might be critical of the diet of people in premodern England, it was generally sufficient for good health. In some ways, it was more healthful than the eating habits of people today as chemical preservatives found in some food, as well as large amounts of sugar, were not present in the diets of premodern people. Nonetheless, for people on the lower rungs of society bad harvests produced food shortages, malnutrition, and even famine.

Diet figured in the medical theories of the time and many remedies for medical problems were dietary in nature. Galen had warned of the danger that gluttony posed as it led to an imbalance in the humors.[37] Following Galen's lead physicians indicated that increasing or decreasing certain foods in patients' diets returned the humors to balance returning them to health. Although they didn't have the advantage of modern biochemical research, premodern physicians did address the relationship between nutrition and infection albeit sometimes with harmful results.

Adequate nutrition is important to good health at any time as it ensures that the body possesses enough energy reserves to go about daily activity as well as helping to produce the right mix of vitamins and minerals in the body that can help ward off various ailments.[38] Today malnutrition is a major cause of immunodeficiency worldwide and there is every reason to expect that malnutrition played the same role in the premodern world.[39] Malnutrition has a variety of causes from political and socioeconomic instability, to poverty, to climatic factors. Malnutrition weakens the body, particularly the immune system, and is especially damaging for children, making it easier for infection to occur. On the other hand, infection and disease can lead to decreased agricultural productivity, poverty, and even political instability creating a circular relationship. Malnutrition of children often has lasting impacts even when it does not lead to immediate death including stunted growth, continued immune deficiencies, and poverty. A major impact of malnutrition is the loss of caloric energy that can lead to reduced productivity and decreased immunity to disease. Malnutrition produces different impacts with different infections. The clinical courses and final outcomes of diseases such as tuberculosis and pneumonia tend to be adversely affected by malnutrition while for other problems such as tetanus it has no impact. For other diseases, such as influenza, the impact of malnutrition is a mixed one although some impact does exist. In the case of plague, one dietary deficiency, iron, may even confer some benefits making it somewhat harder for the *Yersinia pestis* bacteria to infect a person.[40] Iron deficiency causes far more problems such as hampering motor and mental development in children and adolescents. Men and non-menstruating women lose about 1 mg of iron per day, but this loss can generally be overcome with the consumption of meat, beans, or greens. Menstruating and pregnant women lose between 0.6 to 2.5 percent more iron per day, or possibly as much as 10 mg during a menstruation cycle, which often may produce anemia. Iron metabolism is largely controlled by absorption rather than excretion although iron is lost through the loss of cells or by blood loss.[41] At least by 1000, potential iron in the diet had increased so that men could absorb enough iron to compensate for loss, but women's diet was likely to be deficient in the mineral. Anemia that can be the result of an iron-deficient diet does not kill, but it weakens, making a person more susceptible to infection and potentially decreasing the life span for women as well as endangering the health of anyone who was anemic. Iron deficiency is only one example of a dietary problem with large consequences. Overall, dietary deficiency can have mild or very severe health impacts and the impacts of these dietary issues and societal responses may reinforce or mitigate the situation. An infection could lessen a person's ability to work, producing malnutrition. A malnourished person often had a weakened immune system so that further damage to the immune system could be especially harmful. Finally, a weakened immune system could lead to infection. The relationship is not always clear-cut, but when it occurs, it often leads to increased morbidity and mortality rates.[42]

Nutrition has a relationship with infectious disease albeit it is a complex one. Malnutrition can make it easier for a disease to take hold especially in a person with compromised immunity and a malnourished person with a compromised immune system is less likely to survive many diseases. A person who is poorly nourished is likely to suffer more from a bacterial disease than someone who is well-nourished as a synergetic relationship appears to be at work. Poor nutrition does not always worsen a viral disease and may even lead to better results. Some of the diseases considered here seem to display a synergetic relationship with nutrition with poor nutrition leading to a less good outcome for someone infected with leprosy, tuberculosis, measles, or diarrhea. In other cases, there seems to be a minimal relationship: plague, smallpox, malaria, typhoid, tetanus. The relationship of disease and diet is a mixed one in some cases with varying results: influenza, typhus, syphilis.[43]

We know little about diet in the Early Middle Ages.[44] It seems that the food supply was increasing at least from the eleventh century onward. There were still shortages and even famine years, most notably in the early fourteenth century, but famine-induced threats to health were rare by the fifteenth century. People's diet varied by region so, for example, along the coast seafood was more common than inland. Soil quality, access to streams, and latitude also affected what crops were grown and what animals people used for food. As might be expected, the diet of the aristocracy was more varied than that of the peasantry or urban poor and at times included items that clearly might be regarded as luxuries such as peacocks. After the Norman Conquest game, especially venison, was more likely found on the tables of the aristocracy than the peasantry save by poaching. By the Late Middle Ages, the situation was changing with increased consumption of meat by all levels of society. Sumptuary laws and dietary accounts indicated that the diet of the poor should be plain in order to promote good digestion but the trend was one of increasing the amount and variety of food consumed.[45] This trend continued into the sixteenth century although a decline in wages limited the diet of some by then.

Grain provided the staple for many people's diets. Wheat, barley, rye, oats, and peas and beans figured in the diet of almost everyone although the aristocracy were more likely to eat wheat products and the poor barley or rye and for the very poor peas scrounged from the fields. People consumed grain in bread but also in ale and beer. All of these field crops were subject to the vagaries of nature. Too much or too little moisture meant that yields for the year would be down, producing hunger or worse.

Gardens often produced some of the food for the poor although less so for the aristocracy who regarded vegetables as only fit for the poor. In addition, dietary conventions related to humor theory regarded salads and some fruits such as peaches as potentially harmful.[46] Garden produce helped the poor to avert starvation on occasion, but as was the case with cereals, bad weather could limit output.

Meat was a mainstay of the diet of knightly households except during Lent and its consumption was also increasing at other levels of society by the Late Middle Ages. In addition to game, such as deer or rabbits, cattle, sheep, and pigs all served as food sources and also as sources of traction, milk, wool, and manure which limited their availability for food consumption. Cattle provided an important meat source in Saxon England. They declined in importance thereafter for the peasantry because of the need for draught animals and milk production.[47] The situation for members of the aristocracy was different as beef and veal remained staples of their diet throughout the premodern era. The household of John Hales, the fifteenth-century Bishop of Coventry and Lichfield consumed beef, veal, and lamb in large amounts even as poorer members of society struggled to increase their meat consumption.[48] The poor in both the countryside and urban areas relied heavily on preserved meat for what meat they ate, as meat spoiled readily with no refrigeration. Butchering in urban areas created problems for local governments that needed to balance providing cheap meat from nearby butchers with the sanitation problems created by urban butchering.

Cattle provided meat and were the source of cheese, milk, and butter, the staples of many peasants' diets. People at all social levels consumed dairy products. Dairying with cattle varied regionally and gradually became more important in the fourteenth and fifteenth centuries. Sheep also provided a source of cheese (and mutton) but came to be regarded as more a source of wool than milk from the thirteenth century onward. In some areas, goats too contributed to cheese production.

Even though many people did not have a varied diet in the premodern period, they generally did not starve. Starvation was generally uncommon in premodern England except in periods of great agricultural crisis. Malnutrition arising from crop failures was another matter and did lead to health problems. Because of poor transportation and profiteering, a food surplus in one area was not always able to offset dearth in another region. Secular and clerical authorities often tried to react when crop failures occurred but the main societal response to food shortages was for those who had more to become more charitable to those who had not a not always adequate solution.

There is an ongoing debate concerning the causes of famine. The two most common approaches, each with subdivisions are an economic approach and a biomedical approach. The economic approach tends to emphasize one of two explanations. One is to focus on exogenous factors such as climate change or disease, which could be labeled an ecological approach. The other explanation tends to focus on human factors that could be called entitlements such as excess population growth, hoarding, or ownership of property.[49] While advocates of one or the other of the economic arguments often argue for one to the exclusion of the other, there is coming to be a synthesis that emphasizes that they work in complementary fashion.[50] The biological approach focuses on questions of nutrition and diet. In reality, as the Great Famine of the early fourteenth century illustrates, when all of these factors worked together simultaneously, a famine of large proportions could be the result.

Chroniclers sometimes noted a famine either because it had a major impact in their region or in a few instances because dearth was so widespread. Most climatic events that led to harvest failures created short-term food shortages although human action could exacerbate the shortages.[51] A combination of an extended climatic event coupled with human action or inaction could lead to a full-scale famine in a few cases. The authors of the *Anglo-Saxon Chronicle* noted famines in 976, 1005 ("such that no man ever remembered one so cruel"), 1046, 1082, 1086, 1111, and 1125.[52] The author of the Scottish *Melrose Chronicle* also took notice of famine in England in 793, 1005, and 1125.[53] The famines of 1005 and 1125 must have been quite severe in the north of England as observers on both sides of the border noted their occurrence. The author of the *Anglo-Saxon Chronicle* indicated that 1086 was a wet year that led to a cattle plague and the destruction of crops while the winter of 1111 was long and harsh destroying many crops as well as leading to a cattle plague. The Great Famine of 1315–22 received wide attention, because it lasted so long, had several components such as poor grain yield and animal murrains that may have killed sixty percent of bovine animals in England, producing several long-term health issues stemming from lower meat and milk supplies. The Great Famine was quite severe in places and affected most of England leading to starvation.[54] The St. Albans chronicler described the early stages of the famine in extensive detail, pointing out that the poor often suffered starvation, but that the well-off suffered little although they may have had to reduce their household staffs and cut their alms-giving.[55] War with Scotland made the Great Famine worse. In the north of England, raiding across the border led to animal thefts, which produced a decline in food available from cattle as well as a decline in the number of potential draft animals. In the south, royal demands for foodstuffs for the army also produced food shortages.[56] Even though it had initially contributed to the severity of the Great Famine, the government of Edward II did try to alleviate the famine through measures such as prohibiting grain exports and trying to persuade those who had grain to sell it, but these measures proved insufficient to the task.[57] When Parliament passed an ordinance in early 1315, fixing the price of food and even imprisoning butchers who violated it, the result produced more harm than good as producers kept food off the market and Parliament had to repeal the ordinance a year later.[58] Undeterred Parliament tried to regulate the price of ale in 1317.[59] There were lingering health issues for several years thereafter that came from the food energy and nutrient deficiencies arising from the Great Famine such as stunted growth rates for children and immune-compromised individuals.

Bad weather was often the initial culprit when food shortages occurred. Wet weather made it hard to sow and harvest crops and led many crops to rot in the field. Wet weather, especially when combined with cold conditions often led to animal murrains that killed off cattle and sheep. A good example of animal disease that led to a food shortage was the outbreak of rinderpest that spread across

Europe in the early fourteenth century.[60] Usually, these events led to spotty food shortages and malnutrition. When the climate events became extended and forestallers refused to sell stored grain or it was impossible to transport grain from one area to another, more severe problems such as the Great Famine could ensue. An additional complicating factor that helped to produce the Great Famine was the beginning of the transition from the Medieval Climate Anomaly to the Little Ice Age, partially initiated by the Wolf Minimum (1280–1350) and the changing North Atlantic Oscillation and increased volcanic activity such as the eruption of the Indonesian volcano Samalas in 1257. Extreme weather events interacted with societal action, not always in positive ways to affect the impact of food shortages.

The Great Famine of 1315–1322 had impacts that went well beyond the initial dearth. The Great Famine was part of the rapidly worsening situation complicated by outbreaks of plague from 1348 onward so much so that some scholars now speak of the crisis of the fourteenth century. Christopher Dyer goes so far as to indicate that "large numbers of English peasants really did starve" in the worst years of the Great Famine.[61] He goes on to indicate that the situation began to improve even though there would be other famines along the way such as one in the 1430s.

As farming techniques improved, people were less at the mercy of nature, but as the example of the Great Famine illustrates, severe climate conditions coupled with human actions could produce distress. Growing population in the sixteenth century also meant increased demand for food supplies. As late as 1623, northern England felt the ravages of famine as a climate event coming from the Little Ice Age, and the inability of local authorities to act promptly produced further distress.[62]

In addition to leading to health problems resulting from malnutrition, food shortages caused some people to consume crops and animals that they might not have eaten otherwise. Several factors worked to create this situation. Food shortages led some people to turn to whatever food was available even if it smelled and looked unhealthy. Unscrupulous merchants might also try to foist off food that they knew was bad. In 1316, the St. Albans chronicler indicated that spoiled food caused dysentery with the characteristic high fever as well as possibly ergot poisoning. Ergotism can kill quickly, as Trokelowe indicated, as it can cut off circulation to the extremities followed by gangrene, which leads to death if untreated.[63] Any sort of food could pose a problem as when the baker William de Somersete sold bread in London that "was putrid and altogether rotten, and made of putrid wheat so that persons by eating that bread would be poisoned and choked."[64] In a time of no refrigeration, it was also easy for items such as meat to spoil if left out too long even in spite of the good intentions of merchants. Local authorities made stalwart efforts at dealing with "bad" food. Sometimes it was a private group as when the masters of the butchers of St. Nicholas Shambles reported that a pig found at the shop of John Huntyndon "was corrupt and abominable to the human race" in 1364.[65] Sometimes it was government such as when the London recorder's court convicted Thomas Sprothergh on 11 November 1375 of selling a peck of eels "unfit for human beings," and sentenced him to an hour in the pillory and having the eels burnt in front of him (a not uncommon punishment).[66]

Tainted meat could easily lead to various enteric ailments that could kill someone in a weakened condition. Even wine could spoil with potentially harmful effects. In November 1364, the tavern keeper John Penrose was accused of selling wine unfit for human consumption. The court banned him from the vintner trade and ordered: "that the said John Penrose should drink a draught of the same wine which he sold to the common people; and the remainder of such wine shall then be poured on the head of the same John."[67] Gastroenteritis, the "stomach flu," can be spread by eating contaminated food and although it rarely kills, the diarrhea and vomiting that ensue are certainly unpleasant and the ensuing dehydration can lead to further complications. Although adults had developed immunity to many of the viruses likely to produce gastroenteritis, children were only developing immunity and were more severely affected helping to lead to higher child death rates. Rye that grew in wet conditions was often infected by fungal diseases such as ergot that left a red fungal stain on rye and wheat. Ergot poisoning produced several ailments depending on which ergot compound was involved. Even if Piero Camporesi's argument that many peasants experienced hallucinations and hunger because of ergot poisoning is exaggerated, ergotism may have affected some people, especially in bad years.[68]

The relationship between nutrition and disease, and nutrition and climate is a complicated one. Climate events could help to initiate nutritional crises. Human inaction or action made the impact of the event worse or helped to ameliorate it. Forestallers who bought up food supplies with the intent of selling them at high prices could turn a shortage into a famine. Human intervention might ameliorate a food shortage as when an abbey opened its storehouse to the local population or governmental officials helped to move food from one place to another or limit hoarding. Even on a day-to-day basis, selling impure food led to health issues. In any case, nutritional difficulties had an impact on the health of the population even if not that described by the various dietary regime books.

Population size and density

The relationship between the size of a nation or region's population, the density of settlement, and the incidence and impact of disease is a complex one, but one that can be estimated today by epidemiologists. As the size of a population grows and particularly as large numbers of people live close together, it is easier for infectious diseases to spread, increasing their impact.

The size of the population of England before the late eleventh century is nearly impossible to estimate because there were no surveys of population to base estimates on. The population of England before 1000 probably varied between one and two million with few urban centers and even London possessing a population of probably no more than 10,000. Some villages and monasteries were densely populated but by only a few hundred people at most.

The first reasonably accurate estimate of population occurred in 1086 and thereafter it is possible to piece together estimates of the size of the English population. The Domesday survey carried out at the order of William I in 1086, provides a good estimate of population size. Although it has some gaps, it was meticulously carried out and produced an estimate of two million people in England. Christopher Dyer tries to take the gaps into account and estimates a population of between 2.2 and 2.5 million people.[69] Improvements in agriculture, putting more land under the plow, and a favorable climate regime contributed to almost a tripling of the population by 1300, about five to six million people. After a decline arising from the Great Famine, population held steady until the impact of the Second Plague Pandemic starting in 1348, which produced a precipitous decline in the number of people in England to around two million, not to recover to pre-plague levels until the sixteenth century.[70]

In many ways, density of settlement is more important than simply the number of people. England and Western Europe had few urban centers before 1000. London may have numbered as many as 50,000 people in 1300 with Norwich and York lagging far behind with populations between 15,000 and 20,000. All three of these places labeled themselves as cities and had somewhat dense populations as people huddled together inside city walls. Elsewhere there were several towns with populations that hovered around 5,000. People tended to live close together in medieval cities so there would be several places with population densities that could sustain an outbreak of an infectious disease. Even in a village with a population of a few hundred, people tended to crowd together. A densely settled and growing population also introduced additional health problems arising from sanitation issues and the provision of foodstuffs that were harmful. A densely settled population also made it possible for a contagious disease transmitted from one person to another to spread more readily than among a widely scattered population.

Population size and density are also related to human behavior. People who are intensely afraid of a disease and flee at the first signs of an outbreak may be able to escape the disease but they may also serve to spread it if they are already infected. The basic SIR model for the spread of disease described in Chapter 1 does not take human behavior into account. A more sophisticated approach to this issue divides human behavior into two categories: belief-based behavior and prevalence-based behavior and then models human response to the incidence of disease.[71] Belief-based models are dependent on what people believe about how a disease spreads. Prevalence-based models are dependent on the biology of how readily a disease may spread. Awareness of the onset of disease can potentially limit its impact as people self-quarantine or practice better hygiene, reducing the susceptibility to disease.[72] This response is applicable in a modern society, but not in the Middle Ages before an awareness of the role of quarantine. More likely, awareness of the onset of disease led to fear-inspired flight which spread the disease, rather than containing it.[73] Human behavior has an impact on the spread of disease and as information networks improved, some people would follow behaviors that would have an impact on the spread of an infectious disease.

Sanitation and good health

Although evidence from before 1000 is hard to come by, it seems that in cities and towns, at least from the twelfth century onward, individuals and governments took action to deal with potential health problems.[74] Some of this action sprang from the belief that "bad" air, miasmas, caused health problems. Some also sprang from the idea that bad taste was likely to mean harm. The second point resulted in various attempts to ensure the provision of untainted food products. The first might have little authority in fact, but in reality, helped to prevent health problems arising from the need to provide clean water and prevent sewage or animal butchering waste from overwhelming society and contaminating water and the physical environment.

People have long been concerned with obtaining adequate supplies of clean water and people in medieval England were no exception. People who lived in rural areas or small villages turned to local streams or wells for water. While farm waste could contaminate these water supplies, the likelihood was that rural people enjoyed adequate and clean water. Towns and cities such as London or York were another matter, as people might be some distance from a water supply, and the water supply could easily become contaminated by various forms of pollution especially as the population grew. Medieval people made little distinction between the various sorts of pollution of watercourses. Wastes such as dung were obvious pollutants but medieval people also considered natural silting and weed growth as pollution and took action to deal with all three forms.[75] Clean water came to become a sign of a well-run and healthy community.

Although more information is available for London than other towns, it appears that local authorities throughout England took an increasing interest in the provision of adequate and clean water although as towns grew this became more difficult. In the eighth century, Londoners could easily draw clean water from the Thames or local wells, but by the twelfth century, this was becoming more difficult. The Thames remained a source of water for London, but it became polluted, and the small streams that emptied into it, such as Walbrook, were sometimes open sewers. London was not alone with a need to confront polluted waterways as the Ouse, which served as a water and transportation source for York, may have been polluted by the early eleventh century.[76] Wells and cisterns continued to provide water but they too were often polluted. The ready water of a town well often attracted laundresses who took advantage of the available water supply. Proud of their clean water Coventry, Leicester, Sandwich, and Southampton all prohibited laundresses from plying their trade in the vicinity of city wells and streams in the fifteenth century.[77] London authorities began to pipe water into the city from outside sources in the thirteenth century and in the 1230s or 1240s a large system of pipes, called the Great Conduit was constructed. In King's Lynn, a piping system was so well established by 1465 that the mayor and council began leasing rights for homeowners and businesses to tap into the system.[78] In some cases, homeowners tapped into the town's water lines and in other cases, water bubbled up in constructed pools or water carriers sold the water to people. At times local authorities had to confront the issue of over-use by some consumers. In November 1337, the London Common Council ordered that brewers should not use very large tubs to take water from the conduit that piped water into London as this was leading to shortages for other consumers.[79]

If people considered clean water a necessity, they were also concerned by sewage. In some cases, people simply piped sewage into the nearest watercourse, but as towns grew the volume of refuse grew apace creating a smelly, unsightly mess. As early as 1288, London authorities expressed concern that the watercourse of Walbrook was being contaminated by human and animal waste and tried to correct the situation.[80] Throughout the fourteenth century, the government of the city of London fought a continual battle to keep human and animal wastes out of Walbrook and other streams such as the Fleet that flowed into the Thames as well as the Thames itself, although not always successfully. An increase in the volume of waste deriving from larger populations may have motivated this increased concern for both the sight and smell of waste in watercourses. The increased attention may have also arisen from the miasma theory of disease, which indicated that "bad" air produced illness, something of great concern with the coming of the plague in 1348. In September 1357, the London common council received a missive from King Edward III complaining of the sight and smell of "dung, laystalls, and other filth accumulated" along the banks of the Thames encountered by members of the court out for a walk along its bank.[81] While it may have been the courtiers' noses and eyes that were offended, the health hazard was very real even if not originating from the stench and sight of dung. Some people emptied chamber pots in the gutters (at times from upper story windows) or constructed privies that projected out over a watercourse. Some were more inventive as was Alice Wade who ran a wooden pipe from the seat of the privy in her solar to the gutter in the street below.[82] Another attempt at constructing indoor plumbing occurred in 1348 when two men ran a pipe from the privy in their upper story apartment to the cellar below until the volume of filth led them to be discovered.[83] The London city government made strenuous efforts to deal with the sewage problem but often had to repeat prohibitions or prosecute malefactors.

Responsible homeowners constructed privies that piped their wastes to cesspools while latrines including several public ones were scattered about the city. Even so, many urban and rural dwellers relieved themselves wherever they were, either because it was convenient, or because there was no nearby latrine. Archaeological evidence indicates that some of the privies were substantially built with solid rock facing and quite large.[84] The London authorities made a distinction between dirt-lined cesspools and those lined with stone or solid timber facing, requiring the former to be 3.5 feet from walls and the latter to be 2.5 feet away.[85] Unfortunately, not everyone adhered to these rules, and sewage often leaked into adjoining properties, which led to court action to correct the problem.[86] However, others did adhere to the location requirement as in two other cases in which householders were accused of improper locations for their cesspools, but investigation revealed otherwise.[87] It appears that some property owners made a strenuous effort in locating cesspools, while others were more casual, and some tried to ignore the issue entirely. Cleaning these facilities required care and was not an occupation awarding high social standing although it could be profitable. Not all cesspool owners took care of their facilities and some overflowed or as the one noted above were simply illegal facilities that infringed upon their neighbors. Ultimately, some of this sewage found its way into the Thames and other watercourses. Even if the waste from a privy went directly to a watercourse, it might accumulate in the streets along the way as several parish inquisitions indicated in 1427 leading one observer to note "the lane is full of stinking privy filth to the great nuisance of the commonality."[88] In some cases, a stream became noisome in spite of efforts at regulating privies and dumping into it. As early as 1288, the London common council ordered the cleaning of Walbrook but had to repeat the order with some variation in 1374, 1383, 1415, and 1422.[89] The difficulty in keeping Walbrook clean lay in the competing goals of allowing those who lived along it to channel their privies into the stream and keeping it free from filth. Tired of continuing problems of sewage in Walbrook, the London Common Council prohibited latrines dumping into it and ordered it paved over in 1463[90]

As towns grew in size not every dwelling had a privy and some people traveled far from home so that health and decency demanded public facilities. The City government constructed several latrines in London including ones at Temple Bridge, Ludgate, London Bridge, one in the London wall, and another one outside the wall over Walbrook.[91] Like private privies, these public facilities needed cleaning lest they overflow. In January 1422, it was noted that "the common privy of Ludgate is defective and Perilous, and the ordure rots the stone walls, which is likely to be dangerous to the walls and costly."[92] In this case, the situation presented a variety of health and safety standards. Good intentions notwithstanding, the situation remained unremedied, and in December local jurors presented the problem again, this time in stronger language.[93] At least cities that provided public privies were trying to prevent the accumulation of filth in the streets. Human and animal wastes were valuable as fertilizer and so municipal authorities often tried to collect the waste and sell it. In small farming villages, there was a positive incentive to accumulate waste so that it could be used or sold. In the seventeenth century, the Lancashire town of Prescot (population 600) did just that as householders were allowed to pile dung adjacent to their houses for future sale as long as it didn't block the street.[94] Nonetheless, the threat of various intestinal ailments created by encounters with human and animal waste, even if the connection was not directly recognized, assured that the problems of waste remained a constant.

London was not alone in confronting the problem of sewage in the streets and watercourses. In York, Coventry, and Norwich's local authorities struggled with being overwhelmed with sewage or even industrial waste.[95] All three cities faced the ongoing problem of individuals dumping waste in the streets and watercourses, so much at times that streets were blocked or streams were stopped up. For example, the mayor of Coventry issues a strongly worded proclamation in 1421 enumerating these problems and threatening fines for malefactors.[96]

Butchers in London and other towns often created problems of unpleasant odors and offal in the streets leading to efforts at regulating their dumping. Officials ordered offal to be dumped in prescribed places, not dumped in streams, or dumped in streams in only certain locations, and ordered offal to be dumped outside the city or even prohibited butchering within the city. In many ways, the last was the best solution except that it usually caused an increase in the price of meat and municipal authorities had to relent. In 1392, Parliament prohibited butchers from slaughtering animals within the walls of the city. The price of meat increased so that the London Common Council Petitioned Parliament the following year to relax the prohibition. Richard II ordered that one house should be erected near the Thames where butchering could take place. It seems that the concern may have been from the offal found along the banks of the Thames rather than the dumping of waste as the butchers were allowed to load their waste onto boats and dump it mid-stream.[97] At least dumping offal in the middle of the river served to dilute its impact a bit and kept it from rotting along the riverbank.

Tanning and metal working posed special sorts of problems but these industries could easily be contained in a few areas such as the edge of a city, but butchering needed to be carried out in every city, preferably close to customers and was a continuing problem. The stench involved certainly reinforced any views about the health problems of "bad" air. Offal and organic waste produced bad air but also produced material waste that could foul a street or clog a watercourse. Because it often included dung and rotting material, this waste also led to parasite infestations.

Tanning proved to be a particularly problematic business. Tanners had to clean hides they acquired of whatever was on them, such as dung, and then remove the hair from the hide by a chemical process that usually involved sprinkling the hide with urine. In order to make the hides flexible, they were soaked in various chemical solutions, some of which involved the use of dog dung, or an acidic treatment. This treatment before the hide could actually be tanned might take as long as a year producing a stench throughout from the noxious brew that was then dumped into a nearby watercourse. Sections of the river Ouse that flowed through York were centers of tanning activity. Throughout the fourteenth century, local authorities were concerned that wastes from tanners and butchers would foul water downstream that was used for food production. At times the king also became involved, ordering the local government to do something about the problem. Finally, the Crown ordered butchers to dump in a marshy area near St. John Hungate near the river Foss and all dumping in the Ouse was prohibited.[98]

Sewage was only one of the health hazards posed by urban society. Individuals and waste haulers deposited wastes of whatever sort in the street or dumped them in vacant lots. Probably because London was the largest English city as well as the capital, it was the first to try to deal with the problem. The London Common Council waged continual war on this sort of behavior. In 1309, it reminded householders not to place their waste in front of their neighbors' houses and ordered the collection and disposal of "ordure" from houses as well as warning against dumping waste on the King's highway. Sufficiently disturbed by this sort of behavior the Council threatened a fine of 40*d* for offenders.[99] Fines alone were not always a deterrence. In December 1422, jurors from the Farndon Within ward presented "William Emery, poulterer, for throwing goose dung, heron dung, and horse dung on the highway."[100] In spite of severe penalties, people continued to find ways to dispose of waste of all sorts. Some lanes and open spaces such as Tower Hill seemed to be favored spots for dumping. Edward III directed the London city government to clean up "the accumulation of refuse, filth and other fetid matter on Tower Hill whereby the air was foully corrupted and vitiated and the lives of those dwelling or passing there are endangered." Clearly disturbed, King Edward threatened a fine of 100 marks if the waste was not cleaned up.[101] The crown and London government also turned to other means to remove dung and other waste in the streets. In 1357, a number of collectors with carts were ordered to proceed through London to pick up the waste. The situation remained unresolved as people continued to dump their wastes in the streets and in 1372 and 1406 the order had to be repeated but waste disposal in the streets and public places continued to remain a problem.[102] The London Common Council did the best it could and tried to react whenever problems arose. During the parish inquests into local problems in 1421, the aldermen representing the parish of St. Martin presented William atte Wode "for making a great nuisance and discomfort to his neighbors by throwing out horrible filth on to the highway, the stench of which is so odious and infectious that none of his neighbors can remain in their shops, which is a great reproof to all of this honourable city. Because of the lords and other gentlemen and men of the court who go and pass there."[103] Clearly, William's dumping had struck a nerve with his neighbors who wanted the situation resolved and William punished. It also indicates another reason why local authorities wanted to deal with waste in the streets: civic pride that combined appearance with a desire to be known as a salubrious place for business. It wasn't just local governments that wanted to prevent dumping of waste but also those people, such as the offenders' neighbors, who had to deal with the problem on a daily basis. London was not alone and other cities such as York soon followed suit in the collection and the establishment of designated spots for dumping.[104] Providing facilities for the collection of "ordure" from the streets and prohibiting homeowners from using the streets as dumping grounds was somewhat effective. However, there were always those who took the easy path and dumped in the street, perhaps in front of someone else's dwelling. At times, the amount of dung was large enough so that it nearly blocked a street or lane as occurred near Ebbegate in December 1421, which was reported as "abominably stopped up with filth and privies to the great nuisance of the whole community."[105]

Punishing malefactors was one approach to dealing with waste in the streets. London also followed a more proactive approach by providing rakers for every ward whose job was to rake up waste from the streets and cart it away. In addition, the city provided dunghills, or laystalls, that served as collection points for waste. Both contributed to dealing with the waste problem but sometimes things went awry. Richard Mayllour, the raker of Chepe ward, collected the waste from his ward but officials cited him in 1384 for dumping it in the neighboring Colmanstrete ward. This seems to have been an ongoing problem in towns throughout the country as the authorities fined John Plunkett, a waste collector in Ipswitch in the 1440s, for dumping material along the highway instead of the approved dumping site.[106]

Based on the miasma theory of disease, air that smelled bad was deemed a health hazard well into the nineteenth century. Shortly after the first outbreak of plague in England, in 1348, it appears that "bad" air came to be regarded as leading to plague infections, producing another reason to deal with stench in the streets and watercourses. Plague treatises began to make the connection between odor and plague, a connection that gradually seeped down from intellectual discussion to popular culture, as people were encouraged to eschew places with stinking air whether in streets, stables or elsewhere. This argument drew on the authoritative *Canon* of Avicenna in indicating how "bad" air produced an imbalance in the humors leading to pestilence.[107] Although the stench of dung might not produce disease, the bacteria and parasites such as helminths or whipworms within the deposit could lead to various health issues such as diarrheal diseases. Reacting to odors following the dictums of miasma theory did not deal fully with the health problems generated by butchering or human or animal waste. The result of trying to prevent the deposits of dung and clean them up did, however, deal somewhat with the health issues generated by them.

Human excrement also took on another characteristic as Martha Bayless points out because premodern people thought that "excrement was sin made material."[108] People saw excrement as evidence of the corruption that afflicted society, corruption that came from the sinful nature of humankind. As such, dung reflected both cultural and theological attitudes that supplemented the miasma theory in regarding "bad" air as noxious and something that needed to be controlled because it was a symbol of the sin present in society. When combined with arguments arising from civic pride, this approach helped to produce an aversion to dung that went beyond the health concerns of miasma theory.

People deemed air that smelled bad a health hazard, based on the miasma theory of disease well into the nineteenth century. Human and animal wastes generated miasmas, but so did other sources. Air pollution had become a problem in several late medieval cities as people and industry burned sea-coal as wood became harder to acquire. Smiths, lime-burners, and bell founders are only some of the industries that needed the heat of coal as well as appreciating its lower cost relative to wood.[109] Eleanor of Provence, Henry III's queen left Nottingham in 1275 in order to escape the heavy smoke and odor generated by burning sea-coal.[110] The situation was equally bad in London and several nobles complained to Edward I in 1307 about the bad odors arising from burning sea-coal in London.[111] Coal smoke did generate genuine health issues. A comparative study of the remains of 1,042 late medieval individuals from the rural Yorkshire settlement of Wharram Percy and the St. Helen-on-the-Walls parish in York indicated a higher prevalence of sinusitis in the urban setting, which could be attributed to industrial pollution, as well as their occupation.[112] People adversely affected by coal smoke did resort to legal action. In 1377, Thomas and Alice Yonge complained that their neighbors had constructed a forge and the noise disturbed their sleep and the stench from the coal smoke decreased their property value.[113] Coal-burning eventually became a major health issue, but already in the fifteenth century, it could make life uncomfortable for those people with sinusitis or other breathing issues.

Local governments and the Crown clearly had good intentions in trying to deal with the problem of sanitation in late medieval England. Sanitation remained an intractable problem because it involved both the technology of water provision and waste disposal and human action. As cities grew, sanitation issues also grew to present local authorities with conflicting goals. They realized that cleaning up butchers' waste was necessary, but the easiest solution of moving butchering outside the city walls often increased the price of meat. Local authorities often responded with stringent regulation of butchers, but too-stringent regulation encouraged at least some butchers to find ways to evade regulations with secret dumping and other remedies. Sanitation in medieval cities was a tragedy of the common problem in microcosm as what belonged to all was easy to abuse by all.[114] Economists have described the problem as one inherent in trying to prevent misuse of collective goods. Public hygiene was a public good, one that government could not exclude people from enjoying nor was it one that could be depleted, while drinkable water was a common pool resource that could be depleted through pollution. The term negative externality describes this case as people who dumped waste in the streets or watercourses harmed the enjoyment of public health by all.[115]

Governments tried to discourage these negative actions, but it was a never-ending struggle. It was simply too easy to dump a chamber pot in the street, or dump a cart of building material or butchers' waste in a ditch or convenient open space. The obviousness of sanitation issues, especially the resulting "bad" air made it easy for commentators to place the problem within the miasma theory of disease in proclaiming poor sanitation a health problem. Unknowingly, authorities who tried to deal with odors and dirt also dealt with the biological aspects of the problem as they worked to provide clean water, clean food, and even clean air. While the efforts of local officials may not have always had the intended effect, they helped to avert some intestinal ailments. English royal and town governments did try to provide a healthy environment for their people rather than ignoring issues of public health. Their actions were intended to produce a healthy and pleasant environment, one that was also about social control and producing an ideal environment.[116]

Conclusion: Human determinants of health risks

The previous chapter dealt with causative factors for disease in medieval England that were largely beyond human control. This chapter has addressed how individuals, organizations, and governments affected public health. Often the social and political response to a potential health problem was quite positive such as trying to regulate sewage and provide clean water or food shortages. Physicians tried to describe disease and provide for good health. Some of their remedies were helpful, but some such as excessive bleeding or purging could be downright dangerous. Some commentators have gone so far as to say that until the late nineteenth-century medical treatments were at best a placebo effect and at worst actually harmful.[117] These arguments may be overstatements, but they should cause us to look skeptically at medical intervention, if not preventative measures, in the medieval and early modern eras. Many people were their own doctors or turned to a variety of village practitioners for aid. Medical care was better suited to dealing with everyday disease problems as well as external medical problems such as wounds and broken bones. When confronted with an epidemic disease, the medical community tried to respond but their response was often inadequate especially when the disease was a "new" one outside the descriptions inherited from the ancient world. As later chapters indicate, new and changing infectious diseases led to changes in medicine and public health regulation.

Government at all levels did take measures that helped to protect the health of the public. Street cleaning, regulating dumping, dealing with sewage, and taking action to provide clean water all helped to better the lot of the people. The miasma theory meant that governments dealt with the symptoms of the health problems arising from human waste, but at least dealing with "bad" air by trying to control pollution was a start. These efforts did not go far enough so diarrheal diseases continued to trouble society. The arrival of the plague created a new set of problems, one that some European societies tried to deal with already in the fifteenth century by quarantining the afflicted. England would be late in adopting quarantines, but they could be effective if applied correctly.

Good health was difficult to achieve in premodern England. Childhood held many dangers, arising not only from accidents, poor sanitation, and not enough food but also from infectious diseases such as measles. All of this made surviving to age ten a challenge. Even adults faced many everyday ailments that could be fatal. Sanitation measures helped lower the mortality rate, even if undertaken for the wrong reasons. Prevention, when combined with dietary improvements, helped to spur a population increase in the thirteenth century. Infectious disease, however, would remain a limiting factor to population growth throughout the premodern period.

It is easy to be critical of medieval people for inadequate responses to the major health problem presented by infectious disease. Yet, even in the early twenty-first century some of the responses to Ebola and COVID-19 display some of the same sort of ignorance, callousness, and simply bad behavior that medieval people might be accused of as well as complexities arising from the biology of the disease and current climate conditions. Even some preventative public health measures adopted today have come in for criticism at times. The next chapters will deal with some infectious diseases that confronted people in premodern England from the perspectives of the biology of the diseases and how society coped with them and was affected by them.

Notes

1 A good survey of ancient medicine is Vivian Nutton, *Ancient Medicine* (London: Routledge, 2004). Although somewhat dated, Owsei Temkin's two studies provide a sound foundation for understanding the works and long-term impact of Hippocrates and Galen: *Hippocrates in a World of Pagans and Christians* (Baltimore: Johns Hopkins University Press, 1991) and *Galenism: Rise and Fall of a Medical Philosophy* (Ithaca: Cornell University Press, 1973). Susan P. Mattern examines the social context for Galen's career and writings *The Prince of Medicine* (Oxford: Oxford University Press, 2013).

2 The increasing impact of Aristotelian natural philosophy on medical education is detailed in Luis Garcia-Ballester, "The Construction of a New Form of Learning and Practicing Medicine in Medieval Latin Europe," *Science in Context*, 8 (1995), 75–102.

3 The literature of the humor theory is extensive. A brief, well-done introduction can be found in Carole Rawcliffe, *Medicine and Society in Later Medieval England* (Stroud: Alan Sutton, 1995), 32–37.

4 Galen, *A Translation of Galen's Hygiene (De sanitate tuenda)*, R.M. Green, trans. (Springfield, 1951), 35–6.

5 R.R. Sharpe, ed., *Calendar of the Letter Books Preserved among the Archives of the Corporation of the City of London*, 11 vols (London: 1899–1912), "Letter Book G, 1352–1374," 31. The relationship of health and smell is detailed in Dolly Jørgensen, "The Medieval Sense of Smell, Stench and Sanitation," in Ulrike Krampl, Robert Beck, and Emmanuelle Retaillaud-Bajac, eds., *Les cinq sens de la ville du Moyen Âge à nos jours* (Tours: Presses Universitaires François-Rabelais, 2013), 301–13.

6 Bartholomew Anglicus, *On the Properties of Things: John Trevisa's Translation of Bartholomaeus Anglicus' De properietatis rerum*, M.C. Seymour, ed., 3 vols. (Oxford: Oxford University Press, 1975–1988), 1: 116.

7 Andrew Boorde, *A Dietary of Health*, F.J. Furnivall, ed. (EETS, extra ser., 10, 1870), 235, 236. Spelling modernized.

8 E.L. Sabine, "City Cleaning in Mediaeval London," *Speculum* 12 (1937), 19–43.

9 Audrey Meaney, "The Practice of Medicine in England about the Year 1000," *Social History of Medicine*, 13 (2000), 221–237; Peregrine Horden, "What's Wrong with Early Medieval Medicine," *Social History of Medicine*, 24 (2011), 5–25.

10 Anne Van Arsdall mounts a spirited defenses of the value of Anglo-Saxon herbal medicine written from a perspective of modern herblore in "Reading Medieval Medical Texts with and Open Mind," in Elizabeth Lane Furdell, ed., *Textual Healing* (Leiden: Brill, 2005), 9–29, and "Challenging the 'Eye of Newt' Image of Medieval Medicine," in Barbara S. Bowers, ed., *The Medieval Hospital and Medical Practice* (Aldershot: Ashgate, 2007), 195–205. The second piece is a nice corrective to those who argue that medieval medicine was purely superstitious nonsense. See also Linda E. Voigts, "Anglo-Saxon Plant Remedies and the Anglo-Saxons," *Isis*, 70 (1979), 250–68. Extensive testing of medieval remedies that rarely produced positive results is detailed in Barbara Brennessel, Michael D.C. Drout, Robyn Gravel, "A Reassessment of the Efficacy of Anglo-Saxon Medicine," *Anglo-Saxon England*, 34 (2005), 183–95.

11 Vern L. Bullough describes medieval medical study at the two English universities: "Medical Study at Mediaeval Oxford," *Speculum*, 36 (1961), 600–12 and "The Mediaeval Medical School at Cambridge," *Mediaeval Studies*, 24 (1962), 161–68.

12 Two excellent wors that cover the intellectual aspects of medieval medicine are Mirko D. Grmek, ed., *Western Medical Thought from Antiquity to the Middle Ages* (Cambridge: Harvard University Press, 1998) and Roger French, *Medicine before Science* (Cambridge: Cambridge University Press, 2003). Carole Rawcliffe provides excellent coverage of the practical aspects of medical care in Late Medieval England that helps to place the intellectual aspects of medieval medicine into a social context in *Medicine and Society in Later Medieval England*. Faye Getz examines the role of physicians and their writings in the period from 750 to 1450 in *Medicine in the English Middle Ages* (Princeton: Princeton University Press, 1998). Getz also examines the relationship of learned and vernacular medical literature in "Charity, Translation and the Language of Medical Learning in Medieval England," *BHM*, 64 (1990), 1–17. John M. Riddle also relates theory and practice in the Early Middle Ages in "Theory and Practice in Medieval Medicine," *Viator*, 5 (1974), 157–84. Two earlier accounts that are still useful and provide some coverage of the Early Middle Ages and herb lore are C.H. Talbot, *Medicine in Medieval England* (London: Oldborne, 1967) and Stanley Rubin, *Medieval English Medicine* (Newton Abbot: David and Charles, 1974). M.L. Cameron examines Anglo-Saxon medicine in *Anglo-Saxon Medicine* (Cambridge: Cambridge University Press, 1973). The institutional side of Anglo-Norman medicine is detailed in Edward J. Kealy, *Medieval Medicus* (Baltimore: Johns Hopkins University Press, 1981). Also helpful are Sheila Campbell, Bert Hall, David Klausner, eds., *Health, Disease and Healing in Medieval Culture* (New York: St. Martin's 1992) and Luis Garcia-Ballester, Roger French, Jon Arrizabalaga, Andrew Cunningham, eds. *Practical Medicine from Salerno to the Black Death* (Cambridge: Cambridge University Press, 1994). Luke Demaitre discusses the sources that medieval physicians used to identify and treat various diseases in *Medieval Medicine* (Santa Barbara: Praeger, 2013).

13 Michael McVaugh, "Cataracts and Hernia: Aspects of Surgical Practice in the Fourteenth Century," *Medical History*, 45 (2001), 319–40.

14 John Flint Smith, *Memorials of the Craft of Surgery*, D'Arcy Power, ed. (London: Cassells, 1886), xi.; Sidney Young, *The Annals of the Barber-Surgeons of London* (London 1890), 36–38.

15 Sharpe, "Letter Book K, Temp. Henry VI," 11.

16 A study of theraic and its uses from the ancient world into the early modern era is Gilbert Watson, *Theriac and Mithridatium* (London: Wellcome Historical Medical Library, 1966).

17 Young, *Annals of the Barber-Surgeons*, 56.

18 J.K. Mustain, "A Rural Medical Practitioner in Fifteenth-Century England," *BHM*, 46 (1977), 238–73.

19 William Bullein, "The Book of Simples," in *Bulleins Bulwarke of Defence against all Sicknesse, Soarenesse, and Woundes that doe dayly Assaulte Mankinde* (London: Thomas Marshe, 1579), fol. 10.

20 Madeleine Pelner Cosman, "Medieval Medical Malpractice: The Dicta and the Dockets," *Bulletin of the New York Academy of Medicine*, 49 (1973), 22–47; Sara M. Butler, "Medicine on Trial: Regulating the Health Professions in Later Medieval England," *Florilegium*, 28 (2011), 71–94.

21 Riley, *Memorials of London*, 273–74.

22 A.H. Thomas and Philip E. Jones, *Calendar of Plea and Memoranda Rolls, Preserved among the Archives of the Corporation of the City of London at the Guildhall, 1323–1482*, 6 vols. (Cambridge: Cambridge University Press, 1926–1961), 1: "1364–1381," 236.

23 Riley, *Memorials of London*, 465.

24 Thomas, *Plea and Memoranda Rolls*, 4: "1413–1437," 174–75.

25 William Langland, *Piers Plowman*, J. F. Goodridge, trans., rev. ed. (Harmondsworth: Penguin, 1966), 88.

26 "A Poem of the Times of Edward II," in Thomas Wright, ed., *The Political Songs of England from the Reign of John to that of Edward II* (Camden Society, OS, 6, 1839), 252.

27 John Mirfield, *Florarium Bartholomei*, printed in P. Horton-Smith Hartley and H.R. Aldridge, *Johannes de Mirfield of St. Bartholomew's Southfield, His Life and Works* (Cambridge: Cambridge University Press, 1936), 132–33.

28 John de Mirfield, *Surgery*, J.B. Colton, ed. (New York: Hafner Publishing Co., 1969), 19.

29 Lanfranc of Milan, *Lanfrank's Science of Cirurgie*, Robert von Fleishhaker, ed. (EETS, 102, 1894), 9. Lanfranc's Latin treatise was translated into English by 1400. John Arderene, *Treatise of Fistula in Ano*, D'Arcy Power, ed. (EETS, 139, 1910), 5–6, 16. Carole Rawcliffe indicates that some doctors were able to take advantage of their position to further enhance their income. "The Profits of Practice: The Wealth and Status of Medical Men in Later Medieval England," *Social History of Medicine*, 1 (1988), 61–78.

30 Norman Davis, ed., *Paston Letters and Papers of the Fifteenth Century*, 2 vols. (Oxford: Oxford University Press, 1971–6), 1: no. 77.

31 A good starting point for aspects of medical knowledge and treatment in the sixteenth century and beyond can be found in the essays in Charles Webster, ed., *Health, Medicine and Mortality in the Sixteenth Century* (Cambridge: Cambridge University Press, 1979), Margaret Pelling, *Medical Conflicts in Early Modern London* (Oxford: Clarendon Press, 2003), Pelling, *The Common Lot* (London: Longman, 1998), and Andrew Wear, *Knowledge and Practice in English Medicine, 1550–1680* (Cambridge: Cambridge University Press, 2000). If anything, quacks became even more numerous and brazen in with their actions from the sixteenth century onward. Roy Porter, *Quacks* (Stroud: Tempus Publishing, 1989, 2000).

32 Faye Getz, "Medical Education in Later Medieval England," in Vivian Nutton and Roy Porter, eds., *The History of Medical Education in Britain* (Amsterdam: Rodolphi, 1995), 79.

33 Monica H. Greene focuses on the establishment of male authority in the practice of gynecology, but the overall trend, especially in the later Middle Ages and early modern period was to force women out of the medical profession. *Making Women's Medicine Masculine* (Oxford: Oxford University Press, 2008).

34 The literature on miracles and medieval sainthood is extensive. Two works can serve as an introduction. Pierre-André Sigal, *L' homme et le miracle dans la France médiévale* (Paris: Les Éditions du Cerf, 2007) and Robert Bartlett, *Why Can the Dead Do Such Great Things* (Princeton: Princeton University Press, 2013). Iona McCleery provides a discussion of the relationship of miracles and medicine in the Middle Ages. "'Christ More Powerful than Galen'? The Relationship between Medicine and

Miracles," in Matthew Mesley and Louise Wilson, eds., *Contextualizing Miracles in the Christian West, 1100–1500: New Historical Approaches* (Oxford: Medieum Aevum, 2014), 127–154.

35 John Theilmann, "On the Road to Health: Pilgrimage in Medieval England," in Gabriel R. Ricci, ed., *Travel, Discovery, Transformation* (New Brunswick: Transaction Publishers, 2014), 182–84. Health issues involving children and saintly healing are addressed in Eleanora C. Gordon, "Child Health in the Middle Ages as Seen in the Miracles of Five English Saints, A.D. 1150–1220," *BHM*, 60 (1986), 502–22 and "Accidents among Medieval Children as Seen from the Miracles of Six English Saints and Martyrs," *Medical History*, 25 (1991), 145–63, as well as R.C. Finucane, *The Rescue of the Innocents* (New York: St. Martin's Press, 1997). Saintly healing in the modern world is addressed in: Robert A. Scott, *Miracle Cures* (Berkley: University of California Pres, 2010); Jacalyn Duffin, *Medical Miracles* (Oxford: Oxford University Press, 2009) and *Medical Saints* (Oxford University Press, 2013).

36 A good discussion of the concept of health in the late Middle Ages is Carole Rawcliffe, "The Concept of Health in Late Medieval Society," in Simonetta Cavaciocchi, ed., *Economic and Biological Interactions in Pre-Industrial Europe from the 13th to the 18th Centuries* (Florence: University of Florence Press, 2010), 317–34.

37 A selection of some of the works ascribed to Galen dealing with diet and food is Mark Grant, *Galen on Food and Diet* (London: Routledge, 2000).

38 A good introduction to the relationship of diet, population, disease, and economic development is Massimo Livi-Bacci, *Population and Nutrition* (Cambridge: Cambridge University Press, 1991). Ann G. Carmichael cautions against a glib acceptance that food shortages and infection were always related. "Infection, Hidden Hunger, and History," *Journal of Interdisciplinary History*, 14 (1983), 249–64.

39 Ulrich E. Schaible and Stefan H.E. Kaufman, "Malnutrition and Infection: Complex Mechanisms and Global Impacts," *PLoS Medicine*, 4:5 (2007), e115. Peter Katona and Judit Katona-Apte, "The Interaction between Nutrition and Infection," *Clinical Infectious Diseases* 46 (2008), 1582–8.

40 Scott W. Bearden and Robert D. Perry, "The Yfe System of *Yersinia pestis* Transports Iron and Manganese and Is Required for Full Virulence of Plague," *Molecular Microbiology* 32 (1999), 403–14. Because the ability to acquire iron is essential to the establishment of the *Yersinia pestis* bacteria, an iron-deficient person may be less likely to become infected with the plague.

41 Vern Bullough and Cameron Campbell, "Female Longevity and Diet in the Middle Ages," *Speculum* 55 (1980), 317–25. Shersten Killip, John M. Bennett, Mara D. Chambers, "Iron Deficiency Anemia," *American Family Physician* 20 (2007), 671–78.

42 A good, brief discussion of the relationship of infection and nutrition is Alice M. Tang, Ellen Smit, and Richard D. Semba, "Nutrition and Infection," in Kenrad E. Nelson and Carolyn Masters Williams, eds., *Infectious Disease Epidemiology*, 3rd ed. (Burlington MA: Jones and Barlett, 2014), 305–27.

43 Livi-Bacci, *Population and Nutrition*, 36–39; "The Relationship of Nutrition, Disease, and Social Conditions: A Graphical Presentation," *Journal of Interdisciplinary History*, 14 (1983), 506.

44 A survey that is largely focused on the continent is Kathy L. Pearson, "Nutrition and the Early-Medieval Diet," *Speculum* 72 (1997), 1–32.

45 Carole Rawcliffe, *Urban Bodies* (Woodbridge: Boydell Press, 2013), 241–42.

46 C.C. Dyer, "Gardens and Garden Produce in the Later Middle Ages,' in C.M. Woolgar, D. Serjeantson, T. Waldron, eds., *Food in Medieval England* (Oxford: Oxford University Press, 2006). This book is a useful introduction to food in medieval England that encompasses texts and bioarchaeology.

47 N.J. Sykes, From *Cu* and *Sceap* to *Beffe* and *Motton*, in Woolgar et al., *Food in Medieval England*, 57–8.

48 C.M. Woolgar, "Meat and Dairy Products in Late Medieval England," in Woolgar et al., *Food in Medieval England*, 92.

49 A short introduction to this complex topic is Iona McCleery, "Getting Enough to Eat: Famine as a Neglected Medieval Health Issue," in Barbara S. Bowers and Linda Migl Keyser, eds., *The Sacred and the Secular in Medieval Healing* (New York: Routledge, 2016), 116–39. Also see John Walter and Roger Schofield, "Famine, Disease and Crisis Mortality in Early Modern England," in John Walter and Roger Schofield, eds., *Famine, Disease and the Social Order in Early Modern Society* (Cambridge: Cambridge University Press, 1989), 1–73.

50 Philip Slavin, "The Crisis of the Fourteenth Century Reassessed: Between Ecology and Institutions—Evidence from England (1310–1350), *EHA Paper* (2010), 1–10.

51 Philip Slavin, "Climate and Famines: A Historical Reassessment," *Wiley Interdisciplinary Reviews*, 7 (2016), 433–47.

52 Dorothy Whitelock, David C. Douglas, and Susie I. Tucker, eds., and trans., *The Anglo-Saxon Chronicle* (London: Eyre and Spottieswoode, 1961), 79, 87, 109, 160, 162, 182, 192.

53 A.O. Anderson, M.O. Anderson, W.C. Dickinson, eds., *The Chronicle of Melrose Abbey* (London: Percy Lund Humphries and Co., 1936), 5, 18, 32.

54 Philip Slavin, "The Great Bovine Pestilence and its Economic and Environmental Consequences in England and Wales," *EconHistRev*, 65 (2012), 1239–66. Timothy P. Newfield, "A Cattle Panzootic in Early Fourteenth-Century Europe," *Agricultural History Review*, 57 (2009), 155–90; Bruce M.S. Campbell, "Panzootics, Pandemics, and Climate Anomalies in the Fourteenth Century," in Bernd Herrman, ed., *Beiträge zum Göttinger Umwelthistorischen Kölloquium* (Göttingen: Universitatsverlag, 2011), 177–215. The impact of the cattle murrains continued for quite some time although the worst impact of the Great Famine on the human population was over by 1322. William Chester Jordan, *The Great Famine* (Princeton: Princeton University Press, 1996). Jordan provides a Europe-wide perspective. For England see Ian Kershaw, "The Great Famine and Agrarian Crisis in England, 1315–1322," in R.H. Hilton, ed., *Peasants, Knights and Heretics* (Cambridge: Cambridge University Press, 1976), 85–132. A broad-based approach to famine in medieval England is Phillipp R. Schofield, "Approaches to Famine in Medieval England," in Pere Benitoi Montclias, ed., *Crisis Alimentarias en la Edad Media: Modelos, Explicaciones y Representaciones* (Lleida: Milenio, 2013), 71–86.

55 H.T. Riley, ed., *Johannis de Trokelowe et Henrici de Blaneforde chronica et annals* (Rolls Series, 28, 1866), 92–94, 95–96.

56 Slavin "Great Bovine Pestilence."

57 Buchanan Sharp, "Royal Paternalism and the Moral Economy in the Reign of Edward II: The Response to the Great Famine," *EconHistRev*, 66 (2013), 628–47.

58 *Trokelowe*, 89–90, 92–93. Wendy R. Childs and John Taylor, eds., *The Anonimale Chronicle, 1307–1334* (Yorkshire Archaeological Society, 147, 1987), 88–91.

59 *Trokelowe*, 96–98.

60 Newfield, "Cattle Panzootic in Early Fourteenth-Century Europe," Slavin, "Great Bovine Pestilence,"

61 Christopher Dyer, "Did the Peasants Really Starve in Medieval England?' in Martha Carlin and Joel T. Rosenthal, eds., *Food and Eating in Medieval Europe* (London: Hambledon Press, 1998), 66, 53–71.

62 Andrew Appleby, *Famine in Tudor and Stuart England* (Stanford: Stanford University Press, 1978), 133–54.

63 *Trokelowe*, 94.

64 Riley, *Memorials of London*, 90.

65 Thomas, *Calendar of Plea and Memoranda Rolls*, 2: "1364–1381," 12.

66 R.R. Sharpe, (ed.), *Calendar of Letter Books of the City of London*, 11 vols. (London: 1899–1912), "Letter Book H, 1375–1399," 16. Ernest L. Sabine deals with various health issues arising from butchering including the provision of tainted meat in "Butchering in Mediaeval London," *Speculum*, 8 (1933), 335–53.

67 Riley, *Memorials of London*, 318–9.
68 Piero Camporesi, *Bread of Dreams* (Chicago: University of Chicago Press, 1989).
69 Christopher Dyer, *Making a Living in the Middle Ages* (New Haven: Yale University Press, 2002), 95.
70 A good discussion the relationship of population and resources and various issues connected with modeling medieval population size can be found in John Hatcher and Mark Bailey, *Modeling the Middle Ages* (Oxford: Oxford University Press, 2001), 21–63.
71 Sebastian Funk, Marcel Salathé, and Vincent A.A. Jansen, "Modelling the Influence of Human Behavior on the Spread of Infectious Diseases: A Review," *Journal of the Royal Society Interface*, 7 (2010), 1247–56.
72 Sebastian Funk, Erez Gilad, Chris Watkins, and Vincent A.A. Jansen, "The Spread of Awareness and Its Impact on Epidemic Outbreaks," *PNAS*, 106 (2009), 6872–77; S. Funk, E. Gilad, V.A.A. Jansen, "Endemic Disease, Awareness, and Local Behavioral Response," *Journal of Theoretical Biology*, 264 (2010), 501–09.
73 Joshua M. Estein, Jon Parker, Drek Cummings, Ross A. Hammond, "Coupled Contagion Dynamics of Fear and Disease: Mathematical and Computational Explorations," *PLoS One,* 3 (2008), e3955; Sandra Meloni, Nicola Perra, Alex Arenas, Segio Gómez, Yamir Moreno, Alessandro Vespignani, "Modeling Human Mobility Reponses to Large-Scale Spreading of Infectious Diseases," *Nature: Scientific Reports*, 1 (2011), 62.
74 A brief discussion of societal efforts at safeguarding public health and regulating medical practice is J.M. Theilmann, "The Regulation of Public Health in Late Medieval England," in James L. Gillespie, (ed.), *The Age of Richard II* (New York: St. Martin's Press, 1997), 205–23. Carole Rawcliffe's *Urban Bodies* provides extensive information concerning sanitation and safe food and water in urban areas although it does not address medical care. Guy Geltner provides a survey of the literature of what is coming to be called healthscaping in "Public Health and the Pre-Modern City: A Research Agenda," *History Compass*, 10 (2012), 231–45.
75 Dolly Jørgensen, "Local Government Responses to Urban River Pollution in Late Medieval England," *Water History*, 2 (2010), 35–52. Jørgensen's study deals with York, Coventry and Norwich.
76 G.A. King and C.Y. Henderson, "Living Cheek by Jowl: The Pathoecology of Medieval York," *Quaternary International*, 341 (2014), 131–42.
77 Riley, *Memorials of London*, 264–65; Rawcliffe, *Urban Bodies*, 198.
78 Derek Keene, "Issues of Water in Medieval London to c. 1300," *Urban History*, 28 (2001), 176, 173. Carole Rawcliffe details the provision of water in urban England in the late Middle Ages in *Urban Bodies*, 176–228. Further on King's Lynn and London can be found in Christopher Bonfield, "Medical Advice and Public Health: Contextualizing the Supply and Regulation of Water in Later Medieval London and King's Lynn," *Poetica*, 73 (2009), 1–20.
79 Riley, *Memorials of London,* 200–01. It was necessary to again prohibit brewers from wasting the water from the conduit in Cheapside in 1345 (225). This seems to have been an ongoing problem as the order was repeated once again in 1415 (617).
80 Riley, *Memorials of London*, 23.
81 Riley, *Memorials of London*, 295–96.
82 Helena M. Chew and William Kellaway, (eds.), *London Assize of Nuisance 1301–1431, A Calendar* (London Record Society, 1973), no. 214. In this case, the neighbors under whose house the gutter ran complained because it regularly became stopped up, producing a stench.
83 Chew and Kellaway, *Assize of Nuisance,* no. 403.
84 Dave H. Evans, "A Good Riddance of Bad Rubbish? Scatological Musings on Rubbish Disposal and the Handling of 'Filth' in Medieval and Early Post-Medieval Towns," in Koen De Groote, Dries Tys, and Marnix Pieters, (eds.), *Exchanging Medieval Material Culture* (Brussels: Flemish Heritage Institute, 2010), 267–78.

85 Carole Rawcliffe, *Urban Bodies*, 144.
86 For examples, actions e.g., in 1302 (19, 26), 1303 (60), 1304 (69), 1306 (98); Chew and Kellaway, *Assize of Nuisance*.
87 Chew and Kelleway, *Assize of Nuisance*, no, 26, 324.
88 Thomas, *Calendar of Plea and Memoranda Rolls* 4: "1413–1437," 133.
89 Riley, *Memorials of London,* 23, 379–80, 478, 614–15; Thomas, *Plea and Memoranda Rolls,* "1413–1437," 152.
90 Sharpe, *Calendar of Letter Books of London*, "Letter Book L Temp. Edward IV—Henry VII," 21–22.
91 E.L. Sabine, "Latrines and Cesspools of Mediaeval London," *Speculum*, 9 (1934), 307–08.
92 Thomas, *Calendar of Plea and Memoranda Rolls,* 1413–1437, 125.
93 Thomas, *Plea and Memoranda Rolls,* "1413–1437," 157.
94 Walter King, "How High is too High? Disposing of Dung in Seventeenth-Century Prescot," *Sixteenth Century Journal*, 23 (1992), 443–57.
95 Dolly Jørgensen, "Cooperative Sanitation: Managing Streets and Gutters in Late Medieval England and Scandinavia," *Technology and Culture*, 49 (2008), 547–67. Jørgensen, "Local Government Responses to River Pollution." Jørgensen, "'All Good Rule of the Citee': Sanitation and Civic Government in England, 1400–1600," *Journal of Urban History*, 36 (2010), 300–15. Jørgensen, "The Medieval Sense of Smell, Stench and Sanitation;" Nathalie J. Ciecieznski, "The Stench of Disease: Public Health and the Environment in Late-Medieval English Towns and Cities," *Health, Culture and Society*, 4 (2013), 91–104. King and Henderson, "Living Cheek by Jowl: The Pathoecology of Medieval York." Rawcliffe, *Urban Bodies*, 116–228.
96 Jørgensen, "Local Government Responses to River Pollution," 35.
97 Sharpe, "Letter Book H," 392. Health issues related to butchering are detailed in Carole Rawcliffe, "Great Stenches, Horrible Sights, and Deadly Abominations," in Lukas Englemann, John Henderson, and Christos Lynteris, (eds.), *Plague and the City* (London: Routledge, 2019), 18–38.
98 Jørgensen, "Local Government Responses," King and Henderson, "Living Cheek by Jowl."
99 Riley, *Memorials of London*, 140.
100 Thomas, *Plea and Memoranda Rolls,* 4: "1413–1437," 153.
101 Thomas, *Plea and Memoranda Rolls*; 3: "1364–1381," 140.
102 Sabine, "City Cleaning," 23–24; Riley, *Memorials of London*, 249, 367; Thomas, *Plea and Memoranda Rolls*, 3: "1364–1381," 140; Sharpe, "Calendar of Letter Books, I, 1400–22," 45
103 Thomas, *Plea and Memoranda Rolls, 1413–1437*, 129.
104 Rawcliffe, *Urban Bodies,*136–37; Jørgensen, "Cooperative Sanitation," 562.
105 Thomas, *Plea and Memoranda Rolls, 1413–1437*, 133.
106 A.H. Thomas, (ed.) *Calendar of Select Pleas and Memoranda of the City of London Preserved among the Archives of the Corporation of the City of London at the Guildhall, A.D. 1381–1412* (Cambridge: Cambridge University Press, 1932), 7. Rawcliffe, *Urban Bodies*, 139.
107 J.P. Pickett, "A Translation of the 'Cantus' Plague Treatise," in L.M. Matheson, ed., *Popular and Practical Science of Medieval England* (East Lansing MI, 1994), 274. Rawcliffe, "Great Stenches, Horrible Sights, and Deadly Abominations," 20.
108 Martha Bayless, *Sin and Filth in Medieval Culture* (London: Routledge, 2012), xviii.
109 William H. TeBrake, "Air Pollution and Fuel Crises in Pre-Industrial London, 1250–1650," *Technology and Culture*, 16 (1975), 337–59; J.A. Galloway, D. Keene, and M. Murphy, "Fueling the City: Production and Distribution of Firewood and Fuel in London's Region, 1290–1400," *EconHistRev*, 2d ser., 49 (1996), 447–72.
110 Peter Brimblecombe, *The Big Smoke* (New York: Routledge, 1987), 8.

111 Peter Brimblecombe, "Attitudes and Responses towards Air Pollution in Medieval England," *Journal of the Air Pollution Control Association*, 26 (1976), 942–43.

112 M.E. Lewis, C.A. Roberts, and K. Manchester, "Comparative Study of the Prevalence of Maxillary Sinusitis in Later Medieval Urban and Rural Populations in Northern England," *American Journal of Physical Anthropology*, 98 (1995), 497–506.

113 Chew and Kellaway, *Assize of Nuisance,* no. 617. This was a mutual suit as the complainants were being sued by their neighbors because their gutters overflowed and flooded the neighboring property (616).

114 Tragedy of the commons problems are extensively discussed by economists, philosophers, and psychologists. The problem was first enunciated clearly by the biologist Garrett Hardin, "The Tragedy of the Commons," *Science*, 162 (1968), 1243–48.

115 A good discussion, grounded in economic theory, of the problem of public health as a collective good is Ulf Christian Ewert, "Water, Public Hygiene and Fire Control in Medieval Towns: Facing Collective Goods Problems While Ensuring the Quality of Life," *Historical Social Research*, 32 (2007), 222–51.

116 Claire Weeda, "Cleanliness, Civility, and the City in Medieval Ideals and Scripts," in Carole Rawcliffe and Claire Weeda (eds.), *Policing the Urban Environment in Premodern Europe* (Amsterdam: Amsterdam University Press, 2019), 39–68.

117 Arthur K. Shapiro and Elaine Shapiro, *The Placebo Effect* (Baltimore: Johns Hopkins University Press, 1997), 2; David Wootton, *Bad Medicine* (Oxford: Oxford University Press, 2006). The subtitle, Doctors Doing Harm since Hippocrates, is indicative of Wootton's argument.

3

THE EVERYDAY THREAT OF INFECTIOUS DISEASE

Good health was often at a premium for people in premodern England. Everyday health problems such as diarrhea, wounds, cuts, and fevers could lead to life-threatening situations, especially for children and anyone with a compromised immune system. Some diseases appeared to be regional in focus or affected only some segments of the population or were chronic, long-lasting health issues rather than posing immediate threats to life. Other diseases led to major threats to public health but did not do so because of environmental or epidemiological factors that limited their spread.

This chapter first examines health issues arising from everyday living and then turns to four diseases that posed public health threats to premodern people, but did not produce mortality crises. The four diseases are malaria, measles, tuberculosis, and leprosy. All four could and did kill, but they were more threats to overall well-being than major killers in concentrated fashions as was an epidemic disease such as the plague. They also weakened the immune systems, enabling other diseases to harm the victims. How society reacted to the victims of these diseases is telling as leprosy, in particular, could generate a negative social response to those afflicted with the disease.

Leprosy, tuberculosis, measles, and malaria added to the disease burden for many people in premodern England. All four could kill their victims and tuberculosis is still referred to as the "king of death" with good reason. Tuberculosis, leprosy, and malaria were more often chronic diseases that harmed a person's ability to function well in society. In the long run, the prognosis was often death, but the afflicted person might well die of something else before tuberculosis or leprosy had run their course or a particularly serious bout of malaria did the person in. Primarily, a childhood disease, measles can produce a large number of deaths including adults on occasion. The malaria variant *Plasmodium falciparum* is a killer, but it is a disease largely of the tropics as well as medieval Italy. The other

DOI: 10.4324/9781003215219-4

malaria variants, most notably *P. vivax*, are more likely to weaken their victims, making them more susceptible to other medical problems rather than killing them outright. People with other medical issues such as a weakened immune system could die from a malaria attack but otherwise, they survived only to have the disease reappear again and again after the first infection. All four of these diseases interacted with everyday health problems, sometimes in synergistic fashion to worsen health.

Fevers, which include typhus and malaria, were common in the premodern world. People considered fevers a disease itself, not a symptom. By the seventeenth century, some commentators began to identify some fevers as specific diseases, a process that continued into the nineteenth century. Influenza and typhus were probably present in the Middle Ages, but people simply identified them as fevers. Influenza requires a large concentrated population to sustain an epidemic and such was not the case in the Middle Ages. Occasional cases of the flu would have been likely to have been subsumed under the term fever. Typhus, too, often would have been described as a fever although some of its symptoms such as the rash were distinctive. The environmental conditions necessary for a typhus outbreak were certainly present in medieval England. It was not until the fifteenth century, however, when jail fever, a clearly defined disease with discrete symptoms, began to be described. The growth of population in the early modern world made it possible for typhus to emerge as a clear public health threat. Both diseases will be treated later as examples of emerging or re-emerging diseases of the sixteenth century.

The dangers of everyday life

A brief excursion into the dangers of everyday life that influenced the lives of premodern people even when no infectious diseases were present is necessary before turning to more serious health issues. Everyday living often proved hazardous to people's lives in the premodern world. Accidents, violence, childbirth, and childhood itself often threatened people's health. These threats were complicated by sickness and lowered resistance that may have come from dietary insufficiencies.

Even if accidents had been no more common in premodern England than today, resulting infections could kill, and the crippling that often resulted from say a poorly set broken leg, left a person in a weakened condition. Peasant society produced accidents aplenty. A housewife might be scalded by boiling water from a pot while her husband cut himself with an axe or was kicked by a horse. People readily treated minor burns or cuts with ointments and salves some of which proved effective. Major burns were harder to treat and easily led to infection and death. Even a small cut could become infected, but a leg laid open by a misplaced axe stroke was more likely to become infected as well as leading to crippling from cut tendons or ligaments.

Open wounds led to infection and infection often led to tetanus or gangrene—blood poisoning. Some herbal remedies such as Echinacea would have been helpful in treating wounds and burns through its ability to reduce inflammation and possibly limit infection, but the often-used remedy was to cauterize the open wound with a hot iron. Cauterization helped to seal the wound and prevent infection from developing. When poorly done, cauterization left scars or worse led to infection from the burned flesh, not to mention the pain of the operation.

Infections came in many forms, but many originated in the soil. Tetanus is a non-communicable disease that is caused by exposure to the spores of the gram-positive bacteria *Clostridium tetani*. The tetanus organism produces a neurotoxin, tetanospasmin, which is the second most toxic bacterial toxin (botulism is considered the most toxic). Tetanus bacteria are present in soil and manure so it was easy for the spores to enter an open wound. Deep puncture wounds that do not bleed a lot are good sites for a tetanus infection to take hold. Animal bites, stepping on a pitchfork, or a knife produced wounds that were ideal sites for tetanus infections. Once inside the body, the tetanus bacteria interfere with muscular contraction, producing among other symptoms stiffness in the jaw (lockjaw). As early as ten hours after a wound, pain may set in with black or blue discoloration of the skin. The telltale sign of gangrene is the foul odor that comes from the wound. Untreated, which was the case in the past, the disease progressed and produced toxemia (blood poisoning) and interfered with the muscles that control breathing, leading to death from suffocation. Neonatal tetanus follows the same path helping to produce a high infant mortality rate. Cutting the umbilical cord with a rusty knife easily led to infection of the infant and death. People recognized the danger of infection and used cauterization as a remedy to prevent gangrene but it was not always effective.

Local healers often set broken bones and bone-setting could be done quite well by some practitioners. Other, more ham-handed, practitioners left poorly set bones that provided pain and weakness for the afflicted person. Torn ligaments or a torn rotator cuff were nearly impossible to repair save through natural healing so that people often suffered for the rest of their lives. Some people turned to saints for help with these tragedies of everyday life as did parents confronted with the sudden apparent death of a child from an accident. The reality of life was that many peasants and urban poor or even the aristocracy who survived to old age were afflicted with aches and pains that were often made worse by arthritis as they aged.

Axes and farm implements often produced accidental wounds, but so did the use of weapons with the intent to harm. Violence affected all classes of society from knightly warfare to a village brawl. Aside from clubs or maces that crushed a skull or broke an arm, many wounds were inflicted by edged or pointed weapons such as knives, swords, lances, or arrows leading to deep cuts or puncture wounds. Warfare produced wounds but so did simple disputes over straying animals or the result of too much to drink and a hot temper. If not kept clean, such wounds easily led to gangrene. With no antibiotics to treat infection, people tried to reduce the fever, possibly invoked a saint's aid and hoped for the best.

In the Early Middle Ages, various invaders, such as Saxons and Vikings invaded England, bringing death and destruction with them, but after the eleventh-century invasion, except along the Scots border, was no longer much of a threat. Civil war or campaigns abroad by English monarchs produced their share of deaths, wounds, and crippling for those involved. Warfare rarely involved large numbers of men so it was not a major killer. Interpersonal violence arising from the stresses of daily living, however, led to the deaths of many men and women and wounded or crippled many more. Often it was not simply the wound itself that produced the threat to life but the resulting infection. Although premodern English society tried to limit interpersonal violence, it was more successful in dealing with crimes such as murder and less so with lesser hurts.

Everyday diseases that killed

Epidemic diseases killed large numbers of people quickly and received (and still receive) public attention. Other diseases are simply part of everyday life. These diseases might kill only a few people or simply weaken a person so that some other ailment could finish the task. Common colds made people miserable but did not kill. In some cases, colds led to pneumonia. Many people might carry the pneumonia bacteria (*Streptococcus pneumoniae* or other bacteria) in their throat at any time, but it generally takes another infection such as a viral infection like influenza to trigger the pneumonia bacteria. Treatment for pneumonia in the premodern world might be tender loving care if the person was lucky, and bleeding or purging to regain humoral balance if the person was not. A person with a strong constitution could survive a pneumonia attack, but someone with a weakened immune system could die within one to three days of the onset of the disease. By itself, the cold virus was relatively harmless, but when it triggered an attack of pneumonia the result could be deadly.

Other bacterial or viral infections had the same impact as the cold virus. The initial infection was unpleasant, maybe painful, but was not life-threatening. However, if the initial infection led to something worse, lives were at risk. Today, many infections are treated with antibiotics or anti-virals and so do not lead to more serious complications. In a pre-antibiotic society, the person got on with life and tried to ignore the infection, turned to a medical practitioner who might prescribe bleeding or purging to bring the humors back into balance, tried an herbal remedy, or possibly invoked a saint's assistance in order to achieve divine relief. Some herbal remedies were effective but the other treatments might leave the afflicted person worse off than before.

Today, diarrhea remains a major health problem in some countries leading to childhood deaths as well as deaths in the elderly population. The fecal-oral route is the most common process of transmitting diarrheal diseases. Diarrheal diseases are easily preventable through practices such as safe food handling and the proper disposal of human and animal wastes. Rehydration theory helps to cure diarrhea sufferers often without any other medical intervention. Dung in the streets coupled with unsafe food handling practices could easily lead to a host of diarrheal infections through contamination of food and water supplies.

There are several common forms of diarrhea. One of the more common forms of diarrhea, often called travelers' diarrhea today, is caused by a norovirus. Another is transmitted by the *Shigella* bacteria. The *Giardia lamblia* parasite is the source of giardiasis which produces diarrhea symptoms. Another form of often severe diarrhea is caused by the *Entamoeba histolytica* parasite often excreted in the feces of an infected person.[1] Fecal contamination of food and water is the usual means of transmitting all of these agents of disease. Eradicating fecal contamination requires both dealing with the source and hand washing and care in food preparation as well as ensuring clean water, both not always easy to accomplish.

Diarrhea also comes from food poisoning. Eating fecally contaminated meat from animals with the *Salmonella typhimurium* bacteria is the usual means of human infection. Generally, abdominal pain and watery diarrhea for a week or so are the products of food poisoning. Food poisoning could also be caused by the *Staphylococcus aureus* bacteria, the bacteria that cause many cases of food poisoning today as when potato salad is left out in the sun enabling bacteria to multiply and infect people who eat the food. Not as serious as dysentery, bacterial infection resulting from food poisoning was more unpleasant than dangerous unless caused by botulism when it was generally fatal.

Diarrhea was often a common childhood ailment in the Middle Ages but even adults were not immune. By the time they reached adulthood most people had developed some level of immunity to the local flora although dysentery, a serious diarrheal disease, remained a problem for travelers. Left untreated, the fluid loss could lead to other medical problems and death. For a person with a weakened immune system, a bout with diarrhea could lead to complications including death. Dysentery is a catchall term for particularly severe forms of inflammatory diarrhea and was referred to as the bloody flux in the Middle Ages indicating one of its more noticeable and potentially deadly symptoms. Dysentery was often common in army camps and other places where fecal-oral contamination was likely to occur. Left untreated, dysentery could be a major killer, taking, for example, Henry V who died while on campaign in France in 1422.[2]

Improper disposal of human and animal wastes that found their way into water supplies led to parasitic infections from whipworms and roundworms. Human trichiniasis is caused by whipworms and while often asymptomatic it can lead to dehydration, chronic diarrhea, growth retardation in children, and even terminal anemia. Roundworm infections are often asymptomatic but chronic infestations can produce intestinal blockage, respiratory distress, growth retardation, and anemia.[3] Children were more likely to fall victim to worms, something that contributed to high child mortality rates. Both roundworm and whipworm remains have been found at archaeological sites throughout Europe including England leading to an assumption that infections must have been common.[4] The bad odor of dung was actually a signal that potential health problems were present even if people were unaware of their true nature.

Another gastrointestinal infection was not so benign. Even today typhoid fever, the product of the *Salmonella typhi* bacteria, can be life-threatening. Lumped in with other fevers or sometimes confused with typhus in the past, typhoid fever is solely a human disease with no other host. The disease is generally spread by human carriers, people who have recovered from the disease, but who have not eliminated the bacteria from their system. Most often the bacteria continue to grow in the person's gall bladder and are excreted throughout the person's lifetime. Because the infectious dose of the bacteria is very low, typhoid is easily transmitted. The bacteria are readily transmitted through fecal contamination of water or food. The bacteria can also be transmitted by an asymptomatic carrier who handles food, as did the cook Mary Mallon, the "Typhoid Mary," of the early twentieth century, who was responsible for 47 cases of typhoid and at least three deaths in New York. Once ingested, the bacteria pass through the stomach to the small intestine and then through the cells lining the small intestine to the local lymph nodes. Macrophages kill many of the typhoid bacteria at this point but some escape to the bloodstream producing an infection. After a period of malaise lasting about a week, high fever ensues and the infected person becomes increasingly ill, apathetic, and often out of touch with reality. By the third week, the afflicted person is often disoriented and stuporous and toxemia and death often ensues. In the premodern world, there was no remedy for typhoid except to try to keep up the person's strength until the disease passed. Although treatable today, the *Salmonella typhi* bacteria have become resistant to many of the antibiotics that previously were used to treat typhoid fever so that the disease is once again a threat in some parts of the world. A typhoid outbreak was not common in premodern England but when it occurred it could sicken and kill several people, especially those who might be malnourished or suffering from other ailments. Although typhoid could reach epidemic proportions, it was more likely to produce several deaths in an area and then die out although it could continue to infect the population if a carrier was present.

Diseases such as pneumonia or gastrointestinal ailments and wounds and accidents contributed to the mortality rate in society in the past, particularly among children. Wounds and accidents also led to long-term disability. When cross-infections with other ailments, pneumonia or gastrointestinal ailments could kill, especially anyone with a compromised immune system. These health problems are hard to document specifically but were present as an undercurrent in medieval society.

Malaria, ague, or marsh fever

Malaria is rarely considered to be a medical problem anymore in northern countries such as England. The tropics are another matter, and in some parts of Africa, malaria continues to be a major health threat. The *P. vivax* variety of malaria seems to have reached Britain during the Roman occupation and there is archaeological evidence that it was present in England in the years before 1050.[5] Finding solid evidence for the presence of malaria is challenging but, as Timothy Newfield indicates, it is possible to do so. He argues that *P. vivax* was present in Merovingian and Carolingian Europe, appearing in spotty fashion in both time and space.[6] Newfield is careful to point out that many sorts of fevers were present in Early Medieval Europe, but that the descriptions of at least some of them are likely to be malaria. M.L. Cameron goes so far as to argue that malaria was endemic, especially in eastern England, helping to add to the complications of childbirth.[7] During the premodern era, malaria was a health threat almost everywhere in Europe, save possibly in Scandinavia. Because of where the disease was often found, it was often known as marsh fever to distinguish it from other fevers. Existing descriptions of the symptoms of marsh fever are relatively convincing that it and malaria were the same disease. There are four variants of malaria, each with its own characteristics, but only one is of concern here. *Plasmodium falciparum* is probably the oldest species and is a major health threat in the tropical world today but was not found in premodern England. *P. ovale, P. malaria, P. knowlesi,* and *P. vivax* may be found in temperate zones as well as the tropics, but only *P. vivax* was common in the premodern West. *P. vivax* and *P. ovale* produce tertian fevers which occur every two days in an infected person while *P. malaria* produces quartan fever which peaks every 72 hours. All species are subject to periods of remission but may reappear for periods up to ten years. People living in malaria-prone areas are likely to be bitten regularly by the mosquitoes that serve to transmit the disease so that some people continually suffered from malaria as it became a chronic condition.

Malaria is a parasitic disease of humans for which the *Anopheles* mosquito plays an important role in both providing a primary host for the *Plasmodium* protozoa to develop and in transmitting the parasite to humans. *P. vivax*, the most common form of malaria in premodern England, is transmitted by the *Anopheles atroparvus* mosquito. Although the malaria cycle is a complicated one, mosquitoes play a central role. Once the *Plasmodium* parasite infects a mosquito, it develops as the mosquito hibernates over the winter. When mosquitoes become active in spring and summer, they seek a blood meal from mammal sources including humans. When a mosquito bites a human, some of the *plasmodium* may be injected into the person. The malaria parasites incubate in the human host and spread throughout the person's body through the bloodstream producing the symptoms of the disease as the body tries to fight off the infection. Humans also serve to transmit the disease when mosquitoes bite infected people and then bite other people.

Standing water provides a natural habitat for mosquitoes. The marshes and fens of southeastern England provided such a habitat as did backwaters of rivers such as the Thames. Upland bodies of water were less likely to produce the right combination of water quality and temperature that would prove amenable to the growth of a mosquito population but could do so on occasion. Mosquitoes and the *Plasmodium* parasite are temperature sensitive so northern England would be less hospitable to mosquito populations. Climate enters into consideration in two ways. During the period from approximately 1000 to 1400, the climate of Western Europe was slightly warmer than it had been before, a period known as the Medieval Climate Anomaly. Slightly warmer temperatures might have made it possible for malaria to increase its range to north-central England in such areas as the fens surrounding the Isle of Ely in Cambridgeshire. Temperatures were not warm enough so that *P. falciparum* could penetrate into England, but may have increased the range of *P. vivax*. The decline in average temperatures that were characteristic of the Little Ice Age, which stretched from the sixteenth through eighteenth centuries, should concomitantly have produced a decline in the impact of malaria. However, as Paul Reiter has shown, malaria was very much a health threat in southeastern England throughout the Little Ice Age. Reiter's argument is that many factors in addition to temperature are at work with the incidence of malaria, something demonstrated by Mary Dobson who includes elevation, water quality, and human settlement patterns in her explanation of the impact of malaria in the early modern era.[8] Malaria was not a health problem that affected all of England; it was health problem that affected particular areas, most notably the marshy areas of the southeast.

An attack of malaria can lead to death, especially if it is the *P. falciparum* species. The *P. vivax* species was much less likely to produce death among its victims. Children, however, often fell victim to the high fever of an initial bout of malaria.[9] The victim first exhibits chills which turn into recurrent fever. Repeated attacks of malaria or marsh fever often left the person in a weakened condition arising from several bouts with fever and could lead to malaria cachexia, which is characterized by physical weakness, emaciation, and severe anemia which when combined could lead to early death or make the person susceptible to other ailments. Children infected with malaria were more likely than adults to die from the spiking fever that occurred. Women who suffered from anemia were more likely to have complicated pregnancies, give birth to children with low birth weight, and have difficulty in breast-feeding. Surviving several bouts of malaria did give some degree of immunity so those people who encountered it for the first time were more likely to suffer severe consequences. Malaria's primary impact was the cycles of debilitation that it produced and internal impact such as an enlargement of the spleen. Overtime continued bouts of malaria helped shorten the lives of the victims. Weakened workers were likely to be less productive workers and to fall victim to other medical problems more readily than healthy people. The demographic impact of malaria in premodern England is difficult to assess although Dobson argues that it had a substantial impact on the population of southeastern England in the early modern era.[10] Malaria helped to increase the mortality rate in premodern England, but its major impact was the long-term weakness it often produced, weakness that reduced productivity and made people susceptible to other medical problems.

Measles, a childhood disease with deadly implications

Measles has long been assumed to be an old disease and it has been suggested that measles was one of the diseases present during the plague of Athens (430–427 BCE) and particularly the Plague of the Antonine's in 165–80 CE. However, recent work based on molecular clock estimates indicates that measles evolved from rinderpest, a disease of cattle, at some point in the eleventh or twelfth centuries.[11] Measles is a highly communicable disease caused by the measles *Morbillivirus*. It is transmitted by direct contact with nose and throat secretions from infected people as well as airborne transmission and contact with freshly soiled articles. Although measles outbreaks can occur at any time, the disease is primarily a wintertime disease because of the ease of transmission when people are crowded together indoors. It is communicable from slightly before the pro-domal phase to four days after the onset of the disease. During the prodomal stage, small reddened specks, called Koplik's spots, often appear on the mucosal lining of the mouth. The incubation period for measles ranges from eight to thirteen days from the time of exposure to the onset of fever often accompanied by a cough and conjunctivitis. An often painful rash ensues by the fourteenth and may last from three to seven days. The rash first appears on the face and neck and then spreads to the rest of the body. Once the rash subsides, the victim has lifetime immunity. The symptoms are somewhat similar to those of an early stage of smallpox leading to diagnostic confusion. Measles is highly contagious with an R_0 of between 12 and 16.[12] An infected person in a group of people is likely to infect everyone else with the virus who does not possess immunity. Once everyone has been infected with the disease, it burns out as no susceptibles remain. Although generally a fairly mild disease, measles can produce a variety of complications in organ systems and can lead to pneumonia and sometimes encephalitis which can be especially dangerous in people with compromised immune systems.[13]

Measles is usually a childhood disease. Because of its highly contagious nature, measles virus readily infected children who gained immunity. Today a vaccine produces immunity, but as the 2019 epidemic in the United States indicates a large number of unvaccinated children can produce a severe outbreak. As time passes and children are born into a society, a new group of susceptibles arises and the disease cycle repeats itself. Mathematical analysis indicates that a naïve population of at least 250,000 is necessary to maintain a *Morbillivirus* outbreak for an extended period. Infections from the outside can be a source of the disease within a closed population. In this case, the whole population can be susceptible if they possess no immunity and can lead to a high mortality rate as occurred on the Polynesian island of Rotuma in 1911 when a ship visiting the island led to the infection of the island's population. In that case, the measles-related mortality rate was highest among young children (23.4 per 100 person-years) and young adults (17.1 per 100 person-years).[14] Measles epidemics can be exacerbated by overcrowding and malnutrition, leading to higher than usual mortality rates.[15]

Isolated communities in premodern England might avoid a measles outbreak for many years, but their very isolation proved deadly if measles was imported into the community. Particularly in years of food shortages that led to weakened immune systems measles could ravage a community.

Measles appears to have had a limited although important impact on premodern society. As recent research has shown, measles does not appear to have been a problem in the Early Middle Ages. In times of food shortage, especially if coupled with other health problems, measles could have added substantially to the mortality rate especially among the young. The situation in the Americas when Europeans came in contact with the native population was often quite different than in Europe with high mortality rates among a wider range of the population. Measles epidemics added to other health problems and had a lingering demographic impact if enough children died during an outbreak. In the urban centers of Latin America as well as some native American villages in New England, measles helped to produce a dramatic decline in the population in the sixteenth century.

The sometime king of death: *phthisis, consumption, tuberculosis*

In the 1970s, many public health officials indicated that tuberculosis was no longer a public health problem and might soon be eradicated and tuberculosis hospitals repurposed to other uses. Today, tuberculosis is the poster child for what is labeled re-emerging diseases as it has re-emerged with a vengeance, killing more than 5,000 people per day worldwide. Tuberculosis has had a long history, dating back to ancient Egypt and China, of impacting humans and at times has exacted a high toll with its presence, more than earning its title the king of death.[16] Tuberculosis is moderately infectious with an R_0 as high as 4.3 but more often around 2 and as the western world urbanized and people crowded together it became a major everyday health threat.[17] In 1662, John Graunt indicated that the London Bill of Mortality for 1632 had reported that 1,797 of 9,511 deaths were attributable to tuberculosis. By 1799 consumption, as it was then known, accounted for a quarter of the deaths in England.[18] Although it is difficult to ascertain its full impact on medieval England, it is clear that the disease was present in the premodern West.

Tuberculosis is a disease caused by the genus *Mycobacterium*. Although there are many species in the genus, three stand out as affecting human health. *Mycobacterium leprae* gives rise to leprosy and will be dealt with later in this chapter. *Mycobacterium bovis* and especially *Mycobacterium tuberculosis* are potentially lethal to humans. At one point, it was thought that *M. tuberculosis* had evolved from *M. bovis*. Recent work that has examined the molecular structure of a variety of samples indicates that *M. tuberculosis* is an ancient disease that did not evolve from *M. bovis*. Indeed, it is possible that *M. bovis* evolved from tuberculosis several thousand years ago.[19] Humans are infected by *M. tuberculosis* and play a major role in its transmission. Tuberculosis spreads via human-to-human transmission by coughing or spitting. While it spreads readily, tuberculosis requires a large population to sustain continuing infections. The cities of ancient Rome provided a good environment for the spread of tuberculosis. The breakdown of urban society that lasted until the fourteenth century in Italy and later elsewhere meant that the disease had a difficult time sustaining itself as an epidemic disease in the Early and High Middle Ages. Places with several people living in a compact space, such as monastic communities, could remain centers for ongoing tuberculosis outbreaks but the outbreak would soon burn out.

Tuberculosis may spread readily through oral transmission but not everyone becomes infected with the disease. It is generally transmitted by discharges from the nose and mouth although some infections can occur via the gastro-intestinal route such as drinking milk from tuberculosis-infected cows. Often people are exposed to the *M. tuberculosis* bacterium and acquire the disease however, many of those exposed to the disease never exhibit symptoms. Symptoms include coughing that lasts for more than three weeks, coughing up blood, chest pain and trouble breathing, fatigue, fever, and loss of appetite. Those who exhibit symptoms during the first three to eight weeks are said to have primary tuberculosis. During the first three months or so of infection, some victims may develop symptoms of more severe diseases such as meningeal disease. During the first three to four months, some sufferers exhibit symptoms of pleurisy as the disease spreads from the primary lesion into other areas of the lungs. People with compromised immune systems may die at this point. Not all sufferers exhibit severe symptoms and over the next three years, the primary infection subsides although the infection may move into joints and bones. After that period, many victims become asymptomatic as the disease moves into the post-primary phase which will last for the rest of the victim's life. The disease may reappear at a later date spreading to glands such as the lymph nodes of the neck (labeled as scrofula or the King's Evil in the Middle Ages). It may also spread to the spine inducing a curvature of the spine as the vertebrae of the lower back are destroyed, a disease referred to as Pott's Disease today.[20] Ultimately, the disease destroys lung capacity and leaves sufferers coughing up blood as they try to breathe or developing pneumonia. Tuberculosis generally develops in a slow fashion in normally healthy people and is subject to an extended period of remission so that many of its victims may die of some other ailment before they die of tuberculosis. Tuberculosis is an opportunistic disease that easily affects people with compromised immune systems such as HIV-infected individuals today or famine victims in the Middle Ages.

Many of the symptoms of tuberculosis are similar to those of other diseases so it has not always been easy to identify its victims from descriptive material from the past. The skeletons of those people who had the disease settle in their spines are readily identifiable due to the collapsed vertebrae and spinal curvature.[21] The term *phthisis* that once referred to the disease in the ancient world and the Middle Ages literally means wasting, something that tuberculosis did to its victims over time as the body's ability to function normally declined as the disease progressed.

However, this sort of wasting away could also be an indication of other infections so the use of the term *phthisis* is not always be taken as an indication of tuberculosis. Consumption came to be adopted in the Late Middle Ages and was used in the nineteenth century when the disease became almost fashionable because it infected so many artists, musicians, and writers. This term also implied a wasting action but more particularly addressed the declining lung capacity of its sufferers. Again, some other medical problems could produce similar symptoms although it is easier to equate consumption with tuberculosis.

Several factors affect the likelihood of tuberculosis infection in any society. Many of these factors continue to be present in some societies in the twenty-first century helping to explain the continuing incidence of the disease. These same factors were also present in the past. As Roberts and Buikstra indicate, poverty and contact with infected animals had the largest impact in producing tuberculosis infections in the past.[22] The bacteria *M. bovis* is a zoonosis that is readily transmittable from animals to humans. Cattle are readily infected by *M. bovis* and milk from infected cattle can serve as a means for infecting children. Several other domestic animals can also be infected by *M. bovis* and serve as a vector to infect humans. Today control of infected animals is seen as a reliable means for limiting tuberculosis outbreaks in humans, but such an approach would have been unlikely in premodern England.

Poverty is manifested in a variety of ways that can make people susceptible to tuberculosis. Impoverished people often have a diet that is missing several nutrients making them susceptible to a variety of diseases. The poorest levels of English society often exhibited symptoms of malnutrition in even good crop years and during periods of famine even more people would have been vulnerable. The poor were found in both rural and urban environments. Many of the poor were poor all of their lives making it easier for a post-primary tuberculosis infection to return. The poor often lived in the over-crowded and damp conditions in which tuberculosis flourished. Today the poor in urban areas are more likely to live in overcrowded conditions that can make tuberculosis easier to acquire. In the Middle Ages, the members of a rural household lived close together and so even though a village might have few inhabitants, they lived so close together that the advantage of a lower overall population density was negated somewhat. In the Early Middle Ages, many rural dwellers lived in close proximity to their domestic animals making it easier for them to become infected by *M. bovis*. The poor had a less nutritious diet than other people and had to continue to work in order to survive even when sick which made the impact of some of the symptoms of tuberculosis even more harmful.

Other factors influence the incidence of tuberculosis. Children appear to fall victim to the disease more readily than adults. Tuberculosis acquired in childhood can reappear in the post-primary stage much later in life and the damage to the joints and spine takes time to occur. Today, it appears that men rather than women are more likely to develop tuberculosis although other intervening variables such as occupation may also be at work.[23] The impact of climate is harder to trace although it is apparent that people living in wet and cold surroundings are more susceptible to the disease. The transition into the Medieval Warm Anomaly and then into the Little Ice Age is unlikely to have had a direct effect on the incidence of tuberculosis. The ongoing impact of a colder climate during the Little Ice Age may have been one factor that led to the increase of tuberculosis cases in the early modern world. Geography also played a part as living in regions such as the fens of southeastern England could make residents more susceptible to tuberculosis as well as malaria.

Tuberculosis is diagnosed with a skin test often followed by a blood test today. Once diagnosed, the disease is treatable with antibiotics. People with latent tuberculosis may need to receive more than one antibiotic in order to recover. Those patients with active tuberculosis often receive an antibiotic cocktail that may consist of a combination of Isoniazid, Rifampin, Ethambutol, and Pyrazinamide. Some strains of tuberculosis, especially some found in Russia, are partially or nearly completely drug-resistant and other treatments are followed. Drug-resistant tuberculosis is often treated with a combination of antibiotics known as fluoroquinolones and injectable medications such as capreomycin or amikacin. Some strains of tuberculosis are now almost completely drug-resistant forcing the medical community to fall back on palliative care and isolation of the patients as was done in the past.

Some people died soon after becoming infected with the tuberculosis bacteria and others died from complications later in life. Many tuberculosis sufferers had to undergo gradual loss of lung function and crippling that would come to limit their mobility and productivity as well as making everyday life increasingly painful. Writing in the thirteenth century, Bartholomew Anglicus described the wasting nature of the disease as consumption reflecting what the disease was doing to the body.[24] People sought palliative care for tuberculosis including a better diet. Some also turned to the saints for aid. Some of the palliative remedies of the thirteenth-century physician Theodoric of Lucca could even have provided some relief from some of the outward symptoms of the disease.[25] Physicians, such as Gilbertus Anglicus in the thirteenth century also tried to treat *phthisis* with remedies that were intended to return the humors to balance and thus return the sufferer to good health.[26] As late as the sixteenth century, the Italian physician Girolomo Fracastoro continued to prescribe a variety of herbal remedies intended to return the humours to balance as the means for treating *phthisis*.[27] Although tracing the specific symptoms of tuberculosis in the miracles reported at saints' tombs is challenging, clear evidence of tuberculosis is sometimes noted. For example, in 1485, John Angelde of Smallhythe in Kent reported at the tomb of King Henry VI at Windsor Castle that he had suffered from consumption. A voice from Heaven told him to pray to the sainted King Henry. He did and he was cured of the disease.[28] The crippling ensuing from post-primary tuberculosis could also have come from a variety of other causes such as arthritis so it is difficult to determine which pilgrims suffered from tuberculosis. Scrofula, one form of tuberculosis that involved the infection of the cervical lymph nodes, was easier to differentiate from other problems. In England and France, people referred to scrofula as the King's Evil because the royal touch was supposed to lead to its cure. Scrofula is subject to periods of remission so it is possible that the royal touch did appear to cure victims. The first miracle credited to the eleventh century St. Edward the Confessor in the *Vita Edwardi Regis* is for scrofula. In this case, King Edward manipulated the pus-filled sores on a woman's neck to remove the pus and blood and she was pronounced cured.[29] Later English rulers and French kings from the time of Louis IX in the thirteenth century were content with touching the afflicted person on the head as a blessing and at times giving them a token to take with them. In England, the tradition of the royal touch persisted into the early eighteenth century when Queen Anne was the last to touch for the King's Evil.[30]

Tuberculosis was a major health problem in premodern England but one that is difficult to quantify. The growth of population made it a fearful disease by the eighteenth century, one that more people identified. Many sufferers of tuberculosis died of something else long before the disease took its toll. Victims of the crippling that arose from a tuberculosis infection would have been difficult to differentiate from those people with other forms of crippling by medieval people. Paleopathology does reveal numerous medieval skeletal remains from throughout Europe that exhibit the skeletal deformities produced by tuberculosis.[31] For many people, tuberculosis was a long-term ailment that made life miserable rather than something to be feared as was the plague.

Leprosy, fear, and sin?

Like tuberculosis, leprosy is part of the *Mycobacterium* family. The bacteria *Mycobacterium leprae* is the causative agent of leprosy or Hansen's Disease as it is identified today. Today, tuberculosis is often a disease of the poor and disadvantaged and so its victims are sometimes stigmatized because of their social position. That was not the case in the Middle Ages when tuberculosis struck even the elite. Leprosy on the other hand is often considered to be the poster child for a disease that leads its victims to be stigmatized.[32] As Carole Rawcliffe has shown, the stigma surrounding the disease is old, dating from the Old Testament, but it received a good deal of amplification in the nineteenth century.[33] Nineteenth-century writers did much to create the image of the medieval leper as a total outcast, one whose disease was often alleged to have come from the person's sinful nature. The reality of the treatment of lepers in the Middle Ages is far more complex and nuanced than nineteenth-century writers such as Robert Louis Stevenson indicated in his novel of medieval England, *The Black Arrow*. The relationship between leprosy and tuberculosis is also more complex than it was once thought to be and may help to explain the decline of leprosy in the late Middle Ages.

Leprosy takes two very different forms leading it to be labeled a bipolar disease. Lepromatous leprosy can be easily diagnosed by the often-dramatic disfiguring of the skin and seems to have been the most common form in the Middle Ages. In the Middle Ages, someone who exhibited extensive scarring and ulceration of the skin was likely to be diagnosed with leprosy. As affected skin heals, it leaves behind a corrugated scar tissue. Initially, the lesions are highly infective, but as the skin dries and hardens few to no *M. leprae* bacteria remain. The scar tissue gradually loses sensation making it possible for infected people to injure themselves because there is no sensation of pain. Often the combination of scar tissue and ulceration of the limbs and face produce a distinctive appearance that is readily apparent. This appearance may not, however, always be the product of leprosy as syphilis, diabetes, and even frostbite can produce the same disfiguring appearance. In addition, several noninfectious diseases such as pellagra, eczema, and psoriasis can produce secondary infections that can produce many of the same effects as leprosy such as a scaly skin.

A second form of leprosy, the polar opposite of lepromatous leprosy, is tuberculoid leprosy. It too starts with what appears to be a patchy skin infection, but the skin heals readily after the initial infection. New areas of infection appear and often lead to nerve damage in which affected areas are completely desensitized so it is possible for the affected area to be readily harmed. Tuberculoid leprosy often engenders a stronger immune response than lepromatous leprosy which helps to limit its impact and for this reason, it is often considered a milder form of the disease as symptoms are often less apparent. As is the case with any bipolar disease, some people exhibit symptoms that fall between the two poles although this mixed reaction is less common than the two definitive forms.

Leprosy is spread through respiratory discharge and coming in extensive contact with exposed skin of someone in the early stages of the disease although the means of transmission is still not fully understood. The disease is generally only mildly contagious although circumstances such as a compromised immune system can make it possible to acquire the disease more readily. Early symptoms of leprosy often appear three to five years after exposure although symptoms may appear sooner in some individuals. In the past, leprosy was thought to be highly infective so that any contact with someone who had the disease was seen as likely to lead to infection. In reality, it is rather difficult to transmit leprosy. Only people in the early stages of the disease with ulcerating skin are infective. The disfigured victims who are in the later stages of the disease are no longer infective. In addition to the skin lesions and desensitizing of extremities that may occur in some cases, a person suffering from leprosy has a compromised immune system that may lead them to fall victim to a variety of other diseases. It becomes a chronic, long-term medical problem that produces a good deal of pain in the early stages for its victims. Like tuberculosis, leprosy generally does not kill its victims immediately. Many people suffering from leprosy die from other causes including opportunistic infections.

Today leprosy is readily treatable with antibiotics but in the past, there was no treatment except palliative care. No longer present, save for a few isolated cases, in Europe and the United States, leprosy remains a health problem in some parts of the world, especially the tropics. Because the disease was thought to be highly infective in the past and because of the appearance of its victims, many lepers were segregated from society. Special hospitals for the care of victims of leprosy were established to provide palliative care and to remove them from society and continued to be a treatment option well into the twentieth century. Two famous examples are the leper colony of Kalaupapa on the Hawaiian island of Molokai which once had as many as 8000 residents and still is home to six sequestered patients and the leprosaria located in Carville, Louisiana that closed in 1999 although some of its residents continued to live there into the twenty-first century.

Leprosy is notable not just as a medical problem, but also in the way that society perceived its victims in the Middle Ages. It came to have a social stigma and some observers saw leprosy as divine punishment of evil-livers. As such, leprosy became the first of three diseases that carried a social stigma for its victims. Starting in the sixteenth century, syphilis sufferers also came to be stigmatized as "bad" people who were being punished for their sins. In the twentieth century, HIV/AIDS victims were stigmatized as "bad" people meriting their punishment, especially in the early stages of the AIDS epidemic in the 1980s. In all three cases, sexual misbehavior has been seen as the motivating force for the punishment of the victims of the three diseases.

One of the oldest human diseases, leprosy seems to have been present in the ancient Middle East. Some commentators have connected leprosy with the admonition in Leviticus to exclude the "unclean" from the camp of the Jews.[34] India was once thought to be the country of origin for leprosy, but recent work suggests possibly China or the region around Myanmar. Part of the problem in dealing with the origin of the disease is that various strains of leprosy have been transmitted and re-transmitted around the globe.[35] In the ancient world, many other skin diseases such as scabies might be diagnosed as leprosy so it is difficult to ascertain its impact. In the thirteenth century, Theodoric of Lucca warned that a skin rash on the nose and face, which he labeled *Gutta Rosea,* could be confused with the early stages of leprosy.[36] What was sometimes called elephantiasis, corresponds with the symptoms of leprosy as accounts from the third century B.C.E. indicate.[37] Writing in the sixteenth century, the Italian physician Fracastoro describes the confusion surrounding leprosy, confusion that led some contemporaries to confuse it with syphilis. As Fracastoro indicates, elephantiasis was true leprosy and the able physician should have been able to avoid confusing it with other diseases.[38] Evidence from medieval Danish cemeteries seems to bear out Fracastoro's conclusion that leprosy could be identified as cemeteries identified as leper cemeteries have skeletons exhibiting the sort of damage expected from lepromatous leprosy while other cemeteries do not contain skeletons with the same sort of damage.[39] As one modern commentator indicates, medieval medical men may have been overly reluctant to diagnose leprosy, leading to under-diagnoses of the disease.[40] Although it is difficult to determine how common leprosy was in the ancient world and the early Middle Ages, it reached epidemic proportions in medieval Europe, especially in the twelfth and thirteenth centuries. Skeletal evidence exists for the disease in England, Scandinavia, Hungary, Italy, and the Czech Republic.[41] Leprosy cases have been identified from the cemetery at Great Chesterton in England dating from 415–545 C.E.[42] Most of the skeletal evidence for the disease is from lepromatous leprosy. Although there is some debate concerning the origins of medieval leprosy, one explanation is that leprosy entered Europe from the Middle East during the late Greek or Roman era. Subsequent migrations helped to spread the disease throughout Europe and *M. leprae* strains from at least four distinct branches (three in one cemetery) have been discovered.[43] The leprosy epidemic seems to have peaked in the thirteenth century although the disease would continue to be common until the end of the fifteenth century. Carole Rawcliffe indicates that most of the 320 leper hospitals established in England between the eleventh and sixteenth centuries were established before the mid-fourteenth century.[44]

Even though leprosy might be difficult to identify in its early stages, later stages of lepromatous leprosy often produced an almost leonine appearance to the victim's face that could be identified easily. Both medical men and the clergy might participate in the diagnostic process. Some practitioners, such as Guy de Chaulaic, the fourteenth-century papal physician whose work was translated into English, provided an extensive list of symptoms. Guy indicated that the following signs should be present before a diagnosis of leprosy could be made: hardness of flesh, ulceration, a feeble pulse, and black blood. The last symptom was in accordance with Guy's application of humor theory as he indicated that leprosy disturbed the melancholy humor and then spread through the body.[45] John of Gaddesden's (a contemporary of Guy) list of symptoms was similar to Guy de Chaulaic's but he also addressed the mental state of a suspected leper: "He will be anxious and will avoid society, and will fancy that he is a leper. Such a mental state condition should be avoided, for imagination in one disposed to this disease very often actually brings it about."[46] Even if Gaddesden's equation of thinking leprosy equals leprosy is overstated, his addition of the consideration of the mental condition of the patient is perceptive and sympathetic given how many lepers were treated by society. Bernard of Gordon summed up the cause of leprosy as coming from an imbalance in the humors indicating that "melancholic matter spread through the whole body," leading to the onset of the disease.[47] Overall, the medical community was not always inclined to rush to judgment in diagnosing leprosy but to demand clear evidence that the disease was present in the victim and then to try to treat the disease based on accepted medical precepts. The greater involvement of medical men in the diagnosis of leprosy in the fourteenth century may have contributed to the seemingly lower number of cases in the late Middle Ages as they required a higher level of proof before they rendered a diagnosis than did many other people.

The humor theory accounted for leprosy within its own limitations although medical practitioners today would look to the presence of *M. leprae* not melancholy for an explanation of the onset of the disease. Medieval authors went beyond using humor theory to explain leprosy even though they might revert back to it. By the thirteenth century, contagion theory often came to be the means used to explain the onset and spread of leprosy. The understanding of the terms, contagion and infection by medieval authors, is not that of recent scholars, so care must be used in applying the term contagion. In one sense, some medieval authors were describing sin as contagious and so the sinner spread sin (and the resulting disease) by being in contact with others. Theodoric of Cyria may have accepted the idea of infection as he explained leprosy as a hereditary disease, "generated in a womb filled with unclean menses" that produced a corruption of bile, but his argument was thoroughly in the tradition of humor theory.[48] Lanfranc of Milan labeled the disease contagious implying that it could be spread easily.[49] Writing in the late fourteenth century Guy de Chauliac went farther and called leprosy "contagious and infectious" although he is not fully clear in how the disease spread implying physical contact but also the breath of the afflicted person.[50] There seems to be a blurring of infection and contagion as an explanation with both Lanfranc and Guy, a not uncommon occurrence.

Medieval medical writers indicated that the disease was curable once the humors had been brought back into balance. The usual sort of lists of baths, dietary remedies, drugs, and physical manipulation were all prescribed both to bring the humors into balance, remove leprosy from the system, and provide palliative care. Guy de Chaulaic advises medical men to comfort their leprous patients by indicating that the disease provided salvation for the soul.[51] Bartholomew Anglicus even indicated that he had a potion that when ingested would cure the afflicted person. Bartholomew's potion was not for the poor as it included gold as one of its ingredients.[52] During the early stages of the disease, physicians' cures might even appear to work as leprosy is subject to periods of remission. Leprosy generated a good deal of fear leading sufferers to seek out any sort of cure, often falling victim to the wiles of quacks. In September 1408, John of Clotes gave John Luter a leech (medical man of some sort, but most likely a quack) of London jewels worth nine marks, a sword worth 6s. 8d., and gold worth 60s for a cure that promised to be infallible, and when he was not cured, Clotes sued in the mayor's court for the return of his property. Luter argued that he provided a cure for another disease, not leprosy because he didn't think Clotes had leprosy. The mayor did not accept Luter's argument and ordered him to return Clotes' goods.[53]

As was the case with many other diseases in medieval England, people turned to the medicine of the saints for help, especially in the twelfth century. Thirty-six of St. Thomas Becket's 600 miracles were recorded as cures of leprosy. When examined closely, the validity of the cures becomes suspect at times. Walter, a knight, was reported cured at Becket's tomb in Canterbury Cathedral late in the twelfth century, but another cure, reported at the same time, indicates the victim was only partially cured.[54] In 1171, Radulf of Langton sought a cure for his leprosy at the tomb of St. Thomas. He applied some of St. Thomas's water (a reputed mixture of the martyr's blood and water) and called himself cured. Benedict of Peterborough, a compiler of the miracles, describes this cure but notes that a relapse occurred almost immediately, probably coming from Radulf's poor moral character.[55] Other sufferers turned to other saints and seven of the 44 miracles of the early twelfth century St. Osmund of Salisbury are reported as cures of leprosy.[56] The nature of leprosy in its early stages could lead to periods of remission, helping to confirm the validity of saintly cures.

If leprosy was diagnosable and curable within the confines of humor theory according to some medical writers, not everyone agreed. Many writers indicated that leprosy was, to use S.N. Brody's term, a disease of the soul caused by a morally deviant character. Often the sins were spiritual such as envy, wrath, or avarice, but as time passed lechery also came to be the sin that caused a person to be afflicted with leprosy. In such a case, the person should be treated with compassion to assuage their suffering but it was also clear that their poor moral character was contagious so that they needed to at least diminish their contact with society if not be excluded. This approach that saw individual moral failure as the causative factor developed over time and by the late Middle Ages was well in place. Margery Kempe, a housewife, mystic, and pilgrim from King's Lynn in the early fifteenth century was a person greatly concerned with obtaining salvation, which she sought by a life of almost continual pilgrimage. When her son developed symptoms of what appeared to be leprosy such as facial discoloration, pimples, and pustules, she connected these symptoms with what she considered to be his evil-living. After he reformed his conduct, Margery reported that the symptoms went away.[57] Whether Margery's son had leprosy with symptoms that went into remission or some other skin disease is a moot point; Margery made the connection of sin, leprosy, return to moral health, and return to physical health. Margery simply described her son as sinful. Writing at the turn of the fifteenth century, the poet Thomas Hoccleve was quite specific as to what sin led to the affliction of leprosy as he connected sexual misbehavior and leprosy. He indicated that a man who tried to commit incest with his sister-in-law immediately became "as foul a leper as might be."[58] Geoffrey Chaucer, too, seems to connect sin—in this case, anger—with the onset of leprosy in *The Pardoner's Tale*. The pardoner indicates that punishment for the sin should be left to God as the sinner/leper deserved public charity.[59] Thomas Gascoigne made a more telling connection of sin and leprosy with political implications in the early fifteenth century. King Henry IV had Richard Scrope, the Archbishop of York executed in 1405 after Scrope was convicted of treason for his leadership role in a northern rising against the crown. The night after the execution Henry awoke and yelled out "traitors, traitor, you are throwing fire on me," which Gascoigne inferred to be an admission of leprosy. Henry's health was poor for much of his reign, but leprosy was not the cause.[60] Gascoigne with relatives among the traitors of 1405 tried to blacken Henry's reputation with an accusation of something he considered so horrible as to point up Henry's moral guilt. All three of these episodes capture something of popular opinion regarding the relationship between leprosy and sin.

Gascoigne did not impute a carnal sin to Henry IV but Hoccleve saw lechery as leading to the punishment of leprosy. Some writers on the continent went further in this direction. The authors of work such as the *Gesta Romanorum* portrayed lepers as sexually active, often in illicit situations. This often led the non-leprous sexual partner in the illicit relationship to become infected with leprosy, which the author indicated as the just punishment for this sin.[61] Probably one of the more horrifying connections of the lust of lepers, sin, and leprosy can be found in the telling of the story of Tristan and Isolde. In Béroul's version (c 1160–1170), King Mark wants to punish Isolde by giving her to the lepers as a plaything when he finds out about her adultery with Tristan. The leader of the leper band indicates that this is a more fitting punishment than burning because:

> See, I have one-hundred companions; give Isolde to us, and she will be held in common. Never will a woman have a worse end. Sire, there is in us such great ardor that there is not a woman on earth who could endure our intercourse for one day.[62]

Béroul captures the ideas of leprosy as punishment for carnal sin and the reputed unbounded lechery of lepers in this passage. However, this view did not appear in medical writings and even secular English writers tended to not be this explicit. Medical men such as Guy de Chaulaic prohibited sex but not because the disease was sexually transmittable, but because lechery could lead the humors to become unbalanced, leading to disease.[63] Over time leprosy did become more connected with sin but the sin was not always carnal in nature.

Once a person began to exhibit symptoms of leprosy, a diagnosis could be made. Up until the thirteenth century, it was often a local jury that made the determination. Thereafter, a combination of clerics and medical men were often involved. Because many people believed that leprosy was highly contagious, one response to the disease was to try to isolate the afflicted person from the rest of society. Dating from the twelfth-century leprosaria, specialized hospitals for the care of lepers were opened. Already by the end of the eleventh century, charitable individuals were establishing leper hospitals. Eadmer, a Canterbury monk, described how Lanfranc, Archbishop of Canterbury in the eleventh century established a hospital to treat the indigent near Canterbury Cathedral, and

> in a more remote place to the north of the west gate of the city, he built wooden houses on the downward slope of a hill and assigned them for the use of lepers. To these no less he arranged the supply of all things which, because of the nature of their illness, they had to administer for themselves, assigning men of skill, kindness and patience to furnish the supplies.[64]

These institutions served the dual purpose of serving as a hospice, a place of refuge for lepers, and to exclude them from society. The position of the afflicted in these hospitals varied widely. Some were well treated, others were not. Some lepers had difficulty in leaving the facility while other leprosaria allowed their patients to leave. Not everyone who lived in a leper hospital may have a full-blown case of leprosy. The skeleton of a young man, aged eighteen to 25, exhumed from the cemetery of the leprosy hospital at St. Mary Magdalen in Winchester exhibits only minimal skeletal evidence of leprosy. Evidence indicates that he must have been someone of substance, who had visited the shrine of St. James at Compostela in Spain.[65] What is apparent from the comprehensive discussion provided by Rawcliffe is that the old stereotype of automatic and full exclusion of people diagnosed with leprosy is more an invention of the nineteenth and twentieth centuries than the Middle Ages. Nonetheless, some attempts at exclusion did occur as when Edward III ordered that lepers should be banished from the city of London in 1346, and in June 1372, City officials banished John Mayns, a baker from the city because of his leprosy.[66] One medieval relic of leper hospitals often pointed to as an example of the fear of contamination engendered by lepers, is the noisemaking clapper which is often described as means of warning people of the approach of a leper who carried it. François-Olivier Touati advances a different interpretation as he indicates it was used by lepers to attract attention for the begging necessary to support themselves.[67]

There appeared to be a hardening of opinion regarding leprosy in the fourteenth and fifteenth centuries, ironically just as the disease was becoming less prevalent. Late medieval leprosaria often tended to be more restrictive regarding their inhabitants than earlier ones had been. Late medieval determinations of leprosy were also more likely than earlier ones to result in efforts to exclude the leper from society or at least to restrict their movement. The views of physicians such as Guy de Chauliac who grounded a diagnosis of leprosy in humor theory now seemed to be in the minority in society as a whole. The sinful nature of the afflicted was more likely to be seen as the causative factor. How society viewed leprosy changed from the early onslaught of the disease through its peak in the thirteenth century to its decline in the fourteenth and fifteenth centuries. Because of the declining number of cases, society saw leprosy as less of a problem by the fifteenth century. The number of cases declined dramatically and already in the fifteenth-century leprosaria were being converted into regular hospitals or hostels for pilgrims. The trajectory of leprosy as almost an epidemic disease, albeit a chronic one, to one with little impact is difficult to explain.

The rise of leprosy can perhaps be explained as emanating from the not always good hygiene standards, poor diet, and the sometimes weak immune systems of people in the early and high Middle Ages. There did not seem to be a change in the genetic makeup of the disease during the Middle Ages so as to explain its prevalence.[68] Several different strains of leprosy-affected Europe and England, but they were often present at the same time. Climate change does not appear to affect the incidence of leprosy either. Today, the disease is primarily a tropical disease, but as late as the nineteenth century, there were numerous cases in Scandinavia.

The decline of leprosy as a public health problem starting in the fourteenth century is difficult to explain. Genetics and climate change do not seem to have played a role. The increasing urbanization of Europe dating from the late thirteenth century may have played a role, but was more likely to have been a factor in Italy than England which was slower to urbanize. Urbanization may have played a role because of the relationship between *M. leprae* and *M. tuberculosis*. Both leprosy and tuberculosis are part of the *Mycobacterium* family and it seems that infection with one could confer some immunity against the other. Tuberculosis had been a medical problem in urban Rome, but the towns of the early Middle Ages were not large enough to sustain a tuberculosis epidemic. The return of urban growth in the late Middle Ages may have led to an increased onset of tuberculosis which could have crowded out leprosy.[69]

Another disease may also have played a role in the decline of leprosy. Once infected with an active case of leprosy, the person has a weakened immune system thereafter. A variety of diseases could take advantage of weakened immune systems, but this situation existed throughout the Middle Ages. Starting in the mid-fourteenth century plague epidemics had a large impact on European society. Plague can kill even people with strong immune systems, but for those with compromised immune systems, such as lepers, it would be particularly deadly. Even lepers who were not fully symptomatic so as to be diagnosed with leprosy already had a weakened immune system that could cause them to fall victim to the plague. It is impossible to determine just how much the plague epidemics that struck England from 1348 onward affected the leprous population. A safe assumption would be that lepers were more likely to die than other people. The only reservoir for leprosy is the human population and lepromatous leprosy is slightly infective so that the removal of potential hosts who could transmit the disease would decrease the onset of the disease. As diagnosed lepers died there was also less of a need for facilities to treat them.

Another plausible explanation for the decline of leprosy in the Late Middle Ages is a combination of tuberculosis and plague in addition to increased urbanization and the resulting crowding that made it easy to transmit tuberculosis and the plague. In addition, the large number of deaths from plague likely reduced the number of caregivers for lepers. One factor that does not seem to have been at work was a change in the genetic makeup of leprosy. As leprosy came to be less of a medical problem, it became a moral problem and a prototype of how the victim's moral failings explained the onset of the disease and how the person should be treated.

Everyday disease and the disease burden of premodern England

The commonplace ailments as well as the four diseases discussed in this chapter had an impact on the lives of people in medieval England as well as influencing the outlook of people and economic life. Wounds, diarrhea, and fevers claimed lives every year helping to limit population growth. Although impossible to quantify, everyday health problems shaped attitudes and helped maintain a high mortality rate.

The impact of malaria, measles, tuberculosis, and leprosy varied by region and by age. Malaria was a regional disease primarily found in marshy areas of south-eastern England while the other three could be found throughout the country. It killed children, shortened the life span of adults, and weakened many of its sufferers. Measles was usually a disease of childhood, but one that contributed significantly to a high child mortality rate. Tuberculosis was undoubtedly present through the Middle Ages but did not appear to have been not a major health problem because of the necessity for a large population to sustain an ongoing outbreak, but that changed with the growth of towns from the sixteenth century onward. When it struck, it could kill although often slowly and painfully. Leprosy's impact increased up through the thirteenth century. Thereafter the number of leprosy cases declined, but its impact on society remained high because of the fear and moral stigma surrounding the disease. Tuberculosis and malaria sufferers today might be considered as somewhat social outcasts or at least lazy for those people who suffer from repeated malaria infections although that would have been less likely in the Middle Ages. All diseases were seen at times as divine punishment for overall human frailty in the Middle Ages. Many observers came to see leprosy as a disease that came from the moral failings of its victims. Not everyone displayed this perspective and some observers indicated that leprosy provided an opportunity for redemption and sanctification.[70] Some writers noted that Christ washed the feet of lepers and St. Elizabeth of Hungary provided care for lepers in the thirteenth century and in twelfth-century England, Matilda, the queen of Henry I also washed the feet of lepers as well as kissed their hands.[71] As the discussion of the impact of syphilis in Chapter 8 indicates, the moral approach to leprosy became the prototype for the treatment of later victims of diseases that came to be associated with moral failings.

Tuberculosis, leprosy, and malaria had a health impact that went beyond the immediate consequences of the disease. They led to a compromised immune system that made it easier for the victim to become infected with another disease such as pneumonia. Tuberculosis and leprosy sufferers were more likely to die from some other opportunistic infection than from tuberculosis or leprosy. Measles victims who survived the disease in childhood had lifetime immunity to the disease and suffered no lasting impact on their immune system but many children who contracted the disease might die from it or another opportunistic infection while infected by measles. Leprosy and tuberculosis victims often suffered from ongoing weakness that limited their productivity as did malaria victims who lived in an area where continual infection was likely. Today, some observers might call the victims of diseases such as malaria, tuberculosis, and leprosy disabled as they cannot always perform all the tasks that society might expect of them. Medieval people had a concept of the impaired body, but disease victims did not seem to fit the definition.[72] As the discussion of malaria, measles, leprosy, and tuberculosis and everyday health concern indicates, the diseases affecting people in the Middle Ages cannot be treated in isolation. An inter-relationship of various diseases existed which often led to a synergy that produced high death rates especially among children and the elderly. When the impact of these four diseases is examined, our understanding of the medical, social, and economic impact of disease in premodern England is enhanced.

Notes

1 Matthieu Le Bailly and Françoise Bouchet endeavor to trace the early impact of the *Entamoeba histolytica* parasite. "A First Attempt to Retrace the History of Dysentery Caused by *Entamoeba histolytica*," in Piers D. Mitchell, ed., *Sanitation, Latrines and intestinal Parasites in Past Populations* (Farnham: Ashgate, 2015), 219–28.
2 Christopher Allmand is careful to indicate that the cause of Henry's death is unknown but the symptoms he describes as well as contemporary indications suggest that Henry suffered from the flux, lead to the conclusion that dysentery was responsible for the King's death. *Henry V* (Berkeley: University of California Press, 1992), 173.
3 G.A. King and C.Y. Henderson, "Living Cheek by Jowl: The Pathoecology of Medieval York," *Quaternary International*, 341 (2014), 131–42.
4 Piers D. Mitchell, "Human Parasites in Medieval Europe: Lifestyle, Sanitation and Medical Treatments," in *Advances in Parasitology*, 90 (2015), 398–401. Susanna Sabin, Hui-Yuan Yeh, Aleks Pluskowski, Rhrista Clamer, Piers D. Mitchell, Kristen I. Bos, "Estimating Molecular Preservation of the Intestinal Microbiome via Metagenomic Analysis of Latrine Sediments from Two Medieval Cities," *Philosophical Transactions of the Royal Society, B*, 375 (2020), 1812.
5 R.L. Gowland and A.G. Western, "Morbidity in the Marshes: Using Spatial Epidemiology to Investigate Skeletal Evidence for Malaria in Anglo-Saxon England (AD 410–1050)," *American Journal of Physical Anthropology*, 147 (2012), 301–11. Robert Sallares, *Malaria and Rome* (Oxford: Oxford University Press, 2002), 156.
6 Timothy P. Newfield, "Malaria and Malaria-Like Disease in the Early Middle Ages," *Early Medieval Europe*, 25 (2017), 251–300.
7 M.L. Cameron, *Anglo-Saxon Medicine* (Cambridge: Cambridge University Press, 1993), 3, 182. Gowland and Western, "Morbidity in the Marshes," 311.
8 Paul Reiter, "From Shakespeare to Defoe: Malaria in England in the Little Ice Age," *Emerging Infectious Diseases*, 6 (2000), 1–11. Mary J. Dobson, "Malaria in England: A Geographical and Historical Perspective," *Parassitologia*, 36 (1994), 35–60. Dobson, *Contours of Death and Disease in Early Modern England* (Cambridge: Cambridge University Press, 1997).
9 Dobson, *Contours of Death*, 297
10 Dobson, *Contours of Death*, 326–34.
11 Yuki Furuse, Akira Suziki, Hitoshi Oshitani, "Origins of Measles Virus: Divergence from Rinderpest Virus between the 11th and 12th centuries," *Virology Journal* 7 (2010): 52. This argument is amplified by Jennifer Manley who takes historical context into account. "Measles and Ancient Plagues: A Note on New Scientific Evidence," *Classical World* 107 (2013): 393–7.
12 Fiona M. Guerra, Shelly Bolotin, Gilliam Lim, Jane Heffernan, et al., "The Basic Reproductive Number (R_0) of Measles: A Systematic Review," *Lancet Infectious Diseases*, 12 (2017), e420–e428.
13 Robert T. Perry and Neal A. Halsey, "The Clinical Significance of Measles: A Review," *Journal of Infectious Diseases*, 189 (2004), 4–16.
14 G. Dennis Shanks, Seung-EunLee, Alan Howard, and John F. Brundage, "Extreme Mortality after the first Introduction of Measles Virus to the Polynesian Island of Rotuma, 1911," *American Journal of Epidemiology*, 173 (2011), 1211–1222.

15 Peter Aaby, "Malnutrition and Overcrowding/Intensive Exposure in Severe Measles Infection: Review of Community Studies," *Reviews of Infectious Diseases*, 10 (1988), 478–91. Peter Aaby, Jette Bukh, Ida Maria Lisse, and Arjon J. Smits, "Overcrowding and Intensive Exposure as Determinants of Measles Mortality," *American Journal of Epidemiology*, 120 (1984), 49–63.

16 A good summary of tuberculosis in the ancient Greece can be found in Mirko D. Grmek, *Diseases in the Ancient Greek World* (Baltimore: Johns Hopkins University Press, 1989), 177–97. Tuberculosis DNA has been found in Neolithic bone fragments in a submerged village off the coast of Israel and in calcified tissue from 1400 years ago in the remains of a Byzantine temple in the Negev desert. Israel Hershkovitz, Helen M. Donoghue, David E. Minnikin, Gurdyal S. Besra, et al., "Detection and Molecular Characteristics of 9000-Year-Old *Mycobacterium tuberculosis* from a Neolithic Settlement in the Eastern Mediterranean, *PLoS One*, 3 (2008), e3426. H.D. Donoghue, M. Spigelman, J. Zias, A.M. Gernaey-Child, and D.E. Minnikin, "*Mycobacterium tuberculosis* complex DNA in Calcified Pleura from Remains 1400 Years Old," *Letters in Applied Microbiology*, 27 (1998), 265–9.

17 Y. Ma, C.R. Horsburgh, Laura F. White, and Helen E. Jenkins, "Quantifying TB Transmission: A Systematic Review of Reproduction Number and Serial Interval Estimates for Tuberculosis," *Epidemiology and Infection*, 146 (2018), 1478–94.

18 John Graunt, *Natural and Political Observations Made Upon the Bills of Mortality* (London: Gregg International Publishers, 1973, 1662), 9. H.D. Chalke, "The Impact of Tuberculosis on History, Literature and Art," *Medical History*, 6 (1962), 305.

19 Aidan Cockburn, *The Evolution and Eradication of Infectious Disease* (Baltimore: Johns Hopkins University Press, 1963). R. Brosch, S.V. Gordon, M. Marmiesse, et al., "A New Evolutionary Scenario for the *Mycobacterium tuberculosis* Complex," *PNAS*, 99 (2002), 3684–9. A.R. Zink, E. Molnár, N. Motamedi, et al., "Molecular History of Tuberculosis from Ancient Mummies and Skeletons," *International Journal of Osteoarchaeology*, 17 (2007), 380–91. B.M. Rothschild, L.D. Martin, G. Lev, et al., "*Mycobacterium tuberculosis* Complex DNA from an Extinct Bison Dated 17,000 Years before the Present," *Clinical Infectious Diseases*, 33 (2001), 305–11. Anne C. Stone, Alicia K. Wilbur, Jane E. Buikstra, and Charlotte A. Roberts, "Tuberculosis and Leprosy in Perspective," *Yearbook of Physical Anthropology*, 52 (2009), 66–94.

20 A helpful discussion of symptoms can be found in Ethne Barnes, *Diseases and Human Evolution* (Albuquerque: University of New Mexico Press, 2005), 157–72.

21 The wide-ranging paleopathological discussion in Charlotte A. Roberts and Jane E. Buikstra, *The Bioarchaeology of Tuberculosis* (Tallahassee: University of Florida Press, 2003) provides examples from numerous locales throughout Roman and medieval Europe.

22 Roberts and Buikstra, *Bioarchaeology of Tuberculosis*, 85–86.

23 Roberts and Buikstra, *Bioarchaeology of Tuberculosis*, 45–50.

24 M.C. Seymour, ed., *On the Properties of Things: John Trevisa's Translation of Bartholomaeus Anglicus De propietatibus rerurm*, 2 vols. (Oxford: Clarendon Press, 1975), 2: 375. In his description of *phthis*, the fourteenth century layman John de Mirfield also adopted the term consumption to describe the progression of the disease. Percival Horton-Smith and Harold Richard Aldridge, eds. and trans., *Johannes de Mirfield of St. Bartholomew's, Smithfield: His Life and Works* (Cambridge: Cambridge University Press, 1936), 75–89.

25 Theodoric of Lucca, *The Surgery of Theodoric*, Eldridge Campbell and James Colton, trans., 2 vols. (New York: Appleton-Century Crofts, 1955–60), 2: 8–87.

26 Faye Marie Getz, ed. *Healing and Society in Medieval England: A Middle English Translation of the Pharmaceutical Writings of Gilbertus Anglicus* (Madison: University of Wisconsin Press, 1991), 134–41.

27 Fracastoro, *Contagion*, 250–57.

28 Paul Grosjean, ed., *Henrici VI Angliae regis miracula postuma*. (Brussels: Bollandist Society, 1935), 169–71.

29 Frank Barlow, ed. and trans., *The Life of King Edward the Confessor* (London: Nelson's Medieval Texts, 1962), 61–2.

30 Marc Bloch, *The Royal Touch*, J.E. Anderson, trans. (Montreal: McGill-Queens University Press, 1973, 1924). For England, Frank Barlow's "The King's Evil," c. 3 in Frank Barlow, *The Norman Conquest and Beyond* (London: Hambledon Press, 1983) has replaced Bloch as the authoritative treatment for England.

31 Roberts and Buikstra, *Bioarchaeology of Tuberculosis*, 132–61; several of the chapters in György Pàlfi, Olivier Dutour, Judith Deàk, Imre Haas, eds., *Tuberculosis Past and Present* (Budapest: Golden Book Publishers, Ltd., Tuberculosis Foundation, 1999) deal with the paleopathology of tuberculosis in countries such as France, Lithuania, Germany and essentially all of western Europe in the Middle Ages.

32 The connection of leprosy with sin and exclusion in the Middle Ages is stated most strongly by R.I. Moore as part of a construct that he labels the persecuting society in *Formation of a Persecuting Society: Authority and Deviance in Western Europe 950–1250*, 2d ed. (New York: Wiley-Blackwell, 2007). Jeffrey Richards also makes a strong connection of marginalization and leprosy in *Sex, Dissidence and Damnation* (London: Routledge, 1991), c. 8. Moore's and Richards' accounts need to be read in connection with the more nuanced works of Carole Rawcliffe, *Leprosy in Medieval England* (Woodbridge: Boydell Press, 2006) and Luke Demaitre, *Leprosy in Premodern Medicine* (Baltimore: Johns Hopkins University Press, 2007).

33 Rawcliffe, *Leprosy in Medieval England*, 13–43.

34 *Leviticus* 13–14. In *Numbers* 12, leprosy was connected with the sins of envy and pride and led to the exile of Miriam for her sins of trying to usurp the social positions of a man and of a prophet (in this case Moses). The question of how the ancient Hebrews viewed uncleanness is a fraught one. A good introduction is Elinor Lieber, "Old Testament 'Leprosy', Contagion and Sin," in Lawrence I. Conrad and Dominik Wujastyk, eds., *Contagion: Perspectives from Pre-Modern Societies* (Aldershot: Ashgate, 2000), 99–136.

35 Samuel Mark, "The Origin and Spread of Leprosy: Historical, Skeletal, and Molecular Data," *Journal of Interdisciplinary History*, 49 (2019): 367–95.

36 Theodoric of Lucca, *The Surgery of Theodoric*, 2:153–56.

37 An excellent introduction to leprosy and its diagnosis in the ancient Greek world is Mirko D. Grmek, *Diseases in the Ancient Greek World*, Mireille Muellner and Leonard Muellner, trans. (Baltimore: Johns Hopkins University Press, 1989), 152–76.

38 Fracastoro, *Contagion*, 158–69. His treatment involved means directed toward returning the humours to balance (294–9) and nowhere does he argue that the sinful nature of the victim was responsible for the disease.

39 Vilhelm Møller-Christensen, "Evidence of Leprosy in Earlier Peoples," in Don Brothwell and A.T. Sandison, eds., *Diseases in Antiquity* (Springfield, ILL: Charles C. Thomas, 1967), 295–306.

40 Stephen R. Ell, "Plague and Leprosy in the Middle Ages: A Paradoxical Cross Immunity," *International Journal of Leprosy and Other Mycobacterial Diseases*, 2 (1987), 345–50.

41 Verena J. Schuenemann, Charlotte Avanzi, Ben Krause-Kyora, et al., "Ancient Genomes Reveal a High Diversity of *Mycobacterium leprae* in Medieval Europe," *PLoS Pathogens* 14 (2018). Tom A. Mendum, Verena J. Schuenemann, Simon Roffey, et al., "*Mycobacterium leprae* Genomes from a British Medieval Leprosy Hospital: Towards understanding an Ancient Epidemic," *BMC Genmoics*, 15 (2014), 270. V. Mariotti, O. Dutour, M.G. Belcastro, et al, "Probable Early Presence of Leprosy in Europe in a Celtic Skelton of the 4th–3rd century B.C. (Casalecchio di Reno, Bologna, Italy)," *International Journal of Osteoarchaeology*, 15 (2005), 311–25. M. Belcasto, V. Mariotti, F. Facchini, O. Dutour, "Leprosy in a Skelton from the 7th Century Necropois of Vicenne-Campochiaro (Molise, Italy)," *International Journal of Osteoarchaeology*, 15 (2005), 431–48.

42 S.A. Inskip, G.M. Taylor, S.R. Zakrewski, et al., "Osteological Biomolecular and Geochemical Examination of an Early Anglo-Saxon Case of Lepromatous Leprosy," *PLoS One*, 10 (2015).

43 Helen D. Donoghue, G. Michael Taylor, Antónia Marcsik, Erica Molnár et al., "A Migration-Driven Model for the history Spread of Leprosy in Medieval Eastern and Central Europe," *Infection, Genetics and Evolution*, 31 (2015), 250–56; Shueneman, "Ancient Genomes Reveal a High Diversity of *Mycobacterium leprae*."

44 Rawcliffe, *Leprosy*, 106–07. The standard treatment of medieval English hospitals is Nicholas Orme and Margaret Webster, *The English Hospital 1070–1570* (New Haven: Yale University Press, 1995). Rawcliffe focuses on England. For a discussion of leprosy on the continent Luke Demaitre's *Leprosy in Premodern Medicine* compliments Rawcliffe's. Two older accounts also have merit although some of their views are dated and need to be treated with care in light of recent scholarship. S.N. Brody, *The Disease of the Soul* (Ithaca: Cornell University Press, 1974) focuses on the treatment of leprosy in literature. Peter Richards, *The Medieval Leper and His Northern Heirs* (New York: Barnes and Noble Books, 1977) devotes a good deal of attention to leprosy in Scandinavia in the Middle Ages and later.

45 Margaret S. Ogden, ed., *The Cyrurgie of Guy de Chaulaic* (EETS, 265, 1971), 381, 378–9. The thirteenth century physician Lanfranc of Milan also connected leprosy to melancholy although in less convincing fashion than Guy. R. von Fleischhaker, ed., *Lanfrank's Science of Cirurgie* (EETS, O.S., 102, 1894), 196.

46 H.P. Cholmeley, *John of Gaddesden and the Rosa Medicinae* (Oxford: Clarendon Press, 1912), 45–6.

47 Quoted in Luke Demaitre, *Leprosy in Premodern Medicine*, 110. Demaitre provides a useful listing of diagnoses from several medieval commentators (112–13).

48 Theodoric of Lucca, *The Surgery of Theodoric*, 2: 167. Theodoric went on to say that the disease could be passed on by coitus with someone in a leprous condition as it might infect a fetus, even if not the mother (167).

49 Fleishhaker, *Lanfranck's Science of Surgery*, 196. The standard treatment of the development of contagion theory is a trilogy of essays by Vivian Nutton: "Did the Greeks Have a Word for It? Contagion and Contagion Theory in Classical Antiquity," in Conrad and Wujastyk, eds., *Contagion*, 137–62. "The Seeds of Disease: An Explanation of Contagion Theory and Infection from the Greeks to the Renaissance," *Medical History*, 37 (1987), 1–34. With a focus on the sixteenth century medical man, Girolomo Fracastoro in "The Reception of Fracastoro's Theory of Contagion: The Seed that Fell Among Thorns," *Osiris*, 2d ser., 6 (1990), 196–234. Also see: François-Olivier Touati, "Contagion and Leprosy: Myth, Ideas and Evolution in Medieval Minds and Societies," in Conrad and Wujastyk, eds., *Contagion*, 179–201.

50 Ogden, *Churgie of Guy de Chaulaic*, 381.

51 Ogden, *Churgie of Guy de Chaulaic*, 381.

52 Seymour, *On the Properties of Things*, 2: 829.

53 A.H. Thomas, ed., *Calendar of Select Pleas and Memoranda of the City of London, 1381–1412.* (Cambridge: Cambridge University press, 1932), 289.

54 Benedict of Peterborough, *Materials for the History of Thomas Becket*, J.C. Robertson, ed., 7 vols. (Rolls Series, 67, 1875–85), 2: 203.

55 Benedict of Peterborough, 2, 183–84.

56 St. Osmund's miracles are recorded in A.R. Maldon, ed., *The Canonization of Saint Osmund* (Salisbury: Wiltshire Record Society, 1901), 54–90.

57 Barry Windeatt, trans., *The Book of Margery Kempe* (London: Penguin Books, 1985), 266.

58 F.J. Furnivall, ed., *Hoccleve's Works: The Minor Poems* (London: EETS, extra ser., 61, 1892), 164.

59 Geoffrey Chaucer, "The Pardoner's Tale," in *The Complete Poetry and Prose of Geoffrey Chaucer*, John H. Fisher, ed., 2d ed (New York: Harcourt Brace College Publishers, 1989), 221–31.

60 Thomas Gascoigne, *Loci e libro veritatum*, J.H. Thorold Rogers, ed. (Oxford: Oxford University Press, 1881), 228. Peter McNiven provides a discussion of Henry IV's health that indicates that leprosy was not a factor in the king's poor health. "The Problem of Henry IV's Health, 1405–1413," *English Historical Review* 100 (1985), 747–72.

61 Brody provides a discussion of leprosy's appearance in various literary works in *Disease of the Soul*, 143–97. Stephen R. Ell examines the sexual content of medieval writers on leprosy finding that they believed the route of transmission for the disease was venereal. "Blood and Sexuality in Medieval Leprosy," *Janus*, 71 (1985), 153–64.

62 *The Romance of Tristran by Beroul: A Poem of the Twelfth Century*, A. Ewert, ed. (Oxford: Oxford University Press, 1939), lines 1192–1197.

63 Guy de Chaulaic, *Cyrurgie of Guy de Chaulaic*, 385.

64 Eadmer, *Historia Novorum in Anglia*, Martin Rule, ed. (Rolls Series, 81, 1884), 16.

65 The skeleton dates from the late 11th to early 12th century. While the skeletal evidence for leprosy was confined to his legs and feet, molecular testing indicates a strong *M. leprae* infection. Simon Roffey, Kate Tucker, Kori Filpeck-Ogden, et al., "Investigation of a Medieval Pilgrim Burial Excavated from the *Leprosarium* of St. Mary Magdalen Winchester, UK," *PLoS Neglected Tropical Diseases*, 11 (2017).

66 Riley, *Memorials of London*, 230–31, 365–66. In August 1375, the porters of the several London gates swore oaths that they would not admit lepers to the city and that they would detain any suspected lepers (384).

67 Touati, "Contagion and Leprosy," 185.

68 Verena J. Schuenemann, Pushpendra Singh, Thomas A. Mendum, et al., "Genome-Wide Comparison of Medieval and Modern *Mycobacterium leprae*," *Science,* 341 (2013), 179–83. Tom A. Mendum, Verena J. Schuenemann, Simon Roffery, et al., "*Mycobacterium leprae* genomes from a British Medieval Hospital: Towards Understanding an Ancient Epidemic," *BMC Genomics* 15 (2014), 270.

69 Tom Lietman, Travis Porco, and Sally Blower, "Leprosy and Tuberculosis: The Epidemiological Consequences of Cross-Immunity," *American Journal of Public Health,* 87 (1997), 1923–27. Helen D. Donoghue, Antónia Marcsik, Carney Matheson, Kim Vernon et al., "Co-Infection of *Mycobacterium tuberculosis* and *Mycobacterium leprae* in Human Archaeological Samples: A Possible Explanation for the Historical Decline of Leprosy," *Proceedings of the Royal Society B.*, 272 (2005), 389–94. Anne C. Stone, Alicia Wilbur, Jane E. Buikstra, and Charlotte A. Roberts, "Tuberculosis and Leprosy in Perspective," *Yearbook of Physical Anthropology* 52 (2009), 66–94.

70 Touati makes this point with his argument for the need to avoid over-generalization in dealing with medieval leprosy. "Contagion and Leprosy," 198–200.

71 Matthew Paris, *Chronica Majora*, H.R. Luard, ed., 7 vols. (Rolls Series, 57, 1872–83), 2: 130.

72 A good introduction to concepts of physical impairment in the Middle Ages is Irina Metzler, *Disability in Medieval Europe* (London: Routledge, 2006). A treatment of leprosy, tuberculosis, and malaria that questions whether victims of these diseases were considered disabled is John Theilmann, "Disease or Disability? The Conceptual Relationship in Medieval and Early Modern England," in Wendy J. Turner and Tory Vandeventer Pearman, eds., *The Treatment of Disabled Persons in Medieval Europe* (Lewiston: Edward Mellon Press, 2010), 197–229.

4

EPIDEMIC DISEASE AND ITS ARRIVAL IN ENGLAND

Outbreaks of infectious diseases have threatened human populations in the past, but the growth in the size of populations and their concentrations in towns helped to bring about larger outbreaks of disease that posed major health threats. Starting in the Neolithic Age, human population began to increase in size and people began to settle in first villages, then towns, and then cities leading to the first epidemiologic transition.[1] New diseases began to affect human populations as various contagious and vector-borne diseases either evolved from animal hosts to infect humans or a vector, such as flea or mosquito, evolved to enable the infection of humans. The growth of urban populations facilitated epidemics in which a large number of people in a region were infected. Increased human interaction across borders led to pandemics in which diseases affected several countries encompassing a wide area.

Infectious diseases undoubtedly affected the human population during the Bronze Age, but we have little record of the epidemics they produced.[2] Four ancient and early medieval epidemics stand out as the prototypes of epidemics and pandemics to come. The Plague of Athens (430–426 BCE), the Antonine Plague (166–279 CE), the Plague of Cyprian (249–260 CE), and the Plague of Justinian (late sixth century – eighth century) all resulted in large numbers of deaths, had major effects on society, and involved infectious diseases that affected European, and ultimately world, society.[3] Some commentators refer to the Plague of Justinian as the First Plague Pandemic, connecting it to the Second Plague Pandemic (mid-fourteenth century to eighteenth century, and the Third Plague Pandemic, dating from the nineteenth century).[4] The first three epidemics did not appear to have affected England, but from the Plague of Justinian onward, England became part of a larger disease universe.

Population in England grew intermittently for much of the period from the fall of Rome until the High Middle Ages with a steady growth from the twelfth

DOI: 10.4324/9781003215219-5

century onward. The threat of infectious disease always loomed on the horizon though because, without proper medical care based on sound medical knowledge, infectious disease could play havoc with society. One partial public health advantage enjoyed by people in medieval England was the low population density. With few towns that could even pretend to be urban centers, many infectious diseases had a difficult time maintaining themselves and creating epidemics even when they appeared in England.

Some infectious diseases have a long history in Western culture. Zoonotic diseases jumped species from the original animal host and began to infect humans at various points in the past (and are still doing so today, e.g., HIV). For some infectious diseases, it is difficult to trace their origin because so little is known about the disease and how it infects people as is the case for some hemorrhagic fevers such as Ebola. An infectious disease, particularly one that spreads by human contact and that quickly kills its hosts, has little chance of spreading in areas with low population density especially in a society in which far-ranging travel is limited. When an infected population recovers or dies, there are no more susceptibles and an outbreak ends. A disease that has a long incubation period or a long term of illness in which it is also infectious is likely to be more "successful" in infecting many new hosts and continuing to spread the disease.

Infectious diseases played an important but limited role in the ancient world as everyday health problems often were the major health threat. A few infectious disease outbreaks, however, turned into epidemics. There are several potential explanations for this situation, but lack of evidence makes it difficult to assign a certain explanation. Once outside cities such as Athens, Rome, or Alexandria, it was difficult to sustain an epidemic of most infectious diseases in the late Roman world. Another factor, discussed in Chapter 1, has to do with the evolution of disease microbes. Some microbes such as the smallpox virus seem to have been harmful to humans for a long time. Others have evolved to become harmful or have jumped from one species to another and in doing so have become harmful to human beings. Microbial evolution coupled with environmental factors, population growth, and societal organization all contributed to increasing the human disease burden over time.

The first epidemics

In 430 B.C.E., an epidemic struck Athens, continuing for the next three years. It couldn't have come at worse time as Athens was engaged in a war with Sparta. In efforts to escape the war, many people fled the Athenian countryside for the city and its immediate region causing the population of Athens and its adjoining port city of Piraeus to increase to around 400,000 people. The contemporary historian Thucydides, who was struck by the disease but survived, provides a helpful discussion of the symptoms of the disease as well as its impact on Athenian society. Often referred to as the Plague of Athens, the disease was not the plague. People often used the term plague in the past as a generic term to describe a large and deadly pestilence. Most analyses of the disease that infected Athens conclude that it was smallpox, typhus, or measles.[5] One group of researchers using DNA evidence indicates that typhoid fever was the cause of the Plague of Athens, but typhoid fever exhibits few of the symptoms described by Thucydides and it was endemic in ancient Greece and is likely to be found in the dental pulp of many skeletons.[6] Although it is difficult to come by accurate numbers, it seems that between twenty-five and thirty-five percent of the Athenian population perished during the epidemic. Robert Sallares suggests that pregnant women had a particularly high mortality rate contributing to an even more pronounced population downturn over the next few years.[7]

The high mortality rate of the Plague of Athens came from two factors. First, the disease seems to have been a virgin soil epidemic, in that is the population had no previous exposure to the disease and thus little or no innate immunity. Second, the crowded condition of the Athenian population made it easy for a contagious disease to spread readily. Once the disease spread outside the city, it was difficult to maintain the number of contacts necessary for the continuation of the epidemic. Other Greek cities were lucky that the disease did not reach their borders nor did it appear to have infected the besieging Spartan army. Such a situation is indicative of a contagious disease that spread from person to person rather than a vector-borne disease such as one spread by fleas or other parasites.

Smallpox appears to be the most likely culprit for the Plague of Athens. The disease moved so quickly through the Athenian population that it is likely that it spread by airborne or human-to-human contact rather than through an intermediate vector such as a flea or louse. Typhus is spread by lice and so it can likely be ruled out even though many of its symptoms were those described by Thucydides. Bubonic plague is a vector-borne disease spread by fleas making it unlikely given the narrow concentration of the disease within the Athenian city walls and Thucydides describes no buboes, a characteristic of the disease, so it too can be ruled out. Measles is considered relatively harmless today, but it has been a major killer in the past especially when it was a virgin soil epidemic as was the case with the native population of the Americas in the sixteenth and seventeenth centuries and the Fiji Islands in the nineteenth century. However, Thucydides nowhere mentions a rash (the telltale sign of measles) in his description. Moreover, molecular clock analysis now indicates that measles did not evolve from rinderpest (a disease of cattle) until the eleventh or twelfth centuries.[8] Archaeological evidence indicates that smallpox was present in the ancient world and that it had the potential to kill large numbers of people in the right circumstances. A virgin soil epidemic of smallpox would be unusually virulent, a reason why smallpox is considered to be a major threat for bioterrorism today. There seems to be no evidence of smallpox in Athens and possibly even Greece for at least some time before 530 so an outbreak of a contagious disease such as smallpox in densely populated Athens would have wreaked havoc with the city. Smallpox is survivable so that once enough people had been infected and either died or survived with resulting immunity to the disease, it would have burned out unless a continuing outside source of infection had existed.

Thereafter, epidemic disease became a way of life for people in Greece and Rome. The Roman historian Livy reports epidemics in Rome and elsewhere on a nearly eight-year cycle between 490 and 292 B.C.E., a cycle that was reduced to approximately five years for the period from 212 and 165 B.C.E.[9] Thereafter reports of epidemics decline, perhaps suspiciously so as no epidemics are reported from 21 B.C.E. to C.E. 64. Although it is difficult to draw much detail from these accounts, it seems that epidemic disease was a way of life for the Roman and Greek world.

The next major epidemic, the Plague of the Antonines, started in the East among Roman troops in Parthia in 165 C.E. and spread westward to Rome itself by 166, lasting for at least fifteen years. This disease seems to have killed as much as ten percent of the Roman population with army camps and urban areas hard hit. Galen, the great Greco-Roman physician, lived through the epidemic, leaving Rome as the first outbreak of the disease occurred for his home in Pergamum in Greece and left a partial clinical description of the symptoms of the disease and its progression.[10] Although referred to as a plague, this epidemic seems to once again have been largely smallpox in origin. This epidemic had a major impact on all sectors of the economy throughout the Roman Empire although there is no mention of it in Roman Gaul or Britain.[11]

Epidemic disease was a way of life for the urbanized parts of the Roman Empire bordering the Mediterranean in the late Antique world. Many outbreaks of disease were small epidemics that encompassed a town or region but reports of these have generally not come down to us. One epidemic of some note is the Plague of Cyprian that lasted from about 249 to 260 C.E. and spread from Egypt to Rome. Because it spread across the Mediterranean region, it might be labeled a pandemic. Bishop Cyprian of Carthage along with Dionysius of Alexandria provides the best descriptions of the disease although they do not match the detail of Thucydides' description of the Plague of Athens. Based on its symptoms, it seems not to have been smallpox. One diagnosis, based on symptoms and timing has been influenza although there have been no other late antique epidemics identified as influenza which seems to have made its first appearance in the sixteenth century. Another diagnosis is a filovirus such as Ebola. The speed of the transmission of the Plague of Cyprian does indicate human-to-human transmission and much of the pathological and epidemiological evidence could indicate such a disease.[12] However, other evidence for hemorrhagic viruses in the late antique world is not apparent. Because of their severity, hemorrhagic viruses often become the diagnosis of choice when an unknown and deadly disease is encountered but the evidence is not yet convincing for the Plague of Cyprian.

It could be argued that late ancient and early medieval Britain was relatively disease-free in the sense of not encountering major infectious disease outbreaks. While it was part of the Roman Empire, the time to travel from Rome to Britain made it unlikely that disease microbes would survive the trip. The downside of such a situation was that the English people had no acquired immunity to potentially epidemic diseases gained through exposure. Any epidemic would be a virgin soil epidemic likely to produce a high mortality rate.

The plague of Justinian

The disease responsible for the three epidemics noted above has been debated although some consensus is emerging. All three epidemics indicate the difficulties of engaging in retrospective diagnosis but the process involving paying close attention to symptoms and archaeological evidence can yield useful information about the diseases. Plague, not just the generic term plague for pestilence, but plague caused by *Yersinia pestis* was responsible for the Plague of Justinian, often labeled the First Plague Pandemic to relate it to later plague pandemics. Plague is a relatively new disease, one with three main variants: bubonic plague (the most common), pneumonic plague, and septicemic plague. Both pneumonic and septicemic plague can be primary infections but they can also arise as secondary infections resulting from a bubonic plague infection. Plague is caused by the Gram-negative, non-motile, rod-shaped *Yersinia pestis* bacteria, which evolved from *Yersinia pseudotuberculosis* some 5,000 years ago.[13] The newly evolved *Yersinia pestis* bacteria and the plague it caused may have contributed to the decline of Neolithic societies in Eurasia as it branched and spread across the region.[14] The plague bacterium evolved over time and not all strains are present today. Some of the strains that caused the Plague of Justinian were no longer present in the fourteenth century and several new strains arose that composed the Second Pandemic (more discussion of this in the next chapter).[15] Although few cases are reported today, mainly from the Democratic Republic of the Congo, Madagascar, and the southwestern United States, plague has been a major killer with three pandemics: the Plague of Justinian from 541–c.750, the Second Pandemic from 1347 to the late eighteenth century, and the Third Pandemic lasting from the 1770s until 1945.

All three of the *Yersinia* genera (*pseudotuberculosis, pestis,* and *enterocolitis*) have acquired plasmids (floating wheels of genetic material) outside their chromosomes that have encoded a few specialized genes. One plasmid, yPV, is shared by all three species enabling the bacteria to inject specialized proteins into host cells that help to disable the host's innate immunity. The second plasmid, pPCP1, is found only in *Yersinia pestis,* which creates an enzyme that enables the bacterium capable of deep tissue invasion. The third plasmid, pMT1, evolved a gene that codes for a protein called *Yersinia* murine toxin. This toxin protects the bacteria in the mid-gut of fleas, helping lead the digestive path of fleas to become blocked, which leads them to nearly continuous biting in search of blood. Taken together these plasmids enhance the infective and potential killing power of *Yersinia pestis* in a dramatic fashion.[16]

All three major strains of plague can produce very high mortality rates if untreated.[17] Since the mid-twentieth century, practitioners have treated plague successfully with antibiotics such as streptomycin. However, treatment must be started within twenty-four hours of the onset of the disease and the early symptoms of pneumonic and septicemic plague are such that they are often not diagnosed in time. Recently, medical personnel have diagnosed cases of antibiotic-resistant plague from a strain present in Madagascar leading the World Health Organization to list plague as a re-emerging disease in some parts of the world. Untreated, bubonic plague has a case mortality rate between fifty and sixty percent (even when treated, it has a case mortality rate of 5%). When untreated, both septicemic and pneumonic plague have a case mortality rate close to one hundred percent. Surviving a bout with the plague appears to produce only temporary immunity and so survivors might die in a second wave a few years after their first encounter with the disease.

Bubonic plague has both generalized symptoms such as headaches, chills, and fever and some highly noticeable ones. Starting with the Plague of Justinian, commentators noted the swelling of lymph nodes in the neck, groin, or armpits that produced the characteristic buboes that are extremely painful. Many victims also exhibit pustules around the fleabites that served to transmit the disease. If untreated, death often occurs within three to five days after the onset of the disease. If patients survive this initial period, the buboes will burst open during the second week oozing pus. In some cases, the bacteria migrate into the lungs or bloodstream producing secondary pneumonic or septicemic plague which is almost always fatal.

Plague is a zoonotic disease found in animals, particularly black rats, but it can be transmitted readily to humans.[18] Usually, an epizootic among rats or other animals such as marmots occurred, as the rats died from the plague infection and fleas then migrated to nearby hosts such as humans. Rats, however, are not essential for the transmission of plague. Two epidemics ravaged fifteenth-century Iceland and there is no evidence of the presence of rats on the island at the time.[19] Even a primary pneumonic plague outbreak required some starting point and that was not humans.

Flea and possibly lice bites transmit bubonic plague. Human ectoparasites may have also served to transmit plague although the evidence for this is subject to debate.[20] More than 250 species of fleas can transmit the *Yersinia pestis* bacteria, but the most effective is the rat flea, *Xenopsylla cheopis*. Unlike many other types of fleas, these fleas can survive outside of a host by feeding on grain dust, making their transportation across long distances possible. *Yersinia pestis* bacteria multiply within a flea's stomach as it feeds on a host ultimately blocking it. This process keeps the flea from clearing the bacteria through the mid-gut and leads it to regurgitate blood with *Yersinia pestis* in it back into a host when bitten. Over the next four days, the flea bites the host numerous times, as it becomes increasingly hungry and unable to sate its hunger making it more likely that the host will become infected with *Yersinia pestis*. For a long time, the blocked flea thesis governed how scholars saw plague infection taking place. A new approach, called early-phase transmission, emphasizes that some fleas will bite and infect their hosts before becoming blocked. Recent research emphasizes that fleas in this stage can readily transmit plague, making it easier to spread the disease.[21] More than three hundred species of mammals can host fleas, such as domestic cats and dogs, marmots, chipmunks, and humans, and the human flea, *Pulex irritans*, has been shown to be able to transmit the bacteria.

Both primary septicemic and pneumonic plague are much less common than bubonic plague, but when they appear during an outbreak, the results are generally disastrous. Primary septicemic plague occurs when a flea bite occurs on a surface capillary vein enabling the bacteria to immediately enter the bloodstream. Because blocked rat fleas may bite their victims multiple times, the possibility exists for primary septicemic infections. More common are secondary septicemic infections arising from migration of the bacteria to the bloodstream that can occur in about thirty to forty percent of human infections. Pneumonic plague can also arise as a secondary infection from a bubonic plague infection in about five to twenty-five percent of the cases. However, droplets spread by the sneezes or coughs of infected people can serve to transmit primary pneumonic. Primary pneumonic plague is less infective than bubonic plague and outbreaks burn out quickly because of the high death rate, but there is evidence that primary pneumonic plague outbreaks were part of all three pandemics.

The Plague of Justinian was a pandemic that affected first the Mediterranean world, playing havoc in Byzantium and then spreading to Rome and northern Europe.[22] The term Plague of Justinian describes both the first outbreak in the sixth century and the reoccurring outbreaks that lasted well into the eighth century. Commentators have also called it the First Plague Pandemic, emphasizing its widespread coverage and connection to later plague pandemics. The Plague of Justinian came to notice with an outbreak in the Egyptian port of Pelusium in 541 and reached Byzantium by the spring of 542. Scholars dispute its original point of origin with some arguing for the Quinghai-Tibet Plateau in China, others in Africa, and others emphasizing transmission from India.[23] Even the emperor Justinian was not immune although he survived his infection. Thereafter, there would be several more epidemics at approximately twelve-year intervals into the eighth century.[24] The Plague of Justinian so disrupted affairs in Rome, which was already under stress from earlier bouts with disease, financial problems, and invaders, that it hastened the collapse of the western Empire. The historian Kyle Harper places a great deal of emphasis on climatic factors and disease in bringing down the Roman Empire.[25] Not all scholars agree with this interpretation as some indicate that estimates of deaths and the impact of the Junstinianic Plague have been over-exaggerated.[26] At least in Byzantium, the outbreak found an able and fulsome chronicler in the Greek historian Procopius who lived through the outbreak. Some commentators have criticized Procopius and other chroniclers of the plague such as Gregory of Tours (bishop of Tours 573–594) for their use of language that emphasized the dire nature of the pandemic.[27] As Michael McCormick indicates, Gregory considered that the several plague outbreaks he described in the sixth century to be a major threat and that, moreover, archaeological and scientific research collaborates Gregory's judgments.[28] Gregory's descriptions of plague in sixth-century Gaul in *The History of the Franks* are more fulsome than those found in Bede's *Ecclesiastical History of the English* seventh-century epidemics, but taken together they reinforce the view that the Justinianic Plague had a dramatic impact on life in parts of northern Europe. This time the pestilence was indeed the plague, a vector-borne disease caused by the bacteria *Yersinia pestis*. Although the plague diagnosis has been called into question for this outbreak as well as that of the fourteenth century, there is convincing evidence that the Plague of Justinian was indeed the plague with archaeological evidence from throughout Europe including England and not smallpox, anthrax, or some unknown disease.[29] Some of the difficulties of diagnosing disease in past time including the plague are examined in the next chapter where the Black Death, the first outbreak of the Second Plague Pandemic is taken up.

Plague first appeared in Europe in 541 and the last outbreak was recorded in 749 although there is currently no good explanation as to why there were no more cases after this date. The disease was not continuously present everywhere during the two-hundred-year period although individual cases probably occurred outside of major outbreaks. One approach has been to see the outbreaks as waves that swept across Europe. The historian, Dionysios Stathakopoulos records eighteen separate waves for the period indicating that different waves had different impacts and hit different parts of Europe.[30] Implicit in this argument is that plague appeared from the outside and then affected one area on each occasion. Historian, Kyle Harper indicates that plague reservoirs remained after the first outbreak and then through a process of infection and cross-infection plague epidemics broke out. He uses the term amplification to better reflect the continuing presence of the disease and its sudden blossoming into a full-scale epidemic and finds 38 such events.[31] While the evidence for some of the plague events may not always be strong, both approaches, especially Harper's, indicate the periodic nature of the First Pandemic.

Procopius, the great historian of the Byzantine Empire, captured the impact of the First Pandemic with the phrase: "During these times, there was a pestilence, by which the whole human race came near to being annihilated."[32] Certainly, the death toll in Byzantium could have led contemporaries to think that human life was near to extinction, but was the culprit the plague or something else? Here too, Procopius comes to the rescue with an excellent description of the symptoms of the disease, a description that might have been lifted from a twenty-first-century medical textbook.

> [The afflicted person] had a sudden fever, …. But on the same day in some cases, the next day in others, and the rest not many days later, a bubonic swelling developed, and this took place not only in the groin, but also inside the armpits, and in some cases also beside the ears, and at different points on the thighs…. There ensued with some a deep coma, with others a violent delirium… [A]nd in those cases where neither coma nor delirium came on, the bubonic swelling became mortified and the sufferer, no longer able to endure the pain died.[33]

The buboes described by Procopius are a classic sign of bubonic plague and paleopathological evidence confirms his diagnosis. In this case, the high death rates in urban areas probably meant that at least some of the cases were probably primary pneumonic plague in which the plague spread from person to person through nasal or oral discharge. Unlike bubonic plague that did not kill all its victims, witness Justinian, pneumonic plague is invariably fatal.

The first plague pandemic spread by sea and reached Ireland by 544 or 545. The Irish *Annals of Tigernach* referred to it as "blefed."[34] Even though a description of the symptoms of the Irish outbreak is wanting, circumstances point to it being the same disease as what was affecting Byzantium. Ireland had numerous contacts with Gaul in the sixth century so it would have been easy for the fleas that were hosts to the *Yersinia pestis* bacteria and their rat hosts to make the voyage. Ireland continued to be affected by epidemic disease for 30 or so years thereafter, but not all epidemics were the plague. For example, the great mortality of 549, sometimes referred to as "the yellow plague," was most likely smallpox.[35] Plague continued to spare England throughout the sixth century in spite of contact with Ireland and the continent.

English immunity and luck ran out in the summer of 664 when plague visited the island. Several small kingdoms spread across the island and the plague moved across the southern kingdoms first, killing both Earconberht, king of Kent, and Deusdedit, archbishop of Canterbury on 14 July and then spread northward.[36] The monastic chronicler Bede put it simply and eloquently in his *Ecclesiastical History*, "And the pestilence came."[37] Bede completed the *Ecclesiastical History* in 731 and was able to draw on earlier evidence of the epidemic. Unfortunately, there are few other accounts of the English epidemic so we are largely reliant on Bede's observations. He went on to say that the disease raged far and wide and "laid low a great multitude of men."[38] Earlier, in c. 697, Adomnán, abbot of the monastery of Iona, wrote in his biography of St. Columba that "the great mortality that twice in our time has ravaged a large part of the world."[39] In a world in which monastic chroniclers were at pains to recount all the doings of the monastery, the epidemic that swept through Britain made them take notice of events so far beyond their ken and so devastating to the island. Neither the author(s) of the *Anglo-Saxon Chronicle* nor the monastic chroniclers provided numbers of deaths if such had been possible, but they all considered the outbreak of disease a major event not seen before.[40] However, they provided some descriptive material that tells us something about what was a new disease.

The disease arrived from the sea during the summer and the southeast of England was the first area to suffer. Thereafter, it spread through the rest of the island. By autumn of 664, it had reached northern England and struck down Cedd, the bishop of the East Saxons, in his monastery of Lastingham in Northumbria on October 23.[41] Outbreaks of the disease continued into the next year and cases continued to be reported thereafter. At some point, between 666 and 673, there was an outbreak in the double monastery of Barking near London that caused several deaths among the monks and nuns.[42] It seems that the disease became nearly endemic in some parts of England, making it easy for a major epidemic to break out again in 684. Both outbreaks lasted for short periods although the disease lingered so that there were a few cases after the first outbreak. After 687, the disease did not reappear.

Like the first outbreak, the epidemic that lasted from 684 to 687, struck almost all regions throughout England. The abbey at Lindisfarne, an island off the northeast coast of England, was nearly decimated by an epidemic that lasted for nearly a year as was the abbey of Jarrow in Northumberland.[43] Plague outbreaks affected small villages as well as the densely packed monasteries. Bishop Cuthbert of Lindisfarne (bishop 658–687) continually offered comfort to those afflicted during his travels about his diocese.[44] Although the information is lacking for many areas, it seems that both outbreaks affected almost all of England. The monastic clergy were hard-hit by both epidemics, not unsurprising given the closeness of living in monastic communities. Once inside a monastery, the plague was likely to stay until it had killed nearly everyone or burned out.

The disease reached Britain in 664 and lasted through the seventh century with several outbreaks although it found no one as fulsome as Procopius to describe it. As John Maddicott points out, Bede was interested in the disease for its own sake not simply as the working of God on earth.[45] Bede provides one telling description of the disease as he describes how it affected St. Cuthbert when he was struck by the disease at Melrose: "the swelling which appeared in his thigh gradually left the surface of his body, it sank into the inward parts and, throughout almost the whole of his life, he continued to feel some inward pains."[46] Although not as explicit as Procopius' description, this appears to be a description of a bubo, a clear sign of the plague. In addition, the plague seemed to strike hardest during the summer of 664 and summer was a time for fleas to be active, easily spreading the disease as non-human hosts died from infection. As was the case in the East, this outbreak seems to have had a pneumonic component that increased the death rate. Bede indicates that the disease continued through the winter during the second outbreak in the 680s. An outbreak started at Christmas at Lindesfarne Abbey, and Abbot Eosterwine of Wearmouth died in early March.[47] The timing of this outbreak leads to a suspicion that there was a pneumonic component to the English outbreaks increasing mortality rates. Primary pneumonic plague often spreads during the winter when people are cooped up indoors and the coughing of victims is likely to infect those around them.

Much of the evidence concerning the impact of the Justinianic Plague in northern Europe centers on monastic communities. Bede focused on what he knew so much of his discussion of the plague focused on monastic communities. English monasteries in the seventh century often had contact with the continent opening the door to plague. Their residents lived in close quarters making it easy to spread bubonic and pneumonic plague. They also often served as commercial and religious centers for the surrounding area, making it easy to transmit the disease beyond the monastery walls. Evidence concerning the rural communities of England in the seventh century is scarce, but the likelihood is that plague penetrated even isolated villages often from nearby monastic communities that acted as focusing mechanisms for spreading the plague. Studies of the impact of plague in Norway during the Black Death indicate that rural communities were often as hard-hit as towns.[48] It would have been easy to transmit plague in a small village in which everyone regularly came in contact with other villagers. Direct evidence is hard to obtain, but continental comparisons and the number of abandoned villages in some areas such as Northumbria indicate that country dwellers did not escape.[49] The numbers of deaths in England may not have approached the numbers described by Procopius for the eastern Mediterranean, but the population of England was much smaller than in the Byzantine Empire and appears to have had high death rates from the plague.

In part, because monks did the reporting of the plagues, there was a tendency to see divine punishment as the cause of the disease. Bede speaks of "a plague sent from heaven," while Adomnán credits divine protection for protecting St. Columba and his entourage from danger, even though they traveled regularly among the afflicted.[50] Bede spoke of "bad air" as the direct cause of the disease but he was careful to note that this came as the exercise of God's will. People might try to nurse the sick, but this provided scant relief. When plague struck St. Cuthbert in 664, his monks resorted to prayer that Bede reports immediately leading to his recovery.[51] In spite of Cuthbert's saintly example, Christianity did not always have a firm grasp on the island. Bede describes how King Sieghere of the East Saxons and some of his people began "to restore the derelict temples [of the old gods] and to worship images as if they could protect themselves by such means from the plague."[52] The Mercian king Wulfbere, Sieghere's overlord, intervened and the people returned to the Church, much to Bede's relief.

In reality, it is difficult to determine what impact the plague outbreaks of the 660s and 680s had on England. A large number of deaths appear to have occurred, at least in some places and the epidemics clearly affected the mental outlook of some contemporaries and continued to do so well into the eighth century when Bede flourished. Gradually memories of the First Pandemic faded away so that when plague struck again in 1348 people treated it as a new disease. The suddenness of the disease and its high morbidity and mortality rates scared people in a way that other diseases did not. Population figures are impossible to come by and the few accounts tend to focus on monastic communities. It seems that both epidemics hit much of England and generated high mortality rates in at least some of the places struck by disease. Small isolated communities may have escaped the disease, but the death toll in these villages may have simply gone unreported. After 687, there are no reports of the plague so life gradually got back to normal and the population began to regain lost ground.

Epidemic disease in early medieval England and beyond

Although epidemic disease outbreaks likely occurred before the Plague of Athens, including possible plague epidemics in Neolithic Eurasia, it is this epidemic along with the Antonine Plague, the Plague of Cyprian, and the Plague of Justinian that have come to exemplify how we define epidemics.[53] With at least Procopius's, John of Ephesus's, Gregory of Tours' and Bede's descriptions of the Justinian Plague coupled with bioarchaeologic research, other records, chronicles, and art, information about the disease and its impact took a step forward. Although not all scholars agree, there is enough evidence for the spread of the Justinianic Plague and its impact so that it can be labeled a pandemic. An examination of the four epidemics indicates an epidemic or pandemic can be caused by a variety of diseases although smallpox and plague often take pride of place to be challenged by influenza and COVID-19 in the twentieth century. Contemporaries referred to all four epidemics as pestilences or plagues, indicating a non-specific approach to diagnosis that indicated the illness had unbalanced the humors and then commentators described the symptoms.

Increasing population size, density of settlement, and enhanced ability to travel all combined to produce epidemics and then pandemics as diseases spread across the Mediterranean and to northern Europe with the Plague of Justinian. Human behavior helped to either spread or contain a disease. Beliefs about disease and disease causation would affect how a society reacted to a disease and the effectiveness of this reaction. So too did the nature of the disease itself. The method by which a disease was transmitted, e.g., a vector-borne disease or a human-to-human transmission affected how a disease spread. In addition, its morbidity rate (how easily it infected humans) and mortality rate also had impacts on the spread of a disease and its impact on society. Other factors entered in as well such as climate and nutrition. The onset of the Plague of Justinian in England overlapped with the Late Antique Little Ice Age complicating the availability of adequate food supplies. All of these factors have been detailed in the previous two chapters.

Over time, the disease load of the English people increased as old diseases returned, but to different population arrangements or in more or less virulent forms. New diseases also emerged such as syphilis, influenza, and the English Sweat. The concept of syndemics explains a complicating factor that sometimes appeared. Syndemics is the interaction of multiple diseases that produces a negative reaction greater than that produced by one or more diseases.[54] Plague and pneumonia could produce an even more deadly reaction than plague alone. The changing framework of epidemic disease in combination with other factors helped to lead educated people to consider how disease should be defined and how it should be treated. Information about diseases and their impacts increased throughout the Middle Ages and received an enormous boost with the advent of printing in the late fifteenth century. This increased evidence available makes it possible for scholars to develop a more detailed explanation for the role of disease in English society in the centuries beyond the Early Middle Ages.

Several factors influenced how diseases affected English society and how people, government, and the medical community reacted to infectious diseases. The small size of the English population and the rural nature of the country helped to protect it from some epidemic diseases in the early Middle Ages and even into the sixteenth century. As the next two chapters indicate, the vector-borne plague gained traction on the island, largely because it was less reliant on dense population than some other epidemic disease. Even plague may not have caused a large population decline in the seventh century, Bede's contentions notwithstanding, because of the rural nature of the population. Monasteries and what few urban centers existed such as London were vulnerable, but isolated villages might be lucky and escape visitation although many did not. Only with the growth of population and increased trade and travel in the fourteenth century would plague have the potential to be devastating to all of the English population. England was introduced to epidemic disease (although people at the time did not refer to it that way) with the Plague of Justinian. Thereafter, England would be part of the European disease network. A village or a region might experience an outbreak of an infectious disease that might even become large enough to be called an epidemic, but at times infectious disease reached epidemic and even pandemic proportion in the West.

When taken together, the four epidemics described here also help to raise questions about the impact of epidemic and pandemic diseases. While the Plague of Athens may be seen as an epidemic, the other three, especially the Plague of Justinian, were pandemics in their geographical and chronological coverage. They help to address the impact of pandemic diseases on society. The Plagues of the Antonines, Cyprian, and Justinian tended to have a negative impact on society, especially the latter two. Roman society was resilient enough to withstand the Plague of the Antonines, but the next two outbreaks of infectious disease helped to weaken the structure of society, and helped lead to the collapse of the Empire. There were numerous factors that contributed to the Roman collapse, and disease certainly played a role. Each was different though. The disease affecting the society was different: smallpox, plague, and possibly a hemorrhagic fever with the Plague of Cyprian. Leaving aside the Plague of Cyprian because its disease source is still not fully identified, the first two involved smallpox, a disease that would return in the seventeenth century, but which appeared to be absent in the high and late Middle Ages. The Plague of Justinian marked the appearance of plague, a disease with both high morbidity and high mortality rates that continued to pose major public health threats to society from the fourteenth century onward, becoming truly a worldwide pandemic at the turn of the twentieth century. The impact also differed in part because the structure of Roman society was becoming weaker from the third century onward. All three of the post-millennial plagues appeared to have a negative impact on the standard of living although this was due to both the nature of the diseases involved and the structure of society at the time.[55] In many ways, they set the stage for the Second Plague Pandemic that started in the fourteenth century although there would be important differences.

Notes

1   A good introduction to questions of human health and population size in the Neolithic Era is John L. Brooke, *Climate Change and the Course of Global History* (Cambridge: Cambridge University Press, 2014), 213–42. An introduction to the conceptual background of the three epidemiologic transitions is Ron Barrett and George J. Armelagos, *An Unnatural History of Emerging Infections* (Oxford: Oxford University Press, 2013).

2   Some of the difficulties in explaining epidemic disease in the ancient Middle East are detailed in Sergio Sabbatani and Sirio Fiorino, "The Plague of the Philistines and other Pestilences in the Ancient World: Exploring Relations between the Religious-Literary Tradition, Artistic Evidences and Scientific Proofs," *Le Infezioni in Medicina,* 3 (2010), 199–207.

3   A comparative overview of the biological aspects of the three epidemics is Cheston B. Cunha and Burke A. Cunha, "Great Plagues of the Past and Remaining Questions," in Didier Raoult and Michel Drancourt, eds., *Paleomicrobiology* (Berlin: Springer, 2010), 1–20.

4   Merle Eisenberg and Lee Mordechai question the use of the term of First Plague Pandemic, indicating this terminology dates from the plague pandemic at the turn of the twentieth century. "The Justinianic Plague and Global Pandemics: The Making of the Plague Concept," *American Historical Review,* 125 (2020), 1632–1667. This article is part of revisionist effort on their part dealing with the Plague of Justinian and care must be taken with their conclusions.

5   Various commentators have forwarded a variety of diagnoses for the Plague of Athens, but recent work has concentrated on smallpox, typhus, and measles. Robert J. Littman and M.L. Littman, "The Athenian Plague: Smallpox," *Transactions and Proceedings of the American Philological Association,* 100 (1969), 261–75. James Longrigg, "The Great Plague of Athens," *Historical Science,* 18 (1980), 209–25. David M. Morens and Robert J. Littman, "Epidemiology of the Plague of Athens," *Transactions of the American Philological Association,* 122 (1992), 271–304. Burke A. Cunha, "The Cause of the Plague of Athens: Plague, Typhoid, Typhus, Smallpox, or Measles?" *Infectious Disease Clinics of North America* 18 (2004), 29–43. Robert J. Littman, "The Plague of Athens: Epidemiology and Paleopathology," *Mount Sinai Journal of Medicine,* 76 (2009), 456–67.

6   Manolis J. Papagrigorakis, Christos Yapijakis, Philippos N. Synodinos, and Effie Baziotopoulou-Valavani, "DNA Examination of Ancient Dental Pulp Incriminates Typhoid Fever as a Probable Cause of the Plague of Athens," *International Journal of Infectious Diseases,* 10 (2006), 206–14. Littman, "Plague of Athens," provides a telling rebuttal to the typhoid argument.

7   Robert Sallares, *The Ecology of the Ancient Greek World* (Ithaca: Cornell University Press, 1991).

8   Yuki Furuse, Akira Suziki, and Hitoshi Oshitani, "Origins of Measles Virus: Divergence from Rinderpest Virus between the 11th and 12th Centuries," *Virology Journal,* 7 (2010), 52. Jennifer Manley notes these findings and provides a historical context in "Measles and Ancient Plagues: A Note on New Scientific Evidence," *Classical World,* 107 (2013), 393–97.

9   R.P. Duncan-Jones, "The Impact of the Antonine Plague," *Journal of Roman Archaeology,* 9 (1996): 111.

10 R.J. Littman and M.L. Littman, "Galen and the Antonine Plague," *American Journal of Phillology,* 94 (1973), 243–55. Susan P. Mattern discusses reasons why Galen left Rome and describes his experience with the disease in Greece. *The Prince of Medicine* (Oxford: Oxford University Press, 2015), 187–223.

11 Duncan-Jones, "Impact of the Antonine Plague," pp. 121–34. Duncan-Jones provides a fulsome analysis of the disease and its large impact on the Roman world (108–36).

12 Kyle, Harper, "Pandemics and Passages to Late Antiquity: Rethinking the Plague of c. 249–270 Described by Cyprian," *Journal of Roman Archaeology*, 28 (2015), 223–60, and Harper, *The Fate of Rome* (Princeton: Princeton University Press, 2017), 136–49.

13 Yi-Cheng Sun, Clayton O. Jarrett, Christopher F. Bosio, and B. Joseph Hinnebush, "Retracing the Evolutionary Path that Led to Flea-Borne Transmission of *Yersinia pestis*," *Cell Host and Microbe*, 15 (2014), 578–86. Simon Rasmussen, Morten Erik Allentoft, Kasper Nelson, Ludovic Orlando, Martin Sikora, et al., "Early Divergent Strains of *Yersinia pestis* in Eurasia 5,000 Years Ago," *Cell*, 163 (2015), 571–82. B. Joseph Hinnebush, Iman Chouikha, and Yi-Chen Sun, "Ecological Opportunity, Evolution and the Emergence of Flea-Borne Plague," *Infection and Immunology*, 84 (2016), 1932. Aida Andrades Valtueña, Alissa Mittnik, Felix M. Key, Wolfgang Haak, Raili Allmäe, et al., "The Stone Age Plague and its Persistence in Eurasia," *Current Biology*, 27 (2017), 3683–91. Maria A. Spyrou, Rezeda I. Tukbatova, Chuan-Chao Wang, Aida Andrades Valtueña, et al. "Analysis of 3800-Year-Old *Yersinia pestis* Genomes Suggests Bronze Age Origin for Bubonic Plague," *Nature Communications*, 9 (2018), 1–10.

14 Nicolás Rascoven, Karl-Göran Sjögren, Kristian Kristiansen, Rasmus Nielsen, Eske Willerslev, et al., "Emergence and Spread of Basal Lineages of *Yersinia pestis* during the Neolithic Decline," *Cell*, 176 (2019), 295–305.

15 Three recent works describe the state of plague research c. early 2021, but aspects of plague research change rapidly. R. Barbieri, M. Signoli, D. Chevé, C. Costedoat, S. Tzortzis, et al., "*Yersinia pestis*: The Natural History of the Plague," *Clinical Microbiology Reviews*, 34 (2021), e00044–19. Monica H. Green, "The Four Black Deaths," *American Historical Review*, 125 (2020), 1601–31. John Aberth, *The Black Death* (Oxford: Oxford University Press, 2021), 1–13. Both Green and Aberth focus on the Black Death, but provide some discussion of the Plague of Justinian.

16 P.S.G. Chain, E. Carniel, F.W. Larimer, J. Lamerdin, P.O. Stoutland et al., "Insights into the Evolution of *Yersinia Pestis* through Whole-Genome Comparison with *Yersinia pseudotuberculosis*," *PNAS*, 101 (2004), 13826–13831. Daniel L. Zimbler, Jay A. Schroeder, Justin L. Eddy, Wyndham W. Lathem, "Early Emergence of *Yersinia pestis* as a Severe Respiratory Pathogen," *Nature Communications*, 6 (2015), 1–10.

17 There are three rare types of plague, cutaneous, gastrointestinal, and plague conjunctivitis, although finding evidence of them in the premodern literature is difficult. Ruifu Yang, "Plague: Recognition, Treatment, and Prevention," *Journal of Clinical Microbiology*, 56 (2018), e01519–17.

18 Two articles that emphasize the role of rats in the transmission of plague over time are Michael McCormick, "Rats, Communications and Plague: Toward and Ecological History," *Journal of Interdisciplinary History*, 34 (2003), 1–25, and Anne Hardy, "The Under-Appreciated Rodent: Harbingers of Plague from the Middle Ages to the Twenty-First Century," *Journal of Interdisciplinary History*, 50 (2019), 171–85.

19 G. Karlsson, "Plague without Rats: The Case of Fifteenth-Century Iceland," *Journal of Medieval History*," 22 (1996), 263–84. Because rats may have also been scarce in Scandinavia, some other form of transmission may have been necessary. Anne Karin Huffthammer and Lars Walløe, "Rats Cannot Have Been Intermediate Hosts for *Yersinia pestis* during Medieval Plague Epidemics in Northern Europe," *Journal of Archaeological Science*, 40 (2013), 1752–59.

20 One study argues that human fleas (*Pulex irritans*) and human lice (*Pediculus humananus*) may have been responsible for the rapid spread of the Second Pandemic, raising the possibility of a role in the Plague of Justinian. At present, this view does not enjoy wide acceptance. Katherine R. Dean, Fabienne Krauer, Lars Walløe, Ole Christian Lingjaerde, Barbara Bramanti, et al., "Human Ectoparasites and the Spread of Plague in Europe During the Second Pandemic," *PNAS*, 115 (2018), 1304–09.

21 A good brief summary of the role of fleas and rats in the transmission of plague with extensive references is Aberth, *Black Death*, 2–6. See also Barbieri et al., "Natural History of the Plague."

22 Kyle Harper provides the best account of the overall biological, climatological, and political aspects of the Plague of Justinian and its impact on the Roman Empire although not northern Europe in *Fate of Rome*.

23 Kyle Harper, *Fate of Rome*, 210. Barbieri et al., "Natural History of Plague."

24 J.N. Biraben and Jacques Le Goff, "The Plague in the Early Middle Ages," in Robert Forster and Orest Ranum eds, and Elborg Forster and Patricia M. Ranum trans., *Biology of Man in History* (Baltimore: Johns Hopkins University Press, 1975), 58–59.

25 Harper, *Fate of Rome*. Mischa Meier indicates that the Plague of Justinian had a large impact on the economic and cultural aspects of the eastern Roman Empire. "The 'Justinianic Plague': The Economic Consequences of the Pandemic in the Eastern Roman Empire and Its Cultural and Religious Effects," *Early Medieval Europe*, 24 (2016), 267–92, and "The Justinianic Plague: 'An Inconsequential Pandemic'? A Reply," *Medizinhistorisches Journal*, 55 (2020), 172–99.

26 Lee Mordechai and Lee Eisenberg, "Rejecting Catastrophe: The Case of the Justinianic Plague," *Past and Present*, 244 (2019), 3–50, Mordechai, Eisenberg, Timothy P. Newfield, Adam Izdebski, Janet E. Kay, Hendrik Poinar, "The Justinianic Plague: An Inconsequential Pandemic?" *PNAS*, 116 (2019), 25546–54. John Haldon, Hugh Elton, Sabine R. Huebner, Adam Izdebski, Lee Mordechai, Timothy P. Newfield, "Plagues, Climate Change, and the End of Empire: A Response to Kyle Harper's *The Fate of Rome* (1): Climate," *History Compass*, 16:1 (2018), e12508, Ibid, "Plagues, Climate Change... (2): Plagues and a Crisis of Empire," *History Compass*, 16:2 (2018), e12506, Ibid., "Plagues, Climate Change... Disease, Agency, and Collapse," *History Compass*, 16:12 (2018), e125507.

27 Mordechai et al., "Inconsequential Pandemic," 22547.

28 Michael McCormick, "Gregory of Tours on Sixth-Century Plague and Other Epidemics," *Speculum*, 96 (2021), 38–96. Emphasizing that Gregory indicated the importance of plague in several places in his work, McCormick takes aim at Mordechai and Eisenberg ("Rejecting Catastrophe," 15–16) who indicate that Gregory did not consider the plague important in Gaul. Mordechai and Eisenberg's argument is suspect regarding northern Europe, as they appear to misinterpret Gregory of Tours and ignore Bede's *Ecclesiastical History*.

29 The biology of the Plague of Justinian is examined in some of the essays in Little, *Plague and the End of Antiquity*. In particular, see Jo N. Hays, "Historians and Epidemics: Simple Questions, Complex Answers," Robert Sallares, "Ecology, Evolution, and Epidemiology of Plague," and Michael McCormick, "Toward a Molecular History of the Justinian Pandemic." Paleopathology has enabled a definitive diagnosis of *Yersinia pestis* based on analysis of DNA taken from skeletal remains. Michaaela Harbeck, Lisa Seifert, Stephanie Hänsch, et al., "*Yersinia pestis* DNA from Skeletal Remains from the 6th Century AD Reveals Insights into Justinanic Plague," *PLoS Pathogens*, 9 (2013), e1003349; David M. Wagner, Jennifer Klunk, Michaela Harbeck, et al., "*Yersinia pestis* and the Plague of Justinian 541–543 AD: A Genomic Analysis," *Lancet Infectious Diseases*, 14 (2014), 319–26; Michal Feldman, Michaela Harbeck, Marcel Keller, et al., "A High-Coverage *Yersinia pestis* Genome from a Sixth-Century Justinianic Plague Victim," *Molecular Biology and Evolution*, 33 (2016), 2911–2923.

30 Dionysios Ch. Stathakopoulos, *Famine and Pestilence in the Late Roman and Early Byzantine Empire* (Burlington VT: Ashgate, 2004), 113–24. He also provides brief accounts of all recorded instances in the two-hundred-year period (278–386).

31 Harper, *Fate of Rome*, 236, 304–15.

32 Procopius, *History of the Wars* Book II (New York: Cosimo Classics, 2007) 21.

33 Procopius, *History of the Wars, Book* II, 22.

34 W. Stokes, ed., *The Annals of Tigernach, Revue Celtique*, 16–17 (1895–96), 137, 198; Ann Dooley, "The Plague and Its Consequences in Ireland," in Little, *Plague and the End of Antiquity*, 215–28. Maddicott, "Plague in Seventh Century England, p. 173; William MacArthur, "The Medical Identification of Some Pestilences of the Past," *Transactions of the Royal Society of Tropical Medicine and Hygiene*, 53 (1959), 172–73.

35 J.F.D. Shrewsbury, "The Yellow Plague," *Journal of the History of Medicine*, 4 (1949): 34–39. Maddicott, "Plague in Seventh-Century England," (174) agrees with Shrewsbury that the yellow plague was smallpox although MacArthur, "Identification of some Pestilences," 173–75, argues that it was relapsing fever.

36 B. Colgrave and R.A.B. Mynors, eds., *Bede's Ecclesiastical History of the English People* (Oxford, Oxford University Press, 1969), 328.

37 *Bede's Ecclesiastical History*, 564–65

38 *Bede's Ecclesiastical History*, 312–13.

39 *Adomnán's Life of Columba*, A.O. Anderson, M.O. Anderson, eds., and trans. (Oxford: Oxford University Press, 1991), 178–79.

40 An excellent comprehensive account of the seventh century disease is Maddicott, "Plague in Seventh-Century England," in *Plague and the End of Antiquity* 171–214. This work provides excellent coverage of the pandemic as well as useful discussions of the nature of the disease.

41 *Bede's Ecclesiastical History*, 286–89.

42 *Bede's Ecclesiastical History*, 356–59.

43 *Two Lives of Saint Cuthbert,* Bertram Colgrave, trans. (Cambridge: Cambridge University Press, 1940), 244–49. Maddicott, "Plague in England," 176–78.

44 *Two Lives of Saint Cuthbert*, 118–21, 259–61.

45 Maddicott, "Plague in England," 181.

46 *Two Lives of Saint Cuthbert* 180–83.

47 *Two Lives of Saint Cuthbert*, pp. 244–49. Maddicott, "Plague in England," 185.

48 Ole J. Benedictow, *The Complete History of the Black Death* (Woodbridge: Boydell Press, 2021), 401–55.

49 Maddicott, "Plague in Seventh-Century England," 191–205.

50 *Bede's Ecclesiastical History*, 338–39. *Adomnán's Life of Columba*, 178–81.

51 *Two Lives of St. Cuthbert*, 180–81.

52 *Bede's Ecclesiastical History*, 222–23.

53 The evolution of the terms epidemic and pandemic is discussed in: Paul M.V. Martin and Estelle Martin-Granel, "2,500-Year Evolution of the Term Epidemic," *Emerging Infectious Diseases*, 12 (2006), 976–80 and David M. Morens, Gregory K. Folkers, and Anthony Fauci, "What Is a Pandemic?" *Journal of Infectious Disease*, 200 (2009), 1018–21.

54 Merrill Singer and Scott Clair, "Syndemics and Public Health: Reconceptualizing Disease in Bio-Social Context," *Medical Anthropology Quarterly*, 17 (2003), 423–41; Singer, "Pathogen-Pathogen Interaction, *Virulence*, 1 (2010), 10–18.

55 Guido Alfani and Tommy E. Murphy, "Plague and Lethal Epidemics in the Pre-Industrial World," *Journal of Economic History*, 77 (2017), 314–43.

5

THE SECOND PLAGUE PANDEMIC AND THE DEMOGRAPHIC CRISIS IT PRODUCED

Once the Justinian Plague had passed in the late eighth century, the people of Europe soon forgot about it. The plague had not really vanished it had withdrawn to its original habitat, most likely the Tibet-Quinghai Plateau. It would take another epizootic of rats/marmots/gerbils to enable it to spread once again. This happened in the mid-fourteenth century producing what came to be known as the Black Death in Europe. The Black Death was only one of the challenges that confronted English society in the fourteenth century, challenges that produced first a demographic crash and then economic, social, and artistic impacts.

Like much of the rest of Western Europe, England at the end of the thirteenth century was a country with a growing population. England was able to feed its population and the reoccurring famines reported in earlier chronicle accounts had nearly disappeared. The growth of population spurred efforts to put more land under cultivation but there were upper limits to this approach. Agricultural yields remained low so one or more bad harvests raised the specter of dearth if not famine. Even if the country's population did not exceed its carrying capacity, the possibility of a demographic downturn is apparent in retrospect.

Crop failures and famine, especially if coupled with warfare, could lead to a brief short-term decline in population, but it took something far more drastic to produce the massive population decline that occurred in the fourteenth century and continued to affect English and European society until the sixteenth century. Earlier epidemics such as the Plague of Athens or the Plague of Justinian hinted at the impact a highly infectious disease could have in societies with no medical means of coping with it. European society was more integrated by the fourteenth century than ever before. Pilgrims, merchants, and soldiers readily traveled long distances making it easier to spread an infectious disease than in the sixth century. The Plague of Justinian had a dramatic impact on the Byzantine Empire, but as indicated in Chapter 4, the impact of the disease is harder to gauge

DOI: 10.4324/9781003215219-6

for England but did not seem to be nearly as severe as it was in Constantinople or Alexandria.

Plague proved to be uniquely qualified to attack a population and when combined with changing travel patterns and a more urbanized society by the thirteenth century, it could be devastating. The characteristics of fourteenth-century European society and *Yersinia pestis* made it easy for the disease to spread, easy to infect people, and easy to kill its victims, but often not before spreading to others. Other aspects of life in the fourteenth, fifteenth, and sixteenth centuries also made it easier for the disease to have a larger impact than might have been the case earlier.

One approach to the question of population in the fourteenth century can be traced back to the work of Thomas Malthus in the eighteenth century. Malthus argued that past populations often grew in geometric fashion described graphically by a sharply increasing upward shaped curve. The resources to support this population grew arithmetically so that population size would eventually outstrip the ability of a society to feed itself, a situation often described as a Malthusian trap. Scholars have debated Malthus's views and modified the Malthusian argument and there are scholars who describe themselves as neo-Malthusians today. Writing in the years after World War II the historian M.M. Postan argued that Europe's population had outstripped its carrying capacity by 1300.[1] His discussion has served as a useful starting point concerning the late medieval population but the consensus is that developments such as improvements in agriculture made this situation unlikely. Nonetheless, England's population had been growing during the thirteenth century so that declining agricultural productivity brought on in part by climatic changes would be likely to have a harmful impact.

There is an extended debate concerning the impact of the population decline caused by famine and disease in the fourteenth century. After the outbreaks of the plague, land remained uncultivated because there was no one available to work it. Questions remain as to whether this caused wages to rise, food shortages to ensue, or both. It was evident to all Englishmen that a demographic catastrophe, unlike any ever seen before, hit England in the mid-fourteenth century—the Black Death as it eventually came to be known. People were aware at the time that a disease they often called the Great Pestilence was causing changes in their lives and world. The 1348–50 outbreak of the plague was not the only occasion that plague visited late medieval England. As noted in *The Brut*, a fifteenth-century metrical chronicle, the plague pandemic that started in 1347 continued to affect Europe beyond 1348 and eventually into the late eighteenth century, often producing high mortality rates in some years.

> And in this same year [1434] was a great pestilence in London, both of men, women, and children; namely of worthy men, as aldermen and other worthy communers; and also through England the people died sore, both poor and rich, which was great heaviness to all people.[2]

Although exact population counts are impossible to come by, it appears that England's population declined anywhere between forty and sixty percent by the end of the fourteenth century and remained low in number for many years thereafter.

The question of the size of England's population continues to vex scholars. The usual estimate of the country's pre-plague population is five million, but estimates run from Bruce Campbell's low figure of 4 to 4.25 million upward to Richard Smith's 6 to 6.5 million people.[3] Using a mathematical model based on the relationship of population to the marginal product of labor, Gregory Clark computes a figure of slightly over five million when the Black Death first appeared. His model shows the English population continuing to decline after the first outbreak of the plague, reaching a low point of 2.4 million in the decade of 1450–59 and not exceeding three million until the mid-sixteenth century.[4]

Even if people did not understand the cause of the Black Death, they saw it as unprecedented and terrifying. Writing in the reign of Henry VI the chronicler of the Cistercian abbey of Louth Park in Lincolnshire summed up the impact of the pestilence this way:

> This plague slew Jew, Christian and Saracen alike; it carried off confessor and penitent together. In many places not even a fifth part of the people were left alive. It filled the whole world with terror. So great an epidemic has never been seen nor heard of before this time, for it is believed that even the waters of the flood which happened in the days of Noah did not carry off so vast a multitude.[5]

Nineteenth-century historians coined the term Black Death to describe the disease that brought catastrophe to England and most other countries in Europe in the fourteenth century because of some of its symptoms such as the dark-colored buboes that resulted from large pustules of blood near the surface of the skin.[6] People in the fourteenth century usually referred to the *pestis* or *pestilentia generali*, terms that are usually translated as plague, to describe the disease that afflicted them. Today, we use the term plague or refer to the disease and *Yersinia pestis* to refer to the biological agent of the disease.

This chapter provides an examination of the "new" disease that hit England in the fourteenth century and that continued to trouble the island until the late seventeenth century. The examination starts with a look at the demographic situation in England before the plague arrived in 1348. The progress of the disease across the land in 1348–49 will be briefly described as will epidemics through the fifteenth and sixteenth centuries. Although scholars debate the impact of the plague, many consider it a major factor in the transition from the medieval world. More than 40 years ago, the historian William H. McNeill made the case for the impact of disease as driving social and economic change on society.[7] Bruce Campbell, more explicitly, calls the period of demographic change in the fourteenth and fifteenth centuries the Great Transition. He divides it into three phases: the period in which the transition begins, lasting from 1260s/70 to 1330, a period of economic and social transition, lasting from 1340s to 1370s, and an economic and demographic downturn lasting from the 1370s to the 1470s.[8]

Campbell identifies climate change and disease as the main drivers of this period of transition. Not all scholars would impute such a large impact to these factors. Other forces were also at work such as the revival of classical learning that would be part of the Renaissance, the discovery of the western hemisphere at the end of the period, or even the long period of dynastic conflicts throughout the fourteenth and fifteenth centuries that affected Western Europe. Nonetheless, Campbell makes a persuasive argument for considering ecological and biological factors as well as human activity.

The return of famine

Climatic change and famine helped to set the stage for the arrival of the plague in England in 1348. The "good" times of the thirteenth century came to an end in the second decade of the fourteenth century. The reign of Edward II was not a happy one with numerous political problems. Nonetheless, a "Poem on the Evil Times" penned at the beginning of Edward III's reign noted the dearth of Edward II's reign and the resulting famine.[9] Famine struck much of Western Europe in the second decade of the century, not sparing England in the process. Poets often complained of the bad times in the late Middle Ages, but usually spoke to political, social, or religious issues, not natural causes.

Although England's population had grown throughout the thirteenth century, the country's ability to feed its population barely matched the population if any downturn in production occurred. Crop yields varied from place to place but, on average, English agriculture yielded three or four bushels of wheat for every bushel of seed that was sown, oats at 2:1 or 3:1, rye at 4:1 or 5:1, peas and beans at 4:1, and barley from 3.5:1 to 7:1.[10] In essence, England had little room to survive one or more bad years without a great deal of suffering. There are a variety of reasons for the famine that spread across England and Europe from 1315 to 1317 (with some lingering impact until 1322), but much of the cause for the famine came from a climatic turn.[11] During these years, the weather of much of northern Europe, including England, was colder and wetter than usual reducing crop yields substantially. The English people did not have the tools necessary to withstand a prolonged downturn in production without very real suffering and concomitant health and demographic impact. Although the situation improved by 1320, parts of England were visited by drought in the late 1320s and early 1330s which also produced an impact on grain production.[12]

Causes for the "great famine" were many and varied somewhat from country to country, but countries throughout much of Europe felt the negative impact of climatic change. Population pressure, poor farming techniques, problems with the distribution of grain, high taxes, and the impact of war with the Scots all worked to make the situation worse in England. Even taken together these factors did not precipitate the crisis and were not enough to make it as bad as it was for such a long period. The climate anomaly of the second decade of the fourteenth century had an outsize impact on English (and Western European) society. Even today, people are concerned about the potential impact of global warming on agricultural production, and in the Middle Ages people were even more at the mercy of the elements.

Western Europe had been blessed with a somewhat warmer climate in the period from roughly 1000 to the latter part of the thirteenth century, a period generally referred to as the Medieval Climate Anomaly (MCA). The MCA had different impacts in different parts of the world but a strong westerly air-stream generally produced winters over northwest Europe that were mild and wet. Airflow elsewhere did not produce the same results as the westerly air-steam in central Asia maintained conditions of drought which were especially severe in the 1190s and early 1200s.[13] A precipitating factor in the abrupt climate change of the late thirteenth century seems to have been volcanism or changes in the ocean currents. Polar ice core records indicate a volcanic eruption in 1257 or 1258, most likely in the tropics. Recent research has narrowed the source to the Samalas volcano, which is part of a complex of volcanoes on Lombok Island, Indonesia. Estimates indicate a magnitude of 7 (referred to as a super-colossal eruption) on the Volcanic Explosivity Index of 1 to 8 which would rank it as one of the largest Holocene eruptions.[14] Given the delay for a cloud of volcanic dust to reach the northern hemisphere, it would have helped to produce a colder climate regime in northern Europe by the early 1260s. A decline in solar irradiance began in the 1270s producing colder winters in northwestern Europe. This decline did not last but was a sign of what was to come. The Samalas eruption may have triggered a temperature downturn that sea-ice/ocean feedbacks amplified over the next fifty years although some commentators now dispute the impact of the Samalas volcano and focus on possible ozone depletion rather than a depression of global temperature.[15] The North Atlantic Oscillation (the pattern of ocean currents) was largely positive during the MCA helping to send warmer ocean currents toward northern Europe. This pattern changed in the late thirteenth century so that the warmer currents no longer came as close to the European coast producing increased sea ice in the North Atlantic among other impacts.[16] The expansion of sea ice helped expand sea ice in the North Atlantic creating a positive feedback that would help to sustain cold periods such as the Little Ice Age (LIA).[17] Taken together, the decrease in temperature and increase in precipitation sharply curtailed grain yield, had a negative impact on livestock production and even made it difficult to transport food, which was available, from one place to another. In a society that did not enjoy large agricultural surpluses when all of these negative forces came together, short-term famine was likely to result. The continued reinforcement of the progression to a colder climate regime continued to have an effect on the economy and society throughout the fifteenth century and increased thereafter forcing the LIA.

The years 1315, 1316, and 1317 were only slightly colder than usual and did not signal a downward temperature trend. We have no exact measurements of temperatures in those years, but they seem to have been slightly cooler than immediately before or afterward. Cool temperatures that lasted a few days longer in the spring and that appeared a few days earlier in the fall helped shorten the growing season. Summer temperatures were probably somewhat cooler as well so that crops were slower to ripen. Taken together, this reduced the yield for various crops. One bad year produced hardship, but three years running meant that some people had to eat their seed in order to survive leaving little to sow in the spring.

Lower temperatures were only part of the problem. The three years also seem to have had more precipitation than usual. Rain is usually welcome in an agricultural community, but too much rain makes it difficult to harvest crops and leads some crops to rot in the fields. The wetter conditions of 1315–17 also contributed to a decline in grain harvests. Not only did the decline in grain production affect human consumption but it also affected animal consumption so pigs, chicken, geese, sheep, and cattle sickened and died from malnutrition.

Animal disease was also part of the problem that produced an agrarian crisis. Both sheep and cattle were infected and large numbers died.[18] A sheep scab caused the death of many animals as well as led to a decline in wool production. A cattle panzootic spread across central and western Europe during the second decade of the fourteenth century. The chronicler John de Troklowe first reported the cattle plague in Essex about the time of Easter in 1319.[19] Animal diseases were not well-reported in the Middle Ages and even when reported chroniclers tended to not provide symptoms but in this case, rinderpest may have been the culprit.[20] Today, rinderpest is nearly a thing of the past with only a few cases reported in Africa, but in the past, it could be devastating to cattle with close to a one hundred percent mortality rate. The death of a large number of food animals helped to reinforce the dearth that came from the decline in grain production.

A climate-induced shortfall was not able to produce a famine by itself. The climate abnormalities of the early fourteenth century helped to introduce a situation in which famine became possible. The growth of the English population, especially the growing number of poor also made it possible that a food shortage could turn into something worse. Finally, human inaction and action helped to turn the shortfall into a famine. The Crown did little to alleviate the problem, and in some cases, made it worse by purchasing grain to help feed the soldiers going off to war in Scotland. At times, landlords with ample supplies of grain tried to hoard their grain waiting for higher prices.[21] A combination of factors produced famine and near-famine conditions as well as lingering malnutrition.

The decline in agricultural production did not affect everyone in the same way. The well-off still had enough to eat. Peasants, especially those on land holdings that barely supported a family in a good year, faced malnutrition although rarely outright starvation. Not understanding how to cope with the situation, the government of Edward II did little to cope with the situation and baronial landlords were generally no better.[22] In spite of privation, it is difficult to see a Malthusian crisis in which population exceeded carrying capacity producing a decline.[23] There were probably cases of starvation, but malnutrition can have several long-term impacts, unseen at the time as has been detailed in Chapter 2. In this case, malnutrition may have weakened some of the population making them somewhat more susceptible to disease in the future. The relationship between malnutrition and disease is complex and not a simple linear one of malnutrition making people more susceptible to disease. Activation and sustaining an immune response during an infection does require increased energy consumption. The sharp decline in available animal protein that arose from the animal disease of the late 1310s likely produced what is known as protein-energy malnutrition.[24] The long-term impact of the Great Famine on the immunity and health of the English population is difficult to estimate. There may also have been some impact on fertility and child mortality was likely to be exacerbated. Even children who survived the famine may have been somewhat stunted or subject to other diseases later in life.

The agricultural crisis of 1315–22 was very real at the time and caused distress to many people, fostering hostility toward the king in some circles. Like earlier famines, it is difficult to detect a clear impact on the health of the people. The health impact may have more of a long-term issue with the potential for weakened immune systems and children with stunted growth. Even if the rate of population growth had slowed in the early fourteenth century, it seems that England's population was roughly the same size in 1348 as it had been in 1300. Precise estimates of the English population in 1348 are impossible, but a rough estimate of roughly five million people is a useful reference point.

The coming of the Black Death

Even before the plague arrived in England, some chroniclers took notice of it. Henry Knighton, a monk in Leicestershire, had a good grasp of the geographic origin of the disease indicating in his account for 1348: "In this year and the next there was a general plague (*generalis mortalitus*) upon mankind throughout the world. It began in India, then spread to Tartary, and then to the Saracens and finally to the Christians and Jews."[25] Knighton's Indian origin for the disease may have been faulty as it probably originated in central Asia, but it conveys the distance that the disease covered. Most likely, the Second Pandemic originated somewhat in the Mongol Khanate, or the Quinghai-Tibet Plateau in the thirteenth century.[26] It is clear that plague first appeared in the Black Sea region in 1346 with the *Yersinia pestis* bacteria being transported along trade routes from Asia.[27] Connected to a trading system that extended from Asia to the Black Sea and from there across the Mediterranean to northern Europe, England could not escape whatever moved across the trade routes.[28] From 1347 to 1351, the disease spread from central Asia across Europe and back into Russia before dying out only to return periodically for over three hundred years thereafter although never with such a high mortality rate. The disease probably killed from one-third to one-half of the population of Europe in the first outbreak alone. In some places, the death rate was much higher approaching two-thirds of the population. Some older accounts indicate that some regions, such as Poland were spared, but more recent work indicates that no region of Europe escaped the disease.[29]

The variant of *Yersinia pestis* that appeared in Europe in 1347 did not just magically appear. Genomic analysis using samples from medieval cemeteries suggests that the variant that caused the Black Death (Branch 1) branched off from the older plague lineage some time before the fourteenth century, possibly as early as 1170 C.E or by the mid-thirteenth century. What occurred has been labeled the "Big Bang" by some scholars as *Yersinia pestis* mutated in several directions (a polytomy) with Branch 1 producing the Black Death.[30] Branch 1 examples have been found in several medieval cemeteries and have been traced back to Asia. There appears to have been little genetic diversity in the original Black Death outbreak, but analysis of later clades indicates that *Y.pestis* diversified into multiple distinct clades which may have helped to produce multiple disease reservoirs in Europe.[31]

Scholars have mapped the genetic mutation of *Y. pestis* into five major branches and 25 subbranches (or phylogroups).[32] This mutation may occur when one nucleobase on a genome is replaced by a new one and these single nucleotide polymorphisms (SNPs) can then be tracked. Strains on Branch O have been found to be responsible for the Plague of Justinian while Branch 1 contains African Antiqua (1.ANT) and all of the Intermediate (1.IN) and Orientalis (1.ORI) strains that are responsible for the Black Death as well as the Third Pandemic.[33] The strain responsible for the Black Death continued to be the strain infecting Europe until the eighteenth century. It may have gone extinct although a related strain is still present in Africa.[34] As recent work has shown, *Y. pestis* has evolved over time and some strains may have been more virulent than others. Genetics played a major part in how plague-infected England in the fourteenth century and beyond, but other environmental factors, as well as human intervention through trade and pilgrimage routes, also played a role.

The ecology of the period of the various epidemics also played a role in the mortality rate and demographic profile of the plague's victims. Climate change in central Asia helped to foster a situation in which the plague that was endemic in the region became first epidemic and then pandemic. Warmer springs and wetter summers in the region in the early fourteenth century led to an increase in the population of great gerbils, a reservoir host for the fleas carrying the *Yersinia pestis* bacteria. The subsequent expansion of the flea population spread fleas to other animals, humans, and even as stowaways on trade goods to widen the impact of the disease. The plague spread rapidly along trade routes, reaching the Caspian Sea region by 1347 and from there the rest of Europe.[35] One approach indicates that continued climate events in central Asia led to the periodic eruptions of plague that re-infected Europe along sea routes until the early eighteenth century.[36] Other scholars indicate that there may well have been a plague reservoir in Europe that provided for the re-infection of the European population, and that ultimately served to re-infect the central Asian population leading to the Third Plague Pandemic that started in the late eighteenth century.[37]

The plague spread from Asia to Europe by 1347 and continued to spread rapidly across all of Europe by 1351. The widespread incidence of the disease in such a short period has given critics one opening to question the *Yersinia pestis* diagnosis for the Black Death (see Appendix to this chapter). During the Third Pandemic, the plague spread slowly across China and was often a disease of urban areas. The Black Death quickly affected all of Europe although with varying severity. The initial outbreak touched all parts of England and all age groups. Later outbreaks were often centered in London and several seemed to affect children and the poor more than other segments of society. It is apparent that there are differences in the impact of the disease during the Second Pandemic and the Third Pandemic, but as Ole Georg Moseng points out plague has proven to be a versatile disease capable of changing over time, something that those who argue for a strict reading of the documentary record often ignore.[38]

Most scholars indicate that rat fleas (*Xenopsylla cheopis*) were the primary means of transmitting plague, but some speak of human-to-human transmission during the Black Death. Primary pneumonic plague is transmitted from one person to another through aerosol discharges. With primary pneumonic plague the medieval theory of contagion, indicating that plague spread person to person seemed to be upheld. Pneumonic plague has a nearly one hundred percent case mortality rate and is often arises from close human contact as would occur during the winter when people tended to remain indoors. The Black Death may well have included a primary pneumonic plague component, but it is difficult to spread the disease widely because of the short incubation period of pneumonic plague. Recent research, based on London Bills of Mortality, indicates that in the fifteenth- and sixteenth-centuries plague epidemics grew more rapidly than did the Black Death, calling into question whether primary pneumonic plague outbreaks occurred in the fourteenth century.[39] A person infected with primary pneumonic plague quickly became incapacitated and unable to travel. Primary pneumonic plague might account for the quick spread of the disease in a village or neighborhood, but it is not a good candidate for spreading the plague across the country. Rat and human fleas and lice, however, made it possible to spread the disease readily along trade routes.

Arriving in Italy from the Black Sea port of Carfa in 1347, the disease spread northward across Europe over the next few years. The *pestis* reached the southern coast of England in the summer of 1348. The southern ports all engaged in extensive trade with France and so the first case could have appeared in almost any one of them. Henry Knighton indicated that the first case appeared in Southampton while the authors of the *Anonimalle Chronicle* and the *Eulogium Chronicon* both indicated that it was Bristol.[40] Another likely entrée point was

Melcombe Regis (today a suburb of Weymouth) in Dorset. The author of one account indicates:

> In this year 1348, in Melcombe, in the county of Dorset, a little before the feast of St. John the Baptist (24 June), two ships, one of them from Bristol, came alongside. One of the sailors had brought with him from Gascony the seeds of the terrible pestilence and, through him, the men of the town of Melcombe were the first in England to be infected.[41]

Dates for the arrival of the disease also varied from June to late July. Indeed, the plague may have arrived in several ports at different times. Multiple arrivals of plague are likely as most ships departing continental ports during the summer of 1348 likely carried "special" stowaways. Ireland had extensive trade with England and the continent in the mid-fourteenth century and plague made its first appearance in eastern Irish ports in late July or early August, about the same time chroniclers reported it arriving in Bristol.[42] Plague was slower to arrive where waterborne trade routes were less common as it did not reach Scotland until winter 1349 and became widespread in 1350.[43] The chronicler Henry Knighton drew the appropriate moral lesson from how the disease entered Scotland. A Scots army assembled in the forest of Selkirk late in 1349 mocked the England for being struck down by the plague by the avenging hand of God, only to have "a fierce pestilence arose and blew a sudden and monstrous death upon the Scots."[44] Once ensconced in the southern port towns, the plague began to spread via overland trade routes and along the coast from one port to another. It soon spread across Hampshire and was probably at its worst there in early 1349.[45] Late in the fall and early in 1349, cases were being reported in Wiltshire and Berkshire as the disease moved inland from Hampshire and Dorset.[46] Although it is hard to gauge the impact in Wilshire and Berkshire, it seems to have been less than along the coast.

Some observers anticipated the *pestis* before it had arrived on the English coast. As early as May 1348, Edward III had become aware of the spread of plague in France.[47] On 2 September, he suffered a personal loss when Joan, his daughter who was to have married Pedro the heir to the kingdom of Castile, died of the plague in Bordeaux enroute to her husband-to-be. In one of the few instances, in which we can glimpse personal grief over a plague death, Edward's letter to the Queen of Castile displayed the grief of a heartbroken father:

> But see (with what intense bitterness of heart we have to tell your this) destructive Death (who seizes young and old alike, sparing no one, and reducing rich and poor to the same level) has lamentably snatched from both of us our dearest daughter (whom we loved best of all, as her virtues demanded).

> No fellow human being could be surprised if we were inwardly desolated by the sting of this bitter grief, for we are human too.[48]

As the plague became to spread across the countryside, it became evident that some sort of official action was needed. In November, Edward III sent out a call for a meeting of parliament (never held because of the seriousness of the plague epidemic) to discuss "various urgent business and the state of our realm." At the same time, he ordered that no sheriff was to leave his county in an effort to preserve institutional authority to deal with the crisis.[49] As royal and clerical leaders died from the plague, it became difficult to maintain an ongoing response to the disease. A combination of good luck and good leadership was successful overall in preventing a breakdown of order.

Religious leaders also took action before the plague arrived to try to ward off what people often saw as divine punishment. Even as the first cases of plague began to be reported, Archbishop Zouche of York ordered on 28 July 1348 that "devout processions are to be held every Wednesday and Friday" in churches throughout the diocese as well as "a special prayer be said in every mass every day for allaying plague and pestilence."[50] Zouche's order reflected what was happening elsewhere more than what was happening in England, but it presaged a common response of invoking divine intervention in order to ward off the ravages of the plague. Edward III was also alarmed by the account of the plague that reached the royal court and asked the archbishop of Canterbury to provide for prayers against the plague in August. With the death of Archbishop Stratford, it fell to the prior of Christchurch, Canterbury to request the bishop of London to transmit the request to other bishops of the southern province, which he did in October.[51] By late December 1349, as the epidemic had wound its way through southern England. Simon Islip, the new archbishop of Canterbury wrote to the bishops of the southern province ordering a general rejoicing to commemorate the final passage of the disease.[52] As will be seen below, there were other responses to the disease, responses often grounded in efforts to explain it and control it rather than accepting the *pestis* as part of a divine plan.

All paths led to London and probably in November, the disease entered the city. It remained all winter, striking particularly hard from February to July.[53] John of Reading, a Westminster monk, captured the despair verging on nihilism that people must have felt in the winter of 1349: "And there was those days death without sorrow, marriage without affection, self-imposed penance, want without poverty, and flight without escape."[54] Using tax records, Barbara Megson estimates that twenty-five percent of what she calls the well-to-do and at least thirty-five percent of the total population perished.[55] Estimates of the size of London's population and the number of dead, as well as other European cities, vary considerably. Robert Gottfried estimated London's population at 50,000 in 1348.[56] Some estimates of the total number of fatalities range as high as 50,000 which would have been an exaggeration as Britnell points out.[57] A comparative examination of the population of 53 European cities in the mid-fourteenth century indicates, however, that London's population was considerably larger (and cities such as Venice and Florence smaller) than widely accepted estimates such as Gottfried's.[58] A larger population would make the numbers indicated below more plausible. The high number of plague deaths led local authorities to establish two new cemeteries and the possibility exists that most of the plague deaths in 1348–49 were interred in the new East and West Smithfield cemeteries.[59] The Crown appears to have been responsible for opening the West Smithfield cemetery although it seems that a group of leading Londoners was responsible for opening the East Smithfield cemetery in March 1349.[60] Excavations at the East Smithfield cemetery indicate that approximately 12,500 people were interred there with many other victims buried in church yards and other locations. While some of the plague victims interred at the Smithfield sites were accorded a conventional burial with a coffin, others were simply deposited in hurriedly dug plague pits due to the press of time and the lack of manpower.[61] One commentator indicates that the West Smithfield cemetery may have received as many as 50,000 bodies over the course of the outbreak, which was probably an exaggeration but a not unreasonable estimate, if 200 people a day were being buried in London in the spring of 1349 when the worst of the plague had passed, as Robert of Avesbury indicated.[62] We need to treat Avesbury's numbers with care, however. Often medieval writers reported a large round number as exact when they really meant "many, many." Estimates of London's population in the mid–fourteenth century range from 45,000 to 80,000 which would have made a death toll of at least 50,000 truly astounding[63] London's status as an administrative and trade hub made it easy for the disease to spread easily throughout the midlands in early 1349 and probably back to Hampshire and Gloucestershire as well.

The excavations at the East Smithfield site have also helped to address the question of the age and sex of those who died. Chroniclers often based their judgment of the age and sex of the victims on impressionistic evidence but archaeological evidence provides more concrete evidence. The anthropologist Sharon Dewitte argues that the evidence from the London plague pits indicates that the elderly were the more likely victims of the plague, a not unsurprising conclusion as weakened immune systems are often characteristic of the elderly, and that men and women did not exhibit different death rates.[64] Unfortunately, there is less archaeological evidence for later outbreaks so it is currently not possible to test the observations of several chroniclers that more men and children died in the later outbreaks.

Outside of London, the plague exacted differing tolls. In Northamptonshire, the disease seems to have had only a small impact.[65] Based on clerical records, the diocese of Coventry and Lichfield had between a thirty and forty percent death rate with most of the deaths occurring during the summer of 1349.[66] The diocese was northwest of London so the plague had to be transported overland from London and the southern counties. Elsewhere, the story was far more grim. Although the university was closed in Cambridge in response to the plague, possibly as many as half the town died with many bodies flung into a hole in disorderly fashion along what is today, Trinity Street.[67] The rest of East Anglia also had high death rates as well with a large number of deaths in Essex and throughout the diocese of Ely.[68] Plague probably entered East Anglia both overland from London and by sea, increasing its impact. The West Midlands, too, were not spared from the ravages of the plague. Hereford diocese began to record plague deaths in April 1349 and the disease continued to affect the region until October.[69]

Coastal and continental trade in addition to overland trade soon spread the disease to northern England. Probably sea-borne trade served as the means for the disease to enter the north through the ports of Newcastle or Hartlepool. Overland routes made it possible to spread readily throughout Yorkshire as well into Lincolnshire and even remote Durhamshire.[70] Although deadly throughout the north, the disease played havoc with the hilly and remote parts of the diocese of Lincoln.[71] Even Lancashire, one of the most lightly populated counties in the fourteenth century, suffered in late 1349 and early 1350. Although the numbers of reported deaths must always be treated with care, it seems that parts of Lancashire suffered more than almost any part of the country.[72] Unlike what we might expect from some epidemic diseases, the first outbreak of plague often produced higher morbidity and mortality rates in rural rather than in urban areas as it did in remote parts of Lincolnshire, Lancashire, and Durham where small to medium-sized villages suffered greatly.

The rural areas of the northern counties were not alone in reporting death rates close to fifty percent. Parts of Cambridgeshire outside of Cambridge also suffered high mortality rates. London and other towns suffered from the disease, but the *pestis* was also a disease of small villages and isolated monasteries. As long as there was contact with the outside world, the disease had a chance to enter a village and spread. Even when plague was extinguished in a small village, travelers could reintroduce it from a population center such as London. Epidemiologists label such a situation as cycling as the disease seems to spread in almost wave-like fashion.[73] Flight only helped spread the disease from one village to another, as did itinerant traders and other travelers. Fear served to spread the disease in wave-like fashion as people fled as cases developed, causing more cases to occur elsewhere.[74] Fleas could hitch a ride with these travelers and anyone infected with pneumonic plague could carry the disease from one nearby town to another before dying.

Although there were a few stray cases scattered about northern and western counties into 1350, the plague had departed to Ireland, Scotland, and Scandinavia. People probably heaved a sigh of relief once plague cases were no longer being reported, hoping that they had seen the last of it. English society made an effort to get back to a normal life, but this was difficult to do because of a labor shortage and an ensuing food shortage. Nonetheless, marriages occurred and children were born which could have led to the replacement of lost lives over time. Before the country recovered from the first plague outbreak, the disease returned in 1361 and 1362. As occurred before the first visitation in 1348, there were portents of death as the chronicler John of Reading reported an eclipse of the sun on 6 May 1361, a bloody rain that fell in Burgundy, and people saw a bloody cross in the sky over Bologna.[75] The chronicler Ranulph Higden, located in Chester in the west of England, indicated that the plague struck first London around Easter 1361 and then spread across southern England and the rest of country.[76] An anonymous chronicler writing in Canterbury indicated the outbreak was short-lived, lasting four months from the initial outbreak in the summer of 1361.[77] This time the disease seemed to be more discriminating, often killing young people, hence the appellation *pestis puerorum,* children's plague. Henry Knighton, a canon of St. Mary's Leicester, captured both the overall and the personal impact of the outbreak: "In the same year [1361] the people were afflicted by a great mortality, which was called the Second Plague. Both greater and lesser folk died, and especially young people and children. And of our congregation eleven canons died."[78] The death rate for the 1361 epidemic is hard to gauge although Robert Gottfried estimates that twenty percent of the English population died during the epidemic and K. B. McFarlane points out that the death rate of the nobility was higher in the 1361–62 epidemic than in the 1348–50 epidemic.[79] The 1361–63 plague epidemic crisscrossed Europe much as the 1347–50 epidemic had done although with a lower mortality rate. However, even a death rate of only ten to twenty percent on top of the high death rates of the first outbreak continued to reduce the population. The number of deaths in London was such that the cemetery at East Smithfield had to be used once again to inter plague victims, many of whom were children.[80] The economic historian Bruce Campbell goes so far as to indicate that the 1360–63 plague outbreak was second only to the earlier Black Death episode.[81] The combination of the two epidemics produced a block to recovering previous population levels for quite some time.

Although receiving much less attention by the chroniclers when it returned in 1369, the *pestis tertia*, as it was called, also exhibited a high mortality rate, probably killing over ten percent of the population. On this occasion, some of the victims may have died of complications resulting from poor nutrition rather than plague if family breadwinners had died in the 1361 epidemic. The author of the *Anonimalle Chronicle*, for example, pointed out that a large number of the victims were children who might easily have fallen victim to the disease if they were under-nourished because of food shortages.[82] The accounts of the 1369 were brief, however, as the disease had become a way of life to be accorded notice, but no more. The author of the *Anonimalle Chronicle* merely indicates "in 1369 there was third pestilence in England and in several other countries. It was great beyond measure," but provides no detail.[83]

Thereafter, epidemic outbreaks occurred at regular intervals for the rest of the century, sometimes nationally as occurred in 1374–75 and in 1379–80. First reported in southern towns and London, the plague was reported to have killed a large number of people, before moving northward, reaching York by spring of 1375.[84] The epidemic that hit the country as a whole in 1379–80, may have been a combination of bubonic and pneumonic plague. It started in the autumn of 1379, continued throughout the winter and into the autumn of the following year. Bubonic plague that arrived late in the autumn and that did not fully spread to rats and humans might reoccur in the spring with increased flea activity, in what can be called a trans-seasonal epidemic.[85] Thomas Walsingham reported that the 1379 outbreak, which he indicated was caused by a hostile configuration of the planets, was worse in the north of England so "that almost the whole region as rapidly stripped of its best men and among the middle classes it was said that nearly every house was deprived of its residents and standing empty."[86] Walsingham further noted that the Scots took advantage of the English distress and attacked across the border but when local people told them that the plague was God's will they became afraid.[87] This outbreak seems to have killed between ten and twenty percent of the population, matching the mortality rate of the 1361 outbreak although care should be exercised in dealing with the reported number of deaths.[88] Plague returned in 1390 spreading to many parts of England. Walsingham indicated that boys and young men seemed to number many of the victims.[89]

London remained the center for many of the outbreaks subsequent to the 1369 epidemic. After the first outbreak, the plague became more of an urban phenomenon that tended to affect the poor more than the upper elements of society. Localized outbreaks, some producing high death totals such as one that Walsingham noted in and around York in 1391 that reputedly killed eleven thousand people, while others were more limited in impact as those that occurred in Newcastle-on-Tyne in 1409 and Norwich in 1465.[90] In some places, especially monastic communities, the plague settled in leading to almost yearly epidemics. The manorial rolls of Ruthin in Wales reveal that the disease was credited with deaths in 1351, 1354, 1357, 1358, 1359, and 1360.[91] In this case, we might wonder if what appears to have been mini-plague reservoirs served to revive the disease in nearby communities. Even if the plague did not cause all of these deaths, it seems to have come close to becoming endemic in some areas in the late fourteenth and fifteenth centuries.

The Black Death provided a shock to the English demographic system, but if enough time passed population would have begun to recover. The succeeding epidemics of the fourteenth century reduced the population base to a level that reinforced the damage done by the Black Death. After the fourteenth-century outbreaks returned, but on what was close to a ten-year cycle although there were often local outbreaks in intervening years. Because the Black Death was followed almost immediately in 1361 with another epidemic that further decimated the population, it was impossible for the population to recover. Economic historian Mark Bailey places the pre-plague population of England at 5.5 million that was reduced to 2.8 million by 1349 and further reduced to 2.5 million with the 1361 epidemic.[92]

Beyond the Black Death

After the Black Death (1348–50) and its high death rate, plague continued to trouble England the rest of the century and well into the late seventeenth century when the last epidemic occurred. One estimate is that ten large waves of plague afflicted Europe from 1347 to 1453 in addition to numerous local outbreaks.[93] Over time, the respites between national outbreaks grew longer allowing population to start to recover. Small, localized outbreaks, often unrecorded, as well as substantial regional and national outbreaks, continued to occur retarding the growth of population until the sixteenth century. In his history of epidemics in Britain, Charles Creighton indicated a total of 30 in the period from the Black Death to 1485 in which large plague outbreaks occurred.[94] National outbreaks occurred with mortality rates close to ten percent in 1390, 1399–1400, 1405–06.[95] The St. Albans chronicler Thomas Walsingham indicated there was a national epidemic in 1413 although he gave few details.[96] There also seem to have been outbreaks that affected large regions of England in 1433–34, 1471, and 1479–80.[97] The 1433–34 outbreak seems to have affected all of England although London was hard hit. The king prorogued parliament on 13 August 1433 because of the increasing number of deaths which killed "bothe of men, women and children; and namely of worthy men, as aldermen and other worthi communiers.[98] Even localized outbreaks, such as one that struck East Anglia in 1438–39 and may have killed up to twelve percent of the regional population, could have severe consequences. In this case, cold wet weather forced people to huddle close together indoors leading to primary pneumonic plague infecting the population in addition to bubonic plague.[99] The 1479–80 outbreak was so severe in London that the author of *Great Chronicle of London*, who usually concerned himself with only political affairs and the workings of London's economy, spoke of a "huge mortality" in London and the country as a whole with the royal court scattering from London from Easter to midsummer 1480.[100] Although none of these later epidemics produced the mortality rate of the first epidemic, they continued to have an impact often particularly noticeable in small communities afflicted by the disease.

By the end of the fourteenth century, the country's population had declined by approximately sixty percent from the pre-plague level of five million. The continued return of the plague throughout the fifteenth century helped to keep England's population smaller than it had been in 1348. Although deaths might be more scattered or even a large percentage of the population in a small community, some plague epidemics continued to produce high mortality rates. The historian Robert Gottfried estimates that the 1471 outbreak which started in late summer and continued until November may have killed between ten and fifteen percent of the English population.[101] Even when the population began to grow, setbacks such as this continued to make it difficult to recover.

The Black Death and the subsequent outbreaks of the fourteenth century affected both rural and urban communities as geography was no protection. The situation began to change in the fifteenth century. Small communities continued to be afflicted with plague outbreaks, disastrously so in some cases. It was easier for a plague outbreak to sustain itself in urban settings such as London with large numbers of potential victims and so plague was becoming an urban phenomenon so that in the period from 1420 to 1470 there were five national outbreaks, but seven in London alone.[102] In the sixteenth and seventeenth centuries, plague became more urban-centered and London was almost always afflicted by any major epidemic.

Plague epidemics, large and small, continued to break out in England throughout the sixteenth and seventeenth centuries. The accession of the Tudors in 1485 did not end the plague pandemic in England. The disease continued to visit London, but also with national outbreaks throughout the sixteenth century with major outbreaks that affected much of the country in 1544–46, 1563, and 1592–93.[103] Part of the difference from the fourteenth century is that plague had become almost a routine disease with occasional mortality peaks and in doing so had lost some of its ability to generate fear among the people. Whenever urban mortality crises occurred, plague was a major factor although other diseases such as the English Sweat, influenza, and syphilis began to take a hand. At times, plague and another disease stuck at the same time as happened in 1517 with epidemics of first the English Sweat and then plague. The number of plague outbreaks waned in the fifteenth century and did not return in full force throughout the sixteenth century although there were a few severe outbreaks, there would be notably severe plague epidemics in the seventeenth century with outbreaks in 1603–4, 1625–26, and a final visitation in 1665–66.[104] The four major epidemics of 1560, 1603, 1625, and 1665 all had approximately equal mortality rates but the larger population in 1665–66 led to a much larger number of deaths.[105] Appropriately, because it was the death knell of the disease in England, the 1665–66 plague epidemic was unusually severe. The last outbreak severely tried London but the provinces also suffered from the disease.[106] There were no more English plague epidemics after 1665 although a case was recorded in 1679 and there was a scare in 1720–22. There is a possibility that plague persisted in England after 1666 but in such small numbers and isolated settings that it escaped notice. Typhus, for example, was a disease with a presence in the sixteenth century. Some of its symptoms are acute fever, delirium, and petecchiae symptoms that are also present with plague making it difficult to distinguish between the two before the twentieth century when only individual cases are considered. The plague may have trailed off rather than coming to an abrupt halt in 1666.[107] The disease remained active in Western Europe until the early eighteenth century with the Marseilles outbreak of 1720–21 serving as the instigation for Daniel Defoe's *Journal of the Plague Year*. Plague continued to be reported in Russia with the last notice in the 1770s and outbreaks were still being reported in the Ottoman Empire in the early nineteenth century.[108] The Second Plague Pandemic was finally over by the early nineteenth century just in time for its re-emergence in western China by the early nineteenth century.

Most infectious diseases infect a population and once enough people have recovered or died the epidemic is over. The survivors of many diseases such as smallpox or measles have an acquired immunity that will protect them from subsequent outbreaks of the disease. Another epidemic may occur if the disease mutates enough or a different strain is introduced so that acquired immunity is no protection. Over time, as the number of people with acquired immunity declines, it is also possible to reintroduce a disease. An outside reservoir for a disease usually serves as the point of transmission for re-infection. In some cases, no acquired immunity is produced for those people who run the course of the disease, as is the case with the common cold. Influenza, for example, mutates rapidly from year to year so that even vaccines manufactured at the beginning of disease season may not always be completely effective and prevent infection later in the season although it is easier today to tweak vaccines to take into account mutations as pharmaceutical companies have done for COVID-19. Many other diseases may be present in epidemic proportions for a year or two and then seem to disappear for a time as Ebola has done in Africa. Surviving an infection of *Y. pestis* seems to confer immunity for a limited time so that a person could be infected in a later epidemic although people in the fourteenth century may have acquired more lasting immunity.

The accounts of the Black Death generally indicate that the plague was an indiscriminate killer affecting all age groups, men and women, and rich and poor alike. Many of the accounts of the second and third outbreak of plague in the fourteenth century indicate that children were often the victims of the disease. Excavations at the East Smithfield plague cemetery help to provide specific information concerning the victims of the plague as the remains of plague victims can be compared with remains from non-plague cemeteries. When these comparisons are made, it appears that the Black Death killed the same victims, as did many other diseases, i.e., older adults and people in weakened condition with a history of physiological stress.[109] Later outbreaks were also selective. By the late sixteenth century and increasingly in the seventeenth century, plague claimed more live in the poorer sections of London than in the wealthier parishes.[110] Children easily fell victim to plague if they were in a weakened condition. When adults died, this could lead to a decline in food production producing malnutrition that could lower the resistance of children to the plague. Dewitte and Slavin point out that people who survived the Great Famine of 1315–17 may not have been at any increased risk of dying from the plague, but those who survived it or the Bovine Pestilence of 1319–20 may have been in a somewhat weakened condition and less resilient when they encountered the plague.[111] Many survivors were left with a protein deficiency when the milk that had been in their diet was removed by the death of cattle. Environmental conditions played a role both in the spread of the plague with climate conditions affecting the rat population as well as influencing its morbidity and mortality rates.

The First and Second Plague Pandemics each lasted for a few hundred years although not all countries in Europe underwent an epidemic every year, and in some cases, might go 40 or 50 years between outbreaks. Better sources exist for the Second Pandemic than for the First, which, when combined with information about current plague cases, makes it possible to hazard some explanation about why the disease continued for such a long period and to some degree why it vanished in the West in the eighteenth century.

There have been three scholarly phases for explaining the longevity of the plague in England and Western Europe. The first phase often concentrated on the first outbreak, the Black Death of 1347–50 or simply assumed that plague continued to be present in society and included accounts by Philip Zeigler and Robert Gottfried. A more sophisticated explanation is that the disease was periodically transmitted along the same travel paths, via the Silk Road from Central Asia to Europe.[112] Grounded in the process by which the disease first affected Europe, this explanation was often spurred by climate variations that led to a Panzootic that spread the fleas which were the vectors for the *Yersinia pestis* bacteria. This explanation is consistent with the view that the spread of plague occurred in waves coming from maintenance reservoirs, in this case, the population of great gerbils in central Asia.[113] The multiple introduction thesis receives support from a genomic analysis of *Yersinia pestis* that takes historical and climatic data into account as the authors argue for reintroduction from central Asia along traditional trade routes as well as the potential for reintroduction via a northern fur trade route.[114]

Not all epidemics arose from the outside. Plague could also persist in a region, particularly an urban area that provided a home for the hosts for the *Yersinia pestis* carrying fleas such as London in the sixteenth and seventeenth centuries or Ruthin in Wales in the fourteenth century.[115] Eventually, the disease burned itself out and it took an infection from the outside to start a new epidemic. This second explanation intuitively makes sense although for the most part, it leaves unanswered the question of why the disease did not affect Europe after the eighteenth century.

Recently some scholars have begun to question the concept of continual re-infection from the outside. Ann Carmichael indicates that some parts of Europe, most notably some regions of the Alps had been home to substantially greater gerbil populations in the past, providing a maintenance reservoir for the disease in Europe.[116] A central location in the Alps would have made it possible to transmit the disease in periodic epizootics along trade routes. Carmichael concentrates on the cities of northern Italy as the transmission points. It would have been easy once a plague epidemic broke out in Florence, to spread the disease outward, often via sea routes, to other parts of Europe. A genomic analysis of eighteenth-century *Yersinia pestis* genomes taken from the Marseille outbreak in 1722 lends support to Carmichael's argument. The authors indicate that the plague DNA found in the Marseille victims had its ancestry in strains obtained from fourteenth-century plague victims lending support to an argument that the disease may have remained in Europe cycling between human and rodent populations for three centuries.[117] It would have been possible for these regional reservoirs to reinforce local temporary reservoirs continuing to infect people with the same genetic variant of the plague over time.

Two recent studies using ancient DNA (aDNA) from plague victims from the fourteenth through the early eighteenth century indicate that that the *Y. pestis* genome from the beginning and end of the 300-year period was the same, calling into question re-infection with what was likely to be slightly mutated strains from the outside.[118] The presence of plague foci in Europe helps to explain why parts of Europe periodically underwent plague epidemics after the Black Death. The presence of a maintenance reservoir, combined with foci that existed for several years, means that the plague was able to re-emerge especially because surviving a plague infection seems to convey only a temporary immunity. Based on analysis from several European sites, there appear to have been three *Yersinia pestis* genomes with low genetic diversity that contributed to the Second Plague Pandemic. This European plague focus most likely became extinct by the early eighteenth century, but not before enabling the disease to return to Asia via the Silk Road and become the source for the Third Plague Pandemic.[119]

An ambitious analysis of 34 *Yersinia pestis* taken from sites throughout Western Europe from the period from the fourteenth to the eighteenth century shows that at least two distinct clades evolved producing several strains of plague post Black Death. This analysis tentatively argues for more than one reservoir in or close to Europe, but the authors indicate that further analysis particularly of Asian samples is necessary in order to rule out re-infection from central Asia.[120] Plague once appeared to be well-described with a high degree of certainty. This is no longer the case. Advances in paleopathology are contributing to new evidence concerning the Second Plague Pandemic even though there are still some unanswered questions, most notably: why did the genome that produced the Black Death go extinct? A variety of answers have been offered over time such as improved quarantine practices, but quarantine would have been more helpful in dealing with pneumonic rather than bubonic plague. Other changes in public health practices such as improved sanitation may have also played a role. Paleopathology may help to deliver a satisfactory answer, most likely that the clade infecting Western Europe had gone extinct so that an existing reservoir in Europe or Asia could not replace local plague reservoirs.

The impact of the Second Pandemic is not simply the description of death rates and outbreaks. The plague had a human, artistic, and economic impact that is difficult to assess, yet is the real impact of the plague on society. The next chapter will build on the description of the disease provided here in examining how society reacted to the plague pandemic and how it affected society. Understanding the magnitude of the continuing plague outbreaks during the Second Pandemic can help to provide insights into how the plague affected society.

Appendix: Diagnosing the plague

For a time, there was a debate concerning whether the disease that led to the Black Death and millions of deaths was the plague or some other disease. Today that debate has been resolved. The plague was the plague even if the characteristics of the Second Pandemic do not mirror those of the Third Pandemic. Understanding the implications of this debate enables us to understand the role of infectious disease in the past and how modern scholars conceptualize it, and why retrospective diagnosis can play an important role in understanding how various diseases have affected society in the past.

Some historians, such as Robert Gottfried label almost all of the late fourteenth and fifteenth outbreaks of epidemic disease as the plague. Other scholars, such as Samuel K. Cohn Jr., have argued that the causative agent for the First and Second Pandemics could not have been *Yersinia Pestis*.[121] This discrepancy illustrates the difficulty in retrospective diagnosis, but should not be taken as an argument against it.

Part of the problem with retrospective diagnosis is that sources from the past are not always what they could be in terms of accuracy or the detail of information conveyed. As indicated in Chapter 1, terminology has changed over time making it challenging, at times, to know if a medieval writer was talking about the same disease as a modern writer. As was indicated in the Introduction, it is important to take what contemporaries said at face value and not try to interpret their views so that they fit modern frameworks for disease. However, it is possible to parse out lists of symptoms that can be compared to those generated by modern diagnostic tools and by careful reading and comparison of the sources to arrive at some characteristics of diseases as well as demographic information. The tools of paleopathology such as DNA testing can also help to construct a picture of a disease in the past and laboratory tests and fieldwork can often shed insights into how diseases spread. In some cases, laboratory tests of aDNA from different eras can also help to determine how a pathogen evolved over time. More recently mathematical modeling helps to trace the development of genomes over time. These approaches are not the typical tools of the historian but all are useful as historians try to understand aspects of the past.

Descriptions of symptoms in the past can be problematic. Even today, physicians first rely upon the patient's reported symptoms when making a diagnosis, turning to the laboratory for confirmation and medieval medical men were no different. Here, we have a problem as most of the medieval and early modern English accounts contain little concrete information regarding symptoms. Writing in the fourteenth century, Geoffrey le Baker provides the most fulsome list of plague symptoms describing what he calls boils and black pustules on various parts of the body. He indicated that some people went to bed healthy but were dead the next morning.[122] Few diseases can kill this fast although primary pneumonic plague and primary septicemic plague come close as does hemorrhagic smallpox. What is more likely, is that Geoffrey was trying to convey the severity of the disease and was not aware of the early symptoms. A few chroniclers, such as Robert of Avesbury, described how quickly people died once infected as he indicated that often infected people died three or four days after symptoms became evident which is more likely than Geoffrey's timing.[123] Some continental sources are more forthcoming in describing symptoms. Guy de Chauliac, the papal physician in Avignon at the time of the Black Death, indicated that the disease often killed within two days, especially those people who were coughing blood. He also indicated that many victims had what he called carbuncles (buboes), particularly on the groin and armpits.[124] Ironically, it was not a physician but the Italian writer Giovanni Boccaccio in his book the *Decameron* who provided one of the best descriptions of the symptoms of the Black Death. He spoke of tumors in the groin and armpits the size of eggs as the first sign of the disease. Often these tumors were followed by black spots appearing on various parts of the body, often a sign of impending death.[125] Most accounts concentrated on the impacts of the disease, not the symptoms. The descriptions of symptoms seem to indicate a disease that progressed too quickly to have been the plague (or almost any other disease), but these symptoms did not always appear until the disease was well underway. Even though primary pneumonic plague infections kill quickly once symptoms become manifest, pneumonic plague victims rarely died overnight as Geoffrey le Baker indicated. Could this have simply been an exaggeration on Geoffrey's part or misinformation on his part rather than a misdiagnosis? Here too, we must guard against a pedantic and literal interpretation that gives too much precision to inexact sources.

More so than other infectious diseases, the plague has the capability to cause the continuing high mortality rates of the epidemics that comprised the Second Pandemic. Moreover, the pattern of summertime outbreaks fits the usual progression of bubonic plague. If some of the epidemics also included pneumonic plague, mortality rates were likely to increase and large numbers of deaths would occur during the winter. The various local outbreaks of the pest are characteristic of *Y. pestis* when it becomes endemic in a region. Certainly, many people at the time saw no difference in the various outbreaks and people generally labeled the disease *pestis* implying a single disease.

These problems coupled with other issues arising from comparing the Second and Third Pandemics have led some biologists and historians to call into question the plague diagnosis. Their arguments have taken different forms but tend to revolve around questions of mortality rates, the timing of the outbreaks, how rapidly the disease spread, the means of transmission, and the demographic profile of the victims. In constructing their arguments, the plague critics have tended to compare the Second (and by implication the First) Pandemic with the Third Pandemic that affected China and India at the turn of the twentieth century.

Biologists critical of the plague diagnosis for the Black Death question whether the high mortality rate could have been caused by one disease and contrast the course of the Second Pandemic with that of the Third Pandemic as they examine timing, symptoms, and the spread of the disease. J.F.D. Shrewsbury argued that bubonic plague caused most of the deaths during the 1348–49 epidemic, but indicated that typhus alternated with *Y. pestis* in later outbreaks and that smallpox, measles, dysentery, pneumonia, influenza, and enteric fevers were also commonplace in the fourteenth and fifteenth centuries.[126] He, at least, accepted that *Y. Pestis* was present in the fourteenth century and contributed to the death toll. The zoologist Graham Twigg called the plague diagnosis itself into question in his discussion of the Black Death. He based his argument on the discrepancies between the Third Pandemic and the Second Pandemic especially in regard to how fast the plague spread in the fourteenth century and its means of transmission. Twigg also indicated that flea-carrying rats could not have been the means of transmission for *Yersina pestis* in the fourteenth century. The black rat and its flea *X. cheopis* provided the primary means of transmission for the plague in India and China at the turn of the twentieth century. Colder conditions in northern Europe would have made it difficult for *X. cheopis* to sustain itself and the black rat did not seem to be present in northern Europe in the fourteenth century.[127] Twigg argued that anthrax, not plague was the likely culprit although he did not develop this argument. Later critics continued to raise in one way or another the issues that Twigg raised in his commentary.

Twigg fired the opening shot it the attack on the plague diagnosis, but it was not the last. Writing fifteen years after the publication of Twigg's book the demographer, Susan Scott and the zoologist Christopher Duncan expanded the criticism of the plague diagnosis chronologically and scientifically, dealing with the full Second Pandemic in England. They questioned whether fleas could have spread the disease. Grounding their assault in epidemiological theory, Scott and Duncan indicated that plague could not have produced the large number of recorded deaths. They referred to the disease as a hemorrhagic plague, placing it among such hemorrhagic fevers as Ebola and Marburg that were receiving a good deal of attention in the last decades of the twentieth century. In a second book, they took issue with research that cast doubt on their hypothesis and argued that some sort of hemorrhagic plague could reappear.[128] Scott and Duncan focused largely on the biology of the Black Death, but another account examined the spread of the disease. George Christakos, Ricardo A. Olea, Marc L. Serre, Hwa-Lung Yu, and Lin-Lin Wang applied a mathematical approach based in stochastic modeling to examine the spread of the disease. They questioned how previous commentators had conceptualized the spread of the disease as well as the data they used in constructing their assumptions. Shrewsbury and Twigg provided much of the biological ammunition they used for criticizing the plague diagnosis. After constructing their own spatiotemporal stochastic model for the spread of the disease, Christakos and associates tested it and found that plague, as conceptualized from the Third Pandemic, could not have spread as far and as fast as the Black Death of the fourteenth century moved.[129] This novel and sophisticated approach to disease modeling further added to questions concerning the plague diagnosis although it can be criticized for its assumptions regarding the fourteenth-century sources as well as the assumptions drawn from direct comparisons of pandemics in different places and times.

The plague diagnosis critics noted above often focused on one aspect of the Black Death. The historian Samuel Cohn, Jr. has provided a wide-ranging attack on the plague diagnosis well-grounded in historical research, information drawn from accounts of the Third Pandemic, and recent scientific research and has become the critic that all supporters of the plague diagnosis must respond to in developing their arguments.[130] Cohn's and the other critics' arguments against the *Yersinia pestis* may be summarized as follows:

- The symptoms of the Black Death are different than those of modern plague, e.g., buboes in the neck and armpits for medieval plague and in the groin for modern plague.

- The mortality rates and age and sex distribution of victims are different, more children in the post-1348–50 sample than in the Third Pandemic in India and more men than women died during the Second Pandemic. Much higher mortality rate for medieval than modern plague.
- People appeared to exhibit acquired immunity in the Middle Ages, something not present with modern plague.
- The Black Death spread far more rapidly over a large area than did the modern plague.
- The is a lack of evidence for black rats, *Rattus rattus* and their fleas *Xenopsylla cheopis* with medieval and early modern plague, while rat fleas were an important means of transmission during the Third Pandemic.

The plague critics quite correctly highlighted differences between the Second (and First) Pandemic and the Third Pandemic. Taken together these points relate back to other critics, especially the spatiotemporal dimension and the lack of evidence of the presence of fleas that are potentially telling. The plague diagnosis critics have not been without critics who have addressed their points often from the perspective of science.[131]

All of the plague critics are correct in pointing up the differences between the Second and Third Pandemics. These are important differences, but they often do not take into account the five-hundred-year gap between the Black Death and the late nineteenth century or the different environmental and public health conditions of the two eras. The late fourteenth-century outbreaks often claimed more male children and young men among their victims but children were potential victims in any case. The death of adults may have led to food shortages that could have left children somewhat weakened and easy targets for any sort of infectious disease. Cohn and others have pointed out that plague outbreaks quickly followed on one another during the Third Pandemic but that a gap existed from 1350 to 1361 for the first and second outbreaks with similar gaps to follow. Whether human fleas and lice or rat fleas, the death of the infected fleas took away the hosts for *Y. pestis* smaller communities. Cycling meant that the plague reservoirs in larger towns such as London would eventually replenish the host population in the provinces making possible another outbreak but this took time. It might take several years before the plague bacteria that remained in towns spread to other times or the countryside.[132] *Yersina pestis* remained relatively stable from the fourteenth to the eighteenth century although it diversified into several genetically different clades over the centuries.[133] The phenotype of *Y. pestis* had evolved from that of the fourteenth century but overall, there was a low within outbreak diversity of the disease but enough diversity so that local foci could develop.

Transmission of the *Yersinia pestis* bacteria has been a point of contention. Rat fleas were the primary means of transmission during the Third Pandemic. Even during outbreak of plague in India in the early twentieth-century commentators, such as Hankin pointed out that rat fleas were not the only means of transmission.[134] In the early 1940s, Blanc and Baltazard raised the possibility of plague transmission by human fleas, *Pulex irritans* based on their research concerning a plague outbreak in Morocco in 1940.[135] Recent work indicates that human fleas are a likely means of transmission as are human lice so that the lack of black rats and rat fleas in the fourteenth century becomes a non-issue.[136] Recent work indicates that human ectoparasites were the likely means for spreading the plague, at least during the Black Death, rather than rat fleas or human-to-human spread of pneumonic plague.[137] Transmission of plague by human fleas and lice makes it possible for the plague to cover long distances rapidly as human carriers take them from place to place over land and sea. Continued archaeological work and DNA analysis, especially at the East Smithfield site, help to confirm that the skeletons sampled were plague victims.[138]

Part of the difficulty in developing a retrospective diagnosis for the plague as well as other diseases is that historians and scientists often speak past each other. They often consider quite different sorts of evidence and at times are unable to come to grips with arguments outside their own fields. As various scholars such as Michael McCormick have indicated, a consilience of disciplinary perspectives is often necessary for dealing with some questions from the past. The anthropologist Fabian Crespo and the microbiologist Matthew Lawrenz make the point that immunologists need to be aware of environments and social context and historians should be aware of the complexity of the immune system.[139] This multidisciplinary approach makes possible a definitive diagnosis for the causative agent for the First and Second Pandemics and that will help to enhance our knowledge concerning other diseases of the past.

Although Cohn continues to fight a rear-guard action, most scholars have adopted the perspective emphatically put by the historian Monica Green: "The question 'What was the pathogen?' has been decisively resolved."[140] As Green points out, it is now time to turn our attention to questions such as explaining how climatic change affected the initial outbreak as well as later outbreaks of plague, how plague pandemics originated on the Tibetan-Qinghai Plateau, or which animal hosts served as carriers for the initial spread of the disease. It may become possible to apply the lessons learned from the process of developing a retrospective diagnosis for the plague to explaining other epidemics in the past as well as how "new" diseases arise, spread, and affect society. Two of these "new" diseases, the English Sweat and syphilis, will appear in Chapters 7 and 8.

Examination of the debate concerning "what disease was plague?" helps to show some of the difficulties of examining disease in past time. It also illustrates the importance of new tools such as paleopathology for historians. The documentary record is important in understanding the impact of diseases on society and how society reacted to them. The documentary record and the archaeological record taken together give us insights into what diseases people had to cope with, how these diseases affected people, and how they changed over time. This latter point enables comparative work dealing with disease and its impact over time.

Notes

1 M.M. Postan, "Some Economic Evidence of Declining Population in the Late Middle Ages," *Econ.HistRev*, 2d ser., 2 (1950), 221–46. Postan's views on late medieval population have been widely debated. A useful discussion can be found in John Hatcher and Mark Bailey, *Modeling the Middle Ages* (Oxford: Oxford University Press, 2001).
2 F.W.D. Brie, ed., *The Brut*, 2 vols. (EETS, 131, 136, 1906–08), 136: 467.
3 B.M.S. Campbell, *English Seigniorial Agriculture* (Cambridge: Cambridge University Press, 2000), pp. 403–05. R.M. Smith, "Human Resources," in G. Astill and A. Grant, eds., *The Countryside of Medieval England* (Oxford: Basil Blackwell 1988), 189–91.
4 Gregory Clark, "The Long March of History: Farm Wages, Population, and Economic Growth, England 1209–1869," *EconHisRev*, 60 (2007), 120. Not all scholars would agree with deriving population from the marginal product of labor as Clark does.
5 Philip Ziegler, *The Black Death* (New York: Harper, 1969), 179. Edmund Venables, ed., *Chronicon Abbatiae de Parco Ludae*, A.R. Maddison, trans., (Horncastle: Lincolnshire Record Society, 1891), 38–9.
6 J.F.C. Hecker seems to have coined the term Black Death to describe the fourteenth-century epidemic. *The Black Death in the Fourteenth Century*, B.G. Babington, trans. (London, 1833).
7 William H. McNeill, *Plagues and Peoples* (Garden City: Anchor Press, 1976).
8 Bruce M.S. Campbell, *The Great Transition* (Cambridge: Cambridge University Press, 2016).
9 *Thomas Wright's Political Songs of England from the Reign of John to that of Edward II*. Peter Coss, ed., (Cambridge: Cambridge University Press, 1996 [1839]), 239.
10 William Chester Jordan, *The Great Famine* (Princeton: Princeton University Press, 1996), 25.
11 Jordan, *Great Famine*, 21.
12 David Stone, "The Impact of Drought in Early Fourteenth Century England," *EconHistRev*, 67 (2014), 435–62. The years preceding the fourteenth century, often referred to as the Medieval Climate Anomaly, appear to often been characterized by drought conditions. Samuli Helama, Jouko Meriläinen, Heikki Toumenvirta, "Multicentennial Megadrought in Northern Europe Coincided with a Global El Niño-Southern Oscillation Drought Pattern during the Medieval Climate Anomaly," *Geology*, 37 (2009), 175–8.
13 Fa-Hu Chen, J.H. Chen, J. Holmes, et al., "Moisture Changes over the Last Millennium in Arid Central Asia: A Review, Synthesis, and Comparison with Monsoon Region," *Quaternary Science Reviews*, 29 (2010): 1055–68. Michael E. Mann, Z. Zhang, S. Rutherford, Raymond S. Bradley, Malcolm K. Hughes, et al., "Global Signatures and Dynamical Origins of the Little Ice Age and Medieval Climate Anomaly," *Science*, 326 (2009): 1256–60. Michael E. Mann, Z. Zhang, M.K. Hughes, Rayomnd S. Bradley, Sonya K. Miller, et al., "Proxy-based Reconstruction of Hemispheric and Global Surface Temperature Variations over the Past Two Millennia," *PNAS*, 105 (2008): 13252–7.
14 Franck Lavigne, J.P. Degeai, JC. Komorowski, Sébastien Guillet, Vincent Robert, et al., "Source of the Great A.D. 1257 Mystery Eruption Unveiled, Samalas Volcano, Rinjani Volcanic Complex, Indonesia," *PNAS*, 110 (2013): 16742–7. Céline M. Vidal, J.C. Komorowski, N. Métrich, Indyo Pratomo, Nugraha Katadinata et al., "Dynamics of the Major Plinian Eruption of Samalas in 1257 A.D. (Lombok Indonesia)," *Bulletin of Volcanology*, 77:73 (2015): 1–24; Céline M. Vidal, Nicole Métrich, Jean-Christophe Komorowski, Indyo Pratomo, Agnés Michel, et al., "The 1257 Samala Eruption (Lombok, Indonesia): The Single Greatest Stratospheric Gas Release of the Common Era," *Nature: Scientific Reports*, 6 (2016): 34868. It is estimated that there have been ten eruptions of VEI-7 magnitude in the last 10,000 year.

15 B.M.S. Campbell, "Global Climates, the 1257 Mega-Eruption of Samalas Volcano, Indonesia, and the English Food Crisis of 1258," *TRHS*, 6th ser., 27 (2017), 87–121. David C. Wade, Céline M. Vidal, N. Luke Abraham, Sandip Dhomse, Paul T. Griffins, et al., "Reconciling the Climate and Ozone Response to the 1257 CE Mount Samalas Eruption," *PNAS*, 117 (2020), 26651–26659.

16 Valérie Trouet, Jan Esper, Nicholas E. Graham, Andy Baker, James D. Scourse, David C. Frank, "Persistent Positive North Atlantic Oscillation Mode Dominated the Medieval Climate Anomaly," *Science*, 324 (2009), 78–80. Gifford H. Miller, Áslaug Geirsdóttir, Yafang Zhong, Darren J. Larsen, Bette L. Otto-Bliesner, et al., "Abrupt Onset of the Little Ice Age Triggered by Volcanism and Sustained by Sea-Ice/Ocean Feedbacks," *Geophysical Research Letters*, 39 (2012), L02708. Carl-Friederich Schleussner and G. Feulner, "A Volcanically Triggered Regime Shift in the Subpolar North Atlantic Ocean as a Possible Origin of the Little Ice Age," *Climate of the Past*, 9 (2013), 1321–30.

17 Flavio Lehner, Andreas Rorn, Christophy C. Raible, Thomas F. Stocker, "Amplified Inception of European Little Ice Age by Sea Ice-Ocean-Atmospheric Feedbacks," *Journal of Climate*, 26 (2013), 7586–7602.

18 For sheep mortality, see: Ian Kershaw, "The Great Famine and Agrarian Crisis in England 1315–1322," *Past and Present*, 59 (1973): 14–46, as well as Jordan, *Great Famine*.

19 H.T. Riley, ed., *Johannis de Trokelowe, Annales* (London: Rolls Series: 28:3, 1866), 104–5.

20 Timothy P. Newfield, "A Cattle Panzootic in Early Fourteenth-Century Europe," *Agricultural History Review*, 57 (2009): 155–90. Philip Slavin, "The Fifth Rider of the Apocalypse: The Great Cattle Plague in England and Wales and its Economic Consequences, 1319–1350," in Simonetta Cavaciocchi, ed., *Le Interazioni Fra Economia E Ambiente Biologico Nell'Europa Preindustriale Secc. XIII–XVIII* (Florence: University of Florence Press, 2010): 165–79.

21 Philip Slavin, "Climate and Famines: A Historical Reassessment," *Wiley Interdisciplinary Reviews: Climate Change*, 7 (2016): 433–47. Slavin, "Market Failure During the Great Famine in England and Wales (1315–1317)," *Past and Present*, 222 (2014): 9–49.

22 Jordan, *Great Famine*, p. 177.

23 M.M. Postan first presented the argument for a Malthusian crisis in the early fourteenth century (see n.1). Postan's argument has come in for a good deal of criticism as commentators question the evidence for population decline and in the case of Zvi Razi arguing that population in the parish of Halesowen increased from 1310 to 1319. *Life, Marriage and Death in a Medieval Parish* (Cambridge: Cambridge University Press, 1980), 22–34. See also, B.F. Harvey, "The Population Trend in England between 1300 and 1348," *TRHS*, 16 (1966): 23–42.

24 Ann G. Carmichael, "Hidden Hunger, and History," *Journal of Interdisciplinary History* 14 (1983): 249–64. Ulrich E. Schaible and Stefan H.E. Kaufman, "Malnutrition and Infection: Complex Mechanisms and Global Impacts," *PLoS Medicine* 4 (2007), 0806–0812. Peter Katona and Judit Katona-Apte, "The Interaction between Nutrition and Infection," *Clinical Infectious Diseases*, 46 (2008), 1582–8.

25 G.H. Martin, ed. and trans., *Knighton's Chronicle, 1337–1396* (Oxford: Oxford University Press, 1995), 94–95.

26 Two recent works concerning the geographic origin of the Second Plague Pandemic that include relevant bibliography are Monica H. Green, "The Four Black Deaths," *American Historical Review*, 125 (2020), 1601–31, and Ole J. Benedictow, *The Complete History of the Black Death* (Woodbridge: Boydell Press, 2021), 137–52.

27 Hannah Barker, "Laying the Corpses to Rest: Grain Embargoes, and *Yersinia pestis* in the Black Sea, 1346–48," *Speculum*, 96 (2021), 97–126.

28 Janet L. Abu-Lughod, *Before European Hegemony* (Oxford: Oxford University Press, 1989), 33–35.

29 There are numerous general accounts of the Black Death but none that cover all of the Second Pandemic. A good general account of the historical aspects of the Black Death that deals with its origins, its spread, and mortality rates is Benedictow, *History of the Black Death*. John Aberth's, *The Black Death* (Oxford: Oxford University Press, 2021) is a useful, readable account of the Black Death including the scientific debate. Although some of his conclusions may be suspect, J.F.D. Shrewbury provides a comprehensive account of the plague in England from 1348 to the late seventeenth century, including a diocese by diocese narrative for the Black Death. *A History of Bubonic Plague in the British Isles* (Cambridge: Cambridge University Press, 1970).

30 Maria A. Spyrou, Rezeda I. Tukbatova, Chuan-Chao Wang, Aida Andrades Valtueña, Aditya K. Lankapali, et al., "Analysis of 3800-Year-Old *Yersinia pestis* Genomes Suggests Bronze Age Origin for Bubonic Plague," *Nature Communications*, 9 (2018):2234, supplemental table 9. Yujun Cui, Chang Yu, Yamfeng Yan, Dongfang Li, Thibaut Jombart, et al., Historical Variations in Mutation Rate in an Epidemic Pathogen, *Yersinia pestis*," PNAS, 110 (2013), 577–82. Amine Namouchi, Meriam Guellil, Oliver Kersten, Stephanie Hänsch, Claudio Ottoni, et al., "Integrative Approach Using *Yersinia pestis* Genomes to Revisit the Historical Landscape of Plague During the Medieval Period," *PNAS*, 115 (2018), e11790–e11797. Green, "Four Black Deaths."

31 Maria A. Spyrou, Marcel Keller, Rezeda I. Tukhbatova, Christina L. Scheib, Elizabeth A. Nelson, et al., "Phylogeography of the Second Plague Pandemic Revealed through Analysis of Historical *Yersinia pestis* Genomes," *Nature Communications*, 10 (2019), 4470.

32 Yujan Cui, Chang Yu, Yanfeng Yan, Dongfan Li, Yanjun Li, et al., "Historical Variations in Mutation Rate in an Epidemic Pathogen, *Yersinia Pestis*," *PNAS*, 110 (2013), 577–82. A good discussion of the genetics of the plague that relates medieval plague to plague in the modern world may be found in Monica H. Green, "Taking 'Pandemic' Seriously: Making the Black Death Global," *Medieval Globe* 1 (2014), 27–61, at 36–40, and Green, "Four Black Deaths," 1607–15.

33 Michaela Harbeck, Lisa Seifert, Stephanie Hänach, David M. Wagner, Dawn Birsell, et al., "*Yersinia pestis* DNA from Skeletal Remains from the 6th Century AD Reveals Insights into Justinianic Plague," *PloS Pathogens* 9, no. 5 (2013): e1003349. Cui, "Historical Variations in Mutation Rate," In the 1950s, scientists described a three-part approach to describing different strains of the plague: "Antiqua," "Medievalis," and "Orientalis" according to the ability of different strains to reduce nitrate and ferment glycerol. This approach has been shown to be misleading and many scholars have moved away from it although the terms are still used in some circles. Mark Achtman, Giovanna Morelli, Peixuan Zhu, Thierry Wirth, Ines Diehl, et al., "Microevolution and History of the Plague Bacillus, *Yersinia pestis*," *PNAS*, 101 (2004), 17837–42.

34 Green, "Taking 'Pandemic' Seriously," 42. Spyrou, et al. "Historical *Y. Pestis* Genomes, 874. Cui et al., "Historical Variations in Mutation Rate in an Epidemic Pathogen," 577–82.

35 Nils Chr. Stenseth, N.I. Samla, H. Viljugrein,K.L Kausrud, M. Begen, et al., "Plague Dynamics Are Driven by Climate Variation," *PNAS* (2006): 1310–5. Boris V. Schmid, Ulf. Büntgen, W.Ryan. Easterly, Christian Ginzler, Lars Walløe, et al., "Climate-Driven Introduction of the Black Death and Successive Plague Reintroductions into Europe," *PNAS*, 112 (2015): 3020–5.

36 Schmid, et al., "Climate-Driven Introduction of the Black Death."

37 Ann G. Carmichael, "Plague Persistence in Western Europe: A Hypothesis," *Medieval Globe*, 1 (2014): 157–9. Lisa Seifert, Ingrid Weichmann, Michaela Harbeck, Astrid Thomas, Gisela Grupe, et al., "Genotyping *Yersinia pestis* in Historical Plague: Evidence for Long-Term Persistence of *Y. pestis* in Europe from the 14th to the 17th century," *PloS One*, 11 (2015), e0145194. Maria A. Spyrou, Rezeda I. Tukhbatova,

Michel Feldman, Joanna Drath, Sacha Kachi, et al., "Historical *Y. pestis* Genomes Reveal the European Black Death as the Source of Ancient and Modern Plague Pandemics," *Cell Host and Microbe* 19 (2016): 974–81.

38 Ole Georg Moseng, "Climate, Ecology and Plague: The Second and Third Pandemic Reconsidered," in Lars Bisgaard and Leif Søndergaard, eds., *Living with the Black Death* (Odense: University Press of Southern Denmark, 2009), 23–49.

39 David J.D. Earn, Junling Ma, Hendrik Poinar, Jonathan Dushoff, and Benjamin M. Bolker, "Acceleration of Plague Outbreaks in the Second Pandemic," *PNAS*, 117 (2020), 22703–11.

40 *Knighton's Chronicle*, 98–99; V.H. Galbraith, ed., *The Anonimalle Chronicle, 1333–1381* (Manchester, 1927), 30; F. Scott Hayden, ed., *Eulogium Chronicon Sive Temporis*, 3 vols. (Rolls Series, 9, 1858), I: 344.

41 Antonia Grandsden, "A Fourteenth-Century Chronicle from the Grey Friars of Lynn," *English Historical Review* 72 (1957), 274. Robert of Avesbury and Ranulf Higden confirm this entrée point. Edward Maunde Thompson, ed., *Adae Murimuth continuate chronica Robert de Avesbury de gestis mirabilus regis Edwardi Tertii* (Rolls Series, 93, 1893), 406; C. Babington and J.R. Lumby, eds., *Polychronicon Ranulphi Higden monachi Cestrensis*, 9 vols. (London: Rolls Series, 41, 1866), 2: 213. See also, J.M.J. Fletcher, "The Black Death in Dorset (1348–49)," *Proceedings of the Dorset Natural History and Antiquarian Field Club*, 43 (1922): 1–14.

42 Maria Kelly, *A History of the Black Death in Ireland* (Stroud: Tempus, 2001), 22.

43 Karen Jillings, *Scotland's Black Death* (Stroud: Tempus, 2003), 22, 13.

44 *Knighton's Chronicle*, 100–103.

45 Tom Beaumont Jones, "The Black Death in Hampshire," *Hampshire Papers*, 18 (1999), 4.

46 Tom Beaumont Jones, "The Black Death in Berkshire and Wiltshire," *Hatcher Review*, 46 (1998): 11–20.

47 *Calendar of Papal Letters, 1342–62*, W.H. Bliss and C. Johnson, ed. (London, 1897), 3: 37–8.

48 Thomas Rymer, ed., *Foedera, Conventiones, Litterae, et cujuscunque generis acta publica*, 20 vols. (London: Record Commission, 1704–35), 3: 39–40.

49 *Calendar of Close Rolls*, Edward III, 3: viii, 1346-49 (London, 1892–1975) 606–07.

50 James Raine, ed., *Historical Papers and Letters from Northern Registers* (London: Rolls Series, 61, 1873), 395–7.

51 D. Wilkins, *Concilia Magnae Britanniae et Hiberniae*. 4 vols. (London, 1739), 2: 738. The bishops of Exeter and Hereford both received the letter and ordered prayers in their dioceses. C. Hingeston-Randolph, ed., *The Register of John de Grandisson, 1327–1369*. 3 vols. (Canterbury and York Society, 1894–99), 2: 1069–70. J.H. Parry, ed., *Registrum Johannis de Trillek, episcopi Herefordensis, A.D. MCCCXLIV-MCCCLXI* (Canterbury and York Society, 1912), 137–9. This same approach would be followed with later outbreaks as when Simon Sudbury, Archbishop of Canterbury called for prayers during the 1375 outbreak. Wilkins, *Concilia*, 3:100–01.

52 Wilkins, *Concilia*, 2: 752.

53 Robert of Avesbury, *De gestis mirabilus regis Edwardi Terti*, p 407.

54 James Tait, ed., *Chronica Johannis de Reading et Anonymi Cantuarienis* (Manchester: Manchester University Press, 1914), 109.

55 Barbara E. Megson, "Mortality among London Citizens in the Black Death," *Medieval Prosopography*, 19 (1998), 125.

56 Robert S. Gottfried, *The Black Death: Natural and Human Disaster in Medieval Europe* (New York: Free Press, 1983), 64.

57 R. Britnell, "The Black Death in English Towns," *Urban History*, 21 (1994), 185–210, 199.

58 Ricardo Olea and George Christakos, "Duration of Urban Mortality for the 14th-Century Black Death Epidemic," *Human Biology*, 77 (2005), 291–303.

59 Duncan Hawkins, "The Black Death and the New London Cemeteries of 1348," *Antiquity,* 64 (1990): 642.

60 Barney Sloane, *The Black Death in London* (Stroud: The History Press, 2011), 52–57, 90–97.

61 Ian Grainger, Duncan Hawkins, Lynne Cowal, and Richard Mikulski, *The Black Death Cemetery, East Smithfield, London* (London: Museum of London Archaeology Service, 2008), 28. Sloan, *Black Death in London*, 95–98.

62 Britnell "Black Death in English Towns," 198–99. Robert of Avesbury, *De Gestis mirabilibus Regis Edwardi Terti,* 407.

63 D. Keene, "London *circa* 600–1300: The Growth of a Capital," *Franco-British Studies* 17 (1994): 26, 48–49.

64 Sharon N. Dewitte, "Age Patterns of Mortality during the Black Death in London, A.D. 1349–1350," *Journal of Archaeological Science,* 37 (2010), 3394–3400. Dewitte, "The Anthropology of Plague: Insights from Bioarchaeological Analyses of Epidemic Cemeteries," *Medieval Globe,* 1 (2014), 97–123. Dewitte, "Mortality Risk and Survival in the Aftermath of the Medieval Black Death," *PLoS One,* 9 (2014), E96513.

65 Zeigler, *Black Death,* p. 175.

66 R.A. Davis, "The Effect of the Black Death on Parish Priests of the Medieval Diocese of Coventry and Lichfield," *Historical Research,* 62 (1989): 87.

67 Raymond Williamson, "The Plague in Cambridge, *Medical History,* 1 (1957): 51; John Aberth goes so far as to contend that Cambridgeshire had one of the highest death rates in Europe. "The Black Death in the Diocese of Ely: The Evidence of the Bishop's Register," *Journal of Medieval History,* 21 (1995): 286.

68 John L. Fisher, "The Black Death in Essex," *The Essex Review,* 52 (1943): 20; Aberth, "Black Death in the Diocese of Ely," 286.

69 William J. Dohar, *The Black Death and Pastoral Leadership* (Philadelphia: University of Pennsylvania Press, 1995): 37–40.

70 E.A. Bond, ed., *Chronica monasterii de Melsa,* 3 vols. (Rolls Series, 43, 1866-68), 3: 36–37; A. Hamilton Thompson, "The Pestilence of the Fourteenth Century in the Diocese of York," *Archaeological Journal,* 71 (1914): 97–154; A. Hamilton Thompson, "Registers of John Gynewell, Bishop of Lincoln for the Years 1347–1350," *Archaeological Journal,* 68 (1911): 300–60; Richard Lomas, "The Black Death in County Durham," *Journal of Medieval History,* 15 (1989): 127–40.

71 Thompson, "Registers of Gynwell," p. 322.

72 Zeigler, *Black Death,* p. 184.

73 Lisa Sattenspiel, *The Geographic Spread of Infectious Diseases* (Princeton: Princeton University Press, 2009), 86–116.

74 Joshua M. Epstein, Jon Parker, Derek Cummings, Ross A. Hammond, "Coupled Contagion Dynamics of Fear and Disease: Mathematical and Computation Explorations," *PLoS One* 3 (2008), e3955.

75 John of Reading, 148–49.

76 *Polychronicon Ranulphi Higden,* 9: 360.

77 John of Reading, 212.

78 *Knighton's Chronicle,* 84–85. Ranulph Higden indicated that the Second Plague killed more men and women, including Henry, Duke of Lancaster. *Polychronicon,* 9: 360, 411–12. Observing the situation from Scotland the author of the Louth Park Abbey chronicle also noted the larger number of male victims. Edmund Venables, ed., *The Chronicle of Louth Park Abbey,* A.R. Maddison, trans. (Lincolnshire Record Society, 1891), 40–41. The author of the Grey Friars of Lynn chronicle indicated that more men and boys died than women as well as noting that while many people died, fewer died than in the previous epidemic. Gransden, "Fourteenth-Century Chronicle from the Grey Friars of Lynn," 275.

79 Gottfried, *Black Death,* 131. K.B. McFarlane, *The Nobility of Later Medieval England* (Oxford: Clarendon Press, 1973), 168–70. McFarlane bases his conclusion on the *Inquisitions Post Mortem.*

80 Sloane, *Black Death in London*, 136, 142.
81 Campbell, *Great Transition*, 319.
82 *Anonimalle Chronicle,* 77
83 *Anonimalle Chronicle,* 77.
84 *Anonimale Chronicle,* 77, 79, 124.
85 Aberth, *Black Death*, 26.
86 Thomas Walsingham, *Historia Anglicana*, Thomas Riley, ed., 2 vols. (London: Rolls Series, 28, 1863–64), 1: 409.
87 Walsingham, *Historia Anglicana*, 409–10.
88 Gottfried, *Black Death*, p. 133.
89 John Taylor, Wendy R. Childs, and Leslie Watkiss, eds. and trans., *The St. Albans Chronicle, I: 1376–1394* (Oxford: Clarendon Press, 2003), 900–01. Higden, *Polychronicon*, 9: 237.
90 *St. Albans Chronicle, I*, 912–13. The author of the *Polychronicon* (9: 259) also indicated that the north and west of England and especially York was hard-hit by the 1391 outbreak. For Newcastle: *Calendar of Patent Rolls, 1408–13*, 198. For Norwich: W. Hudson and J.C. Tingey, eds, *The Records of the City of Norwich* (Norwich: 1906–10), 2: cxxiii.
91 William Rees, "The Black Death in England and Wales, as Exhibited in Manorial Documents," *Proceedings of the Royal Society of Medicine: Section of the History of Medicine*, 16 (1923), 31.
92 Mark Bailey, *After the Black Death* (Oxford: Oxford University Press, 2021), 135, 234.
93 Nükhet Varlik, *Plague and Empire in the Early Modern Mediterranean World* (Cambridge: Cambridge University Press, 2015), 125.
94 Creighton, *Epidemics*, 202–233. J.M.W. Bean affirms this number. "Population and Economic Decline in England in the Later Middle Ages," *EconHistRev*, n.s., 15 (1963), 427–28.
95 Gottfried, *Black Death*, p. 131. Gottfried drew on the bills of mortality in examining the role of epidemic disease, with a strong focus on plague, in fifteenth century England. *Epidemic Disease in Fifteenth Century England* (New Brunswick: Rutgers University Press, 1978). A good summary of plague and its impact in the late fourteenth and fifteenth centuries that is skeptical of some over-blown claims about its prevalence is Bean, "Population and Economic Decline," 423–37. John Hatcher's "Mortality in the Fifteenth Century: Some New Evidence," *EconHistRev*, 2d ser., 39 (1986): 19–38, draws on the records of Christ Church, Canterbury in indicating that plague was only one among many health problems facing people in the fifteenth century. A useful compilation of national and urban epidemics in England from 1257 to 1530 is found in Carole Rawcliffe, *Urban Bodies* (Woodbridge: Boydell Press, 2013), 360–74.
96 John Taylor, Wendy R. Childs, and Leslie Watkiss, eds. and trans., *The St. Albans Chronicle, II: 1394–1422* (Oxford: Clarendon Press, 2011), 634–5.
97 *The Brut*, 467, Bean, "Population and Economic Decline in England," 429. A.H. Thomas and I.D. Thornley, eds., *The Great Chronicle of London* (London: Library Committee of the Corporation of the City of London, 1938), 226. C.L. Kingsford, *Chronicles of London* (Oxford: Oxford University Press, 1905), 188.
98 *Brut*, 131. 467. Pamela Nightingale provides further evidence of the national character of this outbreak. "Some New Evidence of Crises and Trends of Mortality in Late Medieval England," *Past & Present*, 187 (2005), 48.
99 Gottfried, *Black Death*, 132.
100 *Great Chronicle of London,* 226. The London citizen (and possible author of the *Great Chronicle*) Robert Fabyan echoes this sentiment and he lived through the epidemic. *The New Chronicles of England and France in Two Parts*. Henry Ellis, ed. (London: F.C. and J. Rivington, 1811), 666.
101 Gottfried, *Black Death*, p. 132.

102 Bean, "Population and Economic Decline in England," 430.

103 Slack, *Impact of Plague*, 58.

104 Slack, *Impact of Plague*, 58.

105 Neil Cummins. Morgan Kelly, and Cormac Ó Gráda, "Living Standards and Plague in London, 1560–1665," *EconHistRev.*, 69 (2016), 4.

106 Samuel Pepys wrote extensively about the London outbreak as well as the Great Fire that helped to burn the plague out of the capital. Stephen Porter, *The Great Plague* (Stroud: Sutton Publishing, 1999), A. Lloyd Moote and Dorothy C. Moote, *The Great Plague* (Baltimore: Johns Hopkins University Press, 2004). The term great plague that contemporaries applied to the 1664–65 outbreak helps to indicate both the impact that it had on the population and how short memories were for it had nowhere near the impact of the 1348–50 visitation.

107 Ann G. Carmichael examines this possibility in the context of a fifteenth-century Italian outbreak. *Plague and the Poor in Renaissance Italy* (Cambridge: Cambridge University Press, 1986), 23. Cummins, Kelly, and Ó Gráda, argue the possibly for typhus being mistaken for plague in late seventeenth century England. "Living Standards and Plague," 5.

108 Varlik, *Plague and Empire*, 2.

109 Sharon DeWitte and Philip Slavin, "Between Famine and Death: England on the Eve of the Black Death—Evidence from Paleoepidemiology and Manorial Accounts," *Journal of Interdisciplinary History* 44 (37–60), 37–60. Sharon N. DeWitte, "The Anthropology of Plague: Insights from Bioarchaeological Analyses of Epidemic Cemeteries," *Medieval Globe*, 1 (2016), 97–123.

110 Cummins, Kelly and Ó Gráda, "Living Standards and Plague," 3–34.

111 DeWitte and Slavin, "Between Famine and Death," 57.

112 Schmid, et al., "Climate-Driven Introduction of the Black Death and Successive Plague Reintroductions into Europe," 3020–25.

113 R.J. Eisen and K.L. Gage, "Transmission of Flea-Borne Zoonotic Agents," *Annual Review of Entomology*, 57 (2012): 63.

114 Amine Namouchi, Meriam Guellil, Oliver Kersten, et al., "Integrative Approach Using *Yersinia pestis* Genomes to Revisit the Historical Landscape of Plague during the Medieval Period," *PNAS*, 115 (2018), E11790–E11797.

115 Plague persisted in London from c. 1560 to 1665, driven by continued localized re-infection. Cummins, Kelly, and Ó Gráda, "Living Standards and Plague," 3–34.

116 Carmichael, "Plague Persistence in Western Europe," 162.

117 Kirsten I. Bos, Alexander Herbig, Jason Sahl, Nicholas Waglechner, Mathieu Fourment, et al., "Eighteenth Century *Yersinia pestis* Genomes Reveal the Long-term Persistence of an Historical Plague Focus," *eLIFE* (2016). 11 pp.

118 Seifert et al., "Genotyping *Yersinia pestis* in Historical Plague." Bos, et al., "Eighteenth Century *Yersinia pestis* Genomes." Although both articles argue for a European maintenance reservoir throughout the period, neither indicates where this might have been.

119 Spyrou et al., "Historical *Y. pestis* Genomes Reveal the European Black Death as the Source of Ancient and Modern Plague Pandemics," 874–81.

120 Maria A. Spyrou, Marcel Keller, Rezeda I. Tukhbatova, et al., "Phylogeography of the Second Plague Pandemic Revealed through Analysis of Historical *Yersinia pestis* Genomes," *Nature Communications* 10 (2019), 13 pp..

121 A good summary of the debate is found in Aberth, *Black Death*, 237–49.

122 *Chronica Galfridi le Baker*, 98–99.

123 *Avesbury*, pp. 406–07.

124 Margaret S. Ogden, ed., *The Cyrugie of Guy de Chaulaic*, (EETS, 265, 1971), 155.

125 Giovanni Boccaccio, *The Decameron*, G.H. McWilliams, trans. (Harmondsworth: Penguin Books, 1972), 50.

126 Shrewsbury, *History of Bubonic Plague in the British Isles*, 124–25, 127.

127 Graham Twigg, *The Black Death: A Biological Reappraisal* (New York: Schocken Books, 1985).

128 Susan Scott and Christopher J. Duncan, *Biology of Plagues* (Cambridge: Cambridge University Press, 2001), Scott and Duncan, *Return of the Black Death* (New York: John Wiley, 2004).

129 George Christakos, Ricardo A. Olea, Marc L. Serre, Hwa-Lung Yu, Lin-Lin Wang, *Interdisciplinary Public Health Reasoning and Epidemic Modeling: The Case of the Black Death* (Berlin: Springer, 2005).

130 Building on an article ("The Black Death: End of a Paradigm," *American Historical Review*, 107 (2002), 703–38), Cohn stated his argument with a book-length treatment that was wide-ranging in its treatment of historical sources and guided by his reading of the literature concerning the Third Pandemic in India. He has displayed increasing sophistication in his use of the scientific literature although narrowing his focus to concentrate more on the discrepancies surrounding the spread of the Black Death and the lack of plague carrying fleas in medieval Europe. Samuel K. Cohn, Jr., *The Black Death Transformed: Disease and culture in Early Renaissance Europe* (London: Arnold, 2002), Cohn, "Epidemiology of the Black Death and Successive Waves of Plague," *Medical History* Supp. 27 (2008), 74–100, Cohn, "Changing Pathology of Plague," in Simonetta Cavaciocchi, ed., *Le Interazioni Fra Economia E Ambiente Biologico Nell'Europe Preindustriale Secc. XIII–XVIII* (Florence: University of Florence Press, 2010), 33–56, which focuses particularly on Milan, Cohn, "The Historian and the Laboratory: The Black Death Disease," in Linda Clark and Carole Rawcliffe, eds. *The Fifteenth Century XII, Society in an Age of Plague* (Woodbridge: Boydell, 2013), 195–212. He also developed his criticism in a treatment of the impact of the plague and medical thinking in Renaissance Italy. *Cultures of Plague* (Oxford University Press, 2010).

131 An historian and a pathologist, two historians, and a biologist have provided reasoned arguments why the plague was the plague, often questioning or denying Cohn's points along the way. See: John Theilmann and Frances Cate, "A Plague of Plagues: The Problem of Plague Diagnosis in Medieval England," *Journal of Interdisciplinary History* 37 (2007): 371–93, Ole J. Benedictow, *What Disease was Plague?* (Leiden: Brill, 2010), and J.L. Bolton, "Looking for *Yersinia pestis*: Scientists, Historians and the Black Death," in Clark and Rawcliffe, *The Fifteenth Century*, 15–38. The biologist Lars Walløe focuses more closely than the others on clinical issues, but he, Bolton, and Theilmann and Cate all call for an interdisciplinary approach. "Medieval and Modern Bubonic Plague: Some Clinical Continuities," *Medical History* 27, Supp (2008), 59–73.

132 A good discussion of cycling and the temporal spread of a disease can be found in Sattenspiel *Geographic Spread of Infectious Diseases*.

133 Bos et al., "Eighteenth Century *Yersinia pestis* Genomes." Spyrou, et al., "Phylogeography of the Second Plague Pandemic."

134 E.H. Hankin, "On the Epidemiology of Plague," *Journal of Hygiene* 5 (1905), 48–53. Ole Georg Moseng points out the importance of environmental conditions for fleas to spread disease and emphasizes that only in India did the black rat or *X. cheopis* play a major role in the propagation of plague. "Climate, Ecology and Plague," 23–45.

135 G. Blanc and M. Baltazard, "Recherches sur le mode de transmission naturelle de la peste bubonique et septicémique," *Archives de l'Institut Pasteru de Maroc* 111 (1945), 204–10, 228–71.

136 Didier Raoult and Véronique Roux, "The Body Louse as a Vector of Reemerging Human Diseases," *Clinical Infectious Diseases* 29 (1999), 888–911. Saravanan Ayyadurai, Florent Sebbane, Didier Raoult, and Michel Drancourt, "Body Lice, *Yersinia pestis* Orientalis and Black Death," *Emerging Infectious Diseases* 16 (2010), 892–3, Renaud Piarroux et al., "Plague Epidemics and Lice, Democratic Republic of the Congo," *Emerging Infectious Diseases* 19 (2013), 505–6.

137 Katherine R. Dean, Fabienne Krauer, Lars Walløe, Ole Christian Lingjaerde, Barbara Bramanti, Nils Chr. Stenseth, and Boris V. Schmid, "Human Ectoparasites and the Spread of Plague in Europe during the Second Pandemic," *PNAS*, 115 (2018), 1304–09.
138 DeWitte, "Anthropology of Plague," 97–123.
139 Fabian Crespo and Matthew B. Lawrenz, "Heterogeneous Immunological Landscapes and Medieval Plague: An Invitation to a New Dialogue between Historians and Immunologists," *Medieval Globe*, 1 (2014), 229–57, especially 233.
140 Monica H. Green, "Editor's Introduction to *Pandemic Disease in the Medieval World: Rethinking the Black Death,*" *Medieval Globe*, 1 (2014), 10.

6

RESPONSES TO THE PLAGUE

By itself, the Black Death may have been the worst natural disaster to strike England, but of course, the plague outbreaks kept coming, with great severity in the fourteenth century and at greater intervals, but some still producing mortality crises until the late seventeenth century. The contemporary chronicler John of Reading captured the despair that many people must have felt from plague outbreaks at one point or another from the mid-fourteenth century onward: "And there was those days death without sorrow, marriage without affection, self-imposed penance, want without poverty, and flight without escape."[1]

The previous chapter focused on the demographic impact and touched on various reactions to the disease. This chapter examines the impact of the plague on various aspects of English society. Although people had to get on with their lives after each epidemic, a disease that removed upwards of fifty percent of the population had to have an impact on society. If nothing else, villages and neighborhoods were empty in 1351 with half the population dead. Each of the major epidemics ensured that everyone knew someone who had died from the plague. Death was more common in the premodern world than today, but the suddenness and number of deaths often had the demoralizing impact seen in John of Reading's observation. A natural disaster of this magnitude greatly influences emotional, social, religious, and economic life as well as producing responses in literature and the arts and helping to precipitate changes in medicine. The responses to the onset and continuation of the plague start from the need to explain the disease and expand outward to encompass all of society. Fourteenth-century people in general and medical practitioners, in particular, tried to explain the plague and arrive at some means of dealing with it. Although there had been a plague epidemic in England in the seventh century, it was all but forgotten so people regarded the disease that struck England in 1348 as a new

DOI: 10.4324/9781003215219-7

disease. Already by the fifteenth century, plague was becoming more familiar with numerous descriptions.

Numbers and the impact of the plague

The previous chapter gave some indication of the pre-1348 population of England and the impact of the Black Death and succeeding fourteenth-century epidemics. There are several approaches to counting the dead that has been used in arriving at the demographic impact of the plague each with strengths and weaknesses. None were intended to produce pure demographic information so later scholars have inferred demographic data from the sources producing disagreement over the numbers.

Chroniclers often provided numbers of the dead. Some chroniclers, especially when reporting deaths in their own locality, could be quite accurate. Henry Knighton, a canon of St. Mary's Leicester, indicated that 11 canons died during the 1361 plague, an accounting based on direct personal knowledge.[2] Chroniclers often provided very large, round numbers that had no basis in reality. Often when a medieval chronicler reported that 100,000 people had died in a region, he was really saying many, many people died here. Chronicle accounts often convey a personal touch and can be a starting point for computing the plague's death rate, but more accurate information is needed.

One official accounting that provides useful information is the inquisitions post mortem that authorities conducted after the death of a lord to determine who should inherit an estate. It can be assumed that the Crown conducted the process in a thorough and timely fashion so the numbers of reported deaths should be fairly reliable. Using inquisitions post mortem produces a twenty-seven percent death rate for the 1348–50 period.[3] Inquisitions post mortem contribute precision of process but are lacking in coverage. Only a quite limited part of the population had the lands necessary for the Crown to be interested; the landless poor were ignored. The twenty-seven percent mortality rate is precise, but it underestimates the death rate.

Another sampling of the dead provides broader coverage than inquisitions post mortem for a specific group. Bishops' registers provide a listing of clerical vacancies in the diocese. Parish clergy might have a somewhat higher standard of living than their parishioners, but not always markedly so. The clergy might be more at risk of death from the plague if they were doing their job of comforting their parishioners, but this is hard to assess. Records are present for ten dioceses scattered over all of England, giving a diversity that can encompass differences in local mortality rates. Registers exist for Winchester, Bath and Wells, Ely, Norwich, Worcester, Exeter, Coventry and Lichfield, Hereford, Lincoln, and York, and clerical mortality rates were calculated from them in 1930. More recently, recalculation has been done for Hereford, Coventry and Lichfield, and Ely. These data indicate a mortality rate of fifty percent with some localities suffering from death rates as high as seventy percent.[4] As with the inquisitions post mortem, the bishops' registers do not record cause of death so we cannot be sure if death was always the plague. Clerical vacancies also occurred when a priest ran away so that all not vacancies reflect deaths. Bishops' registers provide better coverage than inquisitions post mortem, but both ignore the poor

When serfs died, their heirs were responsible for paying a death duty, the heriot, to the lord. Records of heriots do not record cause of death, but there are records from several manors scattered across England. Like inquisitions post mortem, heriots may underestimate mortality when an heir died before he could inherit and his death was not recorded. The record from heriots also indicates a death rate between forty and seventy percent with some manors suffering mortalities approaching eighty percent.[5]

In addition to the three large-scale recording efforts, some monastic communities compiled death rates for their monks. The numbers might be small but they provide further confirmatory evidence for a mortality rate that probably exceeded fifty percent for the 1348–50 outbreak. The chronicler of the Cistercian Abbey of Meaux in Yorkshire indicated that when the plague hit in August 1349, the abbot, 21 monks, and six lay brethren out of a total community of 50 monks and lay brothers died in short order. The deaths continued so that finally "only ten monks and no lay brethren were left."[6] Mortality rates were not as high for later outbreaks and obtaining reliable numbers is often challenging, but it appears that some later outbreaks produced mortality rates as high as ten percent in sharply reduced populations. As is the case with inquisitions post mortem and clerical vacancies, there is a question of how representative of the general population monastic communities were.

When we consider the continuing impact of later plague outbreaks, it appears that the population of England continued to decline well into the fifteenth century. The economic historian Gregory Clark has constructed a mathematical model of English population based on the relationship of population to the marginal product of labor. Clark indicates that English population bottomed out at 2.4 million in the decade of 1450–59 and did not reach three million until the mid-sixteenth century.[7] Not all scholars accept Clark's use of marginal product of labor to calculate the size of population. Today most scholars would agree that the continuing impact of the plague produced between a fifty and sixty percent decline in population. Mark Bailey provides numbers that are probably representative of consensus estimates of 5.5 million in the 1340s, 2.8 million in the early 1350s, 2.5 million in 1377, 2.3 million in the 1520s, and only 2.8 million by the mid-sixteenth century.[8]

Without entering into the debate over validity of sources and methodology, it is apparent that the Second Plague Pandemic had a huge impact on the population of England. Much of this impact came with the first outbreak of 1348–50, but the plague kept on killing so the population was unable to grow for a long time. Bailey notes the importance of the 1361 epidemic as it halted what was starting to be modest growth in the 1350s.[9] Such a dramatic decline in population influenced many aspects of England life. The impact of such a large loss of life produced efforts to explain and fight the plague but also touched how people lived their lives and what society could accomplish.

The medical response to the plague

The disease that struck England in 1348 was something new and different for the medical community. In some ways, fourteenth-century medical practitioners were no different than twenty-first-century medical practitioners who confront an emerging disease. They wanted to explain its origin and develop means for treatment. Medieval medical practitioners were limited because their theoretical approach was based on the humor theory of disease traceable back to Galen, as well as by their lack of sophisticated diagnostic tools and empirical knowledge. Their approach was to treat symptoms, not the disease itself, an approach grounded in the teachings of Galen.

Medical men possessed few means of providing a cure for epidemic diseases. They used such methods as dietary remedies, bleeding, and purgatives in efforts to return the humors to balance, none of which were effective in dealing with epidemic diseases. In some ways, however, some medieval medical practitioners were more holistic in their approach than many modern practitioners, as they tried to take environmental factors, broadly defined, and individual patient characteristics into account with their diagnoses and remedies. This broad-based approach provided some opportunities for diagnosis, but also many opportunities for missteps. An obvious question is what did medical practitioners learn from their confrontation with the Black Death, did they learn anything about epidemic diseases and how to treat them from dealing with the Black Death? What did they learn in encountering a new disease even one with many of the symptoms exhibited by other diseases? The same questions might also apply to English society as a whole.

Galen, the second-century Greek physician, was the preeminent authority for medieval physicians. Galen and his intellectual descendants, such as the eleventh-century Persian physician Avicenna, based their approach to disease on the humor theory of disease. Avicenna's views on the remote and direct causes of fevers were particularly important in helping to shape the views of medieval physicians as they tried to deal with the fever that was a symptom of the plague.[10] Good health came from keeping the four humors, blood, phlegm, black bile, and yellow bile in balance. The physician's role was to prescribe preventatives to keep the humors in balance and remedies to return them to balance when they became out of balance. The few university-trained physicians of the fourteenth, fifteenth, and sixteenth centuries approached disease from their existing humorial framework. The Black Death was a "new" disease outside their conceptual framework making it difficult to explain. The symptoms of the plague did not readily fit any nosological category and the enormity of the mortality rate also confounded explanation. Few writers wrote medical treatises concerning the disease during the first outbreak although the number of commentators would increase from the second outbreak of 1361 onward. One, written in Spain in April 1348 by Jacme d'Agramont, first defined what pestilence was and then explained that pestilential air was responsible for the disease. He listed the various factors that led to pestilential air and worked downward from what he called a universal pestilence to one that affected only one dwelling. After describing the origins of the disease, d'Agramont described a preventative regime but was careful not to describe cures as he concluded that people who were not physicians might misuse his cures.[11] D'Agramont describes dietary measures that could be helpful in preventing the change in the air that led to pestilence, advocating cold foods when excessive heat was present and hot foods when excessive cold was present.[12] At first, most medical commentators, such as d'Agramont, tried to force the new disease into their existing framework of divine influence, astrological influences, and the need to return the humors to balance.[13] This approach dealt with the causation of diseases, their symptoms, and how to treat them.

If the plague was universal in that it encompassed the known world, its cause went beyond the explanation offered by the humor theory of disease.[14] Commentators agreed that God was the ultimate origin of disease. However, they offered a variety of often related intermediate causes. In October 1348, the Paris medical faculty indicated that a conjunction of Mars, Jupiter, and Saturn on 20 March 1345 at 1:00 p.m. helped to precipitate the outbreak of the disease. They based their conclusion on Aristotle and argued that a conjunction of the three planets produced great mortality especially when it occurred under a hot, wet sign as occurred in 1345. This planetary conjunction gave rise to powerful winds from the south that raised heat and excess moisture on earth.[15] The climatic change that ensued produced the bad air that led to the epidemic as the authors indicated: "We believe that the present epidemic of plague has arisen from air corrupt in substance, and not changed in its attributes." The corrupted air easily penetrated the heart "and rots the surrounding moisture, and the heat thus caused destroys the life force."[16] In essence, once the humors became unbalanced because of the impact of the bad air, death ensued. People with hot and moist bodies were most likely to fall victim to the ailment, as were women, young people, and those who engaged in too much exercise or sexual activity. Those people who possessed a dry humor and who followed a sensible regime were less likely to fall victim to the disease. After developing an astrological and humor-based explanation for the disease, the authors concluded the chapter by indicating that all diseases flowed from God's will. However, they indicated that did not mean abandoning physicians as God used medical men to cure the sick.[17]

This conjunction of the planets was the universal cause of the disease, but the Parisian medical men went on to argue that it led to a corruption of the air that served as the particular cause of the disease. The astrological and miasma (bad air) explanation was an attractive one although at least one commentator indicated that the corruption of the air was produced by earthquakes in 1347.[18] Physicians fell back on Galen once they had identified the cause for the disease in prescribing how to treat the symptoms of people with various temperaments and how to prevent the disease.

The Paris account was more fulsome than anything produced in England, but English physicians seem to have adopted similar explanations. A typical English tractatus is the translation of a work produced at the University of Montpellier in the fifteenth century. The English treatise followed the usual five-part organizational scheme of medical treatises. It started with the signs of onset of the disease followed by a section dealing with causation—bad air. The third section detailed preventative measures designed to keep the humors in balance with a fourth section dealing with recipes for helping a sick patient to heal. The fifth section, not always found in such treatises, included an abbreviated phlebotomy.[19] By the fifteenth century, plague tracts tended to adopt the sort of conventional style exhibited here and added little to what others had said.

Even today, physicians first rely upon the patient's reported symptoms when making a diagnosis, turning to the laboratory for confirmation. How did commentators go about describing the symptoms of the plague? Here, we have a problem as most of the fourteenth-century English accounts contain little information regarding symptoms. Geoffrey le Baker provides the most fulsome list of symptoms as he describes what he calls boils and black pustules on various parts of the body and indicated that some people went to bed healthy but were dead the next morning.[20] A few chroniclers, such as Robert of Avesbury, described how quickly people died once infected as he indicated that often infected people died three or four days after symptoms became evident.[21] Some continental sources are more forthcoming in describing symptoms. Writing in 1361, Guy de Chauliac, the papal physician at Avignon during the Black Death indicated that one variant of the disease often killed within two days, especially those people who were coughing blood (possibly those with pneumonic or septicemic plague), and another variant took longer. He also indicated that many victims had what he called carbuncles (buboes), particularly in the groin and armpits.[22] Ironically, it was the Italian writer Giovanni Boccaccio who provided one of the best descriptions of the symptoms of the Black Death. He spoke of tumors in the groin and armpits the size of eggs as the first sign of the disease. Often these were followed by black spots appearing on various parts of the body that observers interpreted as a sign of impending death.[23] These reported symptoms remained the commonly reported ones until the last epidemic in the eighteenth century. Many accounts concentrated on the impacts of the disease, not the symptoms. The descriptions of symptoms seem to indicate a disease that progressed too quickly to have been the plague, but these symptoms did not always appear until the disease was well underway. Even though primary pneumonic and septicemic plague infections kill quickly once symptoms become manifest, pneumonic plague victims rarely die overnight as Geoffrey le Baker indicated. Could this have simply been an exaggeration on Geoffrey's part rather than a misdiagnosis? Here, we must guard against a pedantic and literal interpretation that affords too much precision to inexact sources.

Because plague was a new and terrifying disease, it attracted a good deal of attention from medical practitioners. In the early twentieth century, the German medical historian Karl Sudhoff compiled a list of some 281 plague treatises composed from the mid-fourteenth through the fifteenth centuries and probably more were written.[24] English authors scarcely figured in this list, but English authors translated several of the continental treatises into English claiming them as their own work in the process. A few years after the first outbreak of the Black Death, educated people did not lack accounts that attempted to explain the origins of the disease and provide some sort of remedies. The explanations for the disease were grounded in the humor theory of disease and most medical men assigned the cause of the disease to "bad air" i.e., some sort of corruption of the air, often caused by an adverse arrangement of the planets. The underlying cause was of course the will of God. Most of the writers also accepted some sort of contagion theory of disease as they advocated avoiding direct contact with patients or breathing the air around them. An account written around 1400 indicated that:

- The physician should ensure that the sick room was well-ventilated before he entered.
- The afflicted person's room should be aired out before the physician entered else, he should not enter.
- He should avoid touching the patient's clothes when he took the pulse.
- He should try to avoid holding a urinal when taking a urine sample or at least wear gloves.
- The physician should hold a sponge soaked in vinegar to his nose as long as he was in the home of the afflicted person and should not remain with him long.[25]

Such advice indicates that physicians feared contagion, an approach that was helpful in confronting pneumonic plague, but less helpful in dealing with bubonic plague.

In spite of recognition of the plague as a new disease, the medical community's approach to it remains mired in their preconceptions derived from the past. Too much blood—bleed the person. Too much black bile—use a purgative. Application of some approaches such as bleeding or purgatives was likely to further weaken victims of the plague, speeding them to their graves all the more rapidly. Medical responses to the plague were often limited to providing palliative care in the pre-antibiotic era. At least dietary remedies could have had a positive impact on afflicted people, by helping to keep up their strength but were not always well-informed and some may have done harm to the patient. The recommended treatments were rational in light of prevailing knowledge, but what was needed was a new outlook on disease.

Most of the authors of the plague tractates were sincere in their efforts to explain the new disease and tried to provide remedies. The widely translated treatise of John of Burgundy, written around 1365 during the *pestis Secundus*, probably caught this sincerity best as he started his tractate by indicating that he intended his work to help those with no access to medical care to be their own physicians.[26] He concluded the work by indicating that he was "Moved by piety and anguished by an and feeling sorrow because of this calamity ... I have composed and compiled this work not for a price but for your prayers, so that when anyone recovers from the diseases discussed above, he will effectively pray for me to our Lord God."[27] John of Burgundy's treatise commanded attention into the sixteenth century. Thomas Moulton presented it as his own in 1531 with *This is the Myrour or Glasse of Helth Necessary and Needfull for Euery Person to Loke in, that Wyll Kepe Theyr Body from the Syckenes of the Pestylence* and Moulton's pamphlet was reprinted several times.[28] Although numerous quacks also provided plague remedies for a price, the medical community tried to do what it could. Some produced plague accounts, such as that of Guy de Chaulaic, who continued to treat patients during the first outbreak and fell ill with the plague although he survived, made a point of indicating that the physician should stay at his post rather than flee.[29]

Overall, the remedies provided in the plague treatises were not very helpful, nor could they be when antibiotics are the recognized treatment for *Y. pestis* and antibiotics were not available to medieval practitioners. The historian Philip Zeigler's assessment is a negative one. He concludes that the writers knew their remedies were worthless so their remedies were designed to boost morale.[30] Yet, maintaining the victims' strength, as some of the remedies did, at least gave those with a strong constitution a chance at survival. In light of the antibiotic treatments for the plague developed in the twentieth century, Zeigler is correct; any other treatment could only help patients keep their strength up, giving them a better chance of survival. In another sense, Zeigler's view is anachronistic and displays the triumphalist view once found in the history of medicine; it was impossible to prescribe antibiotics in a pre-antibiotic world and physicians prescribed the remedies they knew. Medieval and early modern writers tried to explain the plague and provide cures within the medical mindset of the day. Darrel Amundsen provides a more nuanced view of the plague tractates. He concludes that the medieval writers generally had faith in the remedies they prescribed and tried to incorporate new remedies in their works.[31] Almost any epidemic disease proved difficult for the medical profession before the late nineteenth century. Even smallpox for which Edward Jenner found a preventative in the late eighteenth century was not fully understood until the twentieth century.

Because many physicians thought that bad air helped to spread the plague, they advocated a variety of means for avoiding the miasmas that cause disease. Individuals could build their houses in healthful places, not those that were sources of bad air, such as marshes. As is indicated in Chapter 2, even before the Black Death local governments tried to deal with such sources of "bad" air as dung in the streets. The Black Death gave an additional push to efforts to clean up English towns. Dealing with waste remained an ongoing problem throughout the premodern era and beyond. Removing human and animal wastes from the streets had a positive impact on preventing diarrheal diseases but had a minimal impact on preventing the plague. Full-scale cleaning efforts that helped to remove rat habitat had an impact but this was more a response to the Third Pandemic than the Second Pandemic. Royal and some municipal governments began to see a role for themselves in protecting the health of the population. Later quarantine efforts grew out of this increased activity.

Another remedy or more accurately a preventative did have some success as the exhortations to physicians not to flee the plague indicate. If the plague could not be cured, it could at least be prevented. Fleeing a disease-ridden locality always had merit. Boccaccio captured this approach in the *Decameron* as his storytellers have fled Florence in order to escape the plague. Unfortunately for them, they brought the plague with them to their country retreat. Flight only worked when people did not take the disease with them, something difficult to do without an understanding of fleas as the disease vectors. Only flight at the first whiff of an epidemic disease or avoidance of an infected area had a chance. Nonetheless, flight remained a preventative for the plague as well as other diseases such as yellow fever into the twentieth century. The problem remained that flight could actually have a negative impact as it served to spread the disease faster than it might otherwise have spread.

The other side of avoidance was quarantine. Preventing plague victims from coming in contact with the healthy population had merit as long as the disease was transmitted from human to human although rigorous isolation might also prevent the movement of fleas or lice. British authorities in Hong Kong in 1894 applied a rigorous quarantine of plague victims and their families as part of their efforts to halt the spread of the disease. The disadvantage of quarantine from the victims' standpoint was that they were often separated from those people who might look after them and, in some cases, denied almost any contact with the outside world. The hospital quarantine wards that would later be used were not present as a treatment option for medieval diseases. Instead, an infected household would be shut off from the rest of the community until the disease passed or everyone inside was dead. No wonder that families tried to hide evidence of disease to avoid such actions. A different form of quarantine, more like an embargo, was to prevent outsiders from entering a community until it was known that they were disease-free. This form of quarantine survives today in ports of entry. In order to be effective, a village would have to cut itself off fully from any outside contact with neighbors, traders, or anyone, something difficult to enforce. The lack of understanding of the flea vector of disease helped to make this approach to quarantine difficult to accomplish. Inadvertent quarantines of this sort did seem to happen as there is evidence of villages or even whole regions bypassed by the plague. Although some Italian cities such as Florence and Milan established quarantines during fifteenth-century epidemics, England did not follow suit until the late sixteenth century.

English authorities turned to continental responses to the plague in the sixteenth century as they tried to prevent the spread of the disease. In 1518, a royal proclamation tried to control contagious diseases by marking houses that were infected.[32] Local governments followed this up with ordinances of their own that were designed to identify and stop the spread of the disease. As the 1518 proclamation indicates, opinion was also turning to contagion, either from individuals or miasmas, as the means by which plague was spread. The views of royal and local officials tended to run ahead of those of medical men who continued to rely on miasma theory as their explanation for the plague. Ann Carmichael makes this point in connection with Milan that was one of the first cities to adopt quarantine policies based on contagion theory in the latter part of the fifteenth century.[33] Local governments followed the royal proclamation up with ordinances of their own that were designed to identify and stop the spread of the disease. Humor theory continued to be used to explain individual cases, but the impact of plague as an exceptional disease helped to change medical opinion.

Plague of course, was not contained and the country suffered another mortality crisis with the 1563 epidemic and smaller outbreaks as well as an outbreak of typhus in 1577. The time was ripe for full-scale intervention. The Privy Council issued the Plague Orders in 1578 intended to stop the spread of epidemic diseases. They were rooted in contagion theory, not miasma theory as the disease was described as spreading from person to person rather than through the air. The 1578 Orders contained 17 clauses specifying how plague should be controlled as well as a summary of various medical remedies prepared by the London College of Physicians.[34] The Orders would be reissued with minor alterations in 1592, 1593, 1603, and 1625. In addition, they were issued as a part of statute and order collections in 1609, 1630, 1636, and 1646, finally to be issued in a revised form in 1666 after the Great Plague. Local justices of the peace carried much of the burden of enforcing the orders. They had to find observers to check bodies for plague. These searchers then identified the houses of the victims and closed them up for a period of up to six weeks after the last case was reported. In addition, the searcher marked the houses with a sign that disease was present inside. The authorities also burned the clothing and bedding of the victims. One of the orders did make provision for providing food for households that had no means of obtaining it. In essence, the Plague Orders provided a thoroughgoing system of quarantine of plague victims, a system that did help to limit the spread of the disease. The Plague Orders were a change in focus for England from an individual approach to a societal one. Various continental authorities had long followed some form of quarantine, and while the English came late to this approach, an increased reliance on governmental action, which had started with waste removal actions in the fourteenth century and was being implemented to deal with other problems such as the poor laws of 1572 and 1576.

The medical remedies printed with the Plague Orders were conventional ones that included blood-letting, purging, dietary remedies, and perfuming the air to ward off "bad' air. Nonetheless, the thrust of the Plague Orders was a change from what had long been accepted ideas. The Orders indicated that contagion was behind how the plague spread. Miasmas were still accepted as a means for spreading the disease, but the focus had changed to individual interaction. Thomas Moulton's *Glass of Health* had first been published in 1531 and continued to circulate when the Plague Orders were implemented. Moulton saw sin as the cause for the disease, but the immediate cause was "bad" air that came from a conjunction of Saturn and Jupiter.[35] Society did not completely jettison his ideas, which had been rooted in humor and miasma theory, but medical men had come to the realization that they needed a better explanation for how the disease spread. The contagion theory they adopted missed the mark in many ways, as humans did not transmit the disease, save for pneumonic plague, but quarantine did help to deal with the problem of rats and fleas to a limited degree.

Moulton's *Glass of Health* was not the only available work dealing with the plague from the fifteenth century onward. Paul Slack estimates that 23 of 153 different books dealing with medicine between 1486 and 1604 dealt exclusively with the plague.[36] Some were warmed over translations of continental authors as was Moulton's but there were several original works in addition to plague chapters in other medical books. Publishers often reissued successful plague tracts several times as interest in combating the disease remained high. The thought behind the plague tracts was not always that original. Conjunctions of the planets, miasmas, contagion, imbalance of the humors, and of course, a sinful society were all seen as the causes for plague although in different combinations. Forced by the deadly uniqueness of plague, medical opinion began to shift away from a strictly Galenic view in the sixteenth century, but vestiges of Galen's views continued to predominate. Gradually, the continued impact of the plague began to force at least some medical writers to focus on plague as an entity in its own right, worthy of attention instead of the Galenic focus on individuals and their symptoms. This changing focus made it easier to see diseases as something that came from the outside and their spread was explained by contagion theory. Care must be taken not to infer a too neat picture of contagion theory in the premodern world. Individual definitions differed and it is difficult to find a writer whose definition of contagion would match that of a modern medical practitioner.

Older views continued to hang on throughout the sixteenth century. William Bullein, physician and staunch Puritan, wrote a typical plague treatise in 1564: *A Dialogue Both Pleasant and Pitiful wherein is a Goodly Regiment against the Fever Pestilence.* He also dealt with plague in his more general works *The Government of Health* (1558) and *The Bulwark of Defense against All Sickness, Soreness and Wounds* (1562). Opinions differ as to his motivation. Margaret Healy accuses Bullein of writing Puritan propaganda masquerading as medical tracts.[37] Aspects of Bullein's Puritanism certainly came through in his writing, but so too his mastery of contemporary medical views. Bullein uses various speakers to deal with a variety of issues in the *Dialogue*, but plague weaves through the discussion by the characters with medical opinion being represented by the character Medicus.[38] Plagues symptoms were well known by the mid-sixteenth century and Medicus identifies fever as an early symptom as well as buboes although he indicates that they may not always appear.[39] Medicus is conventional with his warnings to avoid "bad" air and the need to keep the humors in balance as well as seeing planetary conjunctions as a causative factor for the disease.[40] Bullein is unoriginal in his advocacy of blood-letting as a remedy ("four ounces or a little more") especially at the onset of the disease. He is aware that blood-letting may be harmful to some and so advocates pills made with myrrh, aloe, and saffron, as well as a theriac potion, and even a different potion for someone with a weak stomach.[41] There is much more in the *Dialogue* than the plague however, as Bullein condemns greed and idleness and advocates charity toward the deserving poor. He also expressed a typical Protestant complaint in his advocacy of charity: "Riches hath poisoned the church and transformed the clergy, especially in Rome among the popes and many great men."[42] Bullein wrote in English and his dialogue approach was approachable for the non-medically trained. His medical views were typical of sixteenth-century medical views of the plague, as well as much that had been written before.

What was changing was that plague was becoming more of an urban phenomenon, a disease that struck hard at the poor. The Plague Orders spoke of quarantine for all, but the suspicion remains that the authorities applied quarantine more harshly to the poor than the upper crust.[43] William Bullein is critical at times of the immorality of society, which he relates to the poor. Social control of the poor, who were often seen as immoral and a force of disorder, was being expressed in a variety of ways in the late sixteenth century as the discussion of the response to syphilis in Chapter 8 will indicate.

Plague did help to force some medical writers to think in different ways about causation and treatment. Most writers saw plague as different and did not apply the lessons learned to their views of the treatment of other diseases. When taken with some of the challenges to Galenic medicine expressed by commentators such as Paracelsus, the impact of plague was gradually beginning to open the door to new views of medicine that would be expressed in the seventeenth century.

The religious response

As most contemporary commentators pointed out, the plague came from the will of God, often in response to a sinful society. Jacme d' Agramont, a Spanish author, advocated various medical approaches to the presence of disease, building on his contention that bad air was responsible for pestilence and that it could be prevented. However, he then noted: "because if the corruption and putrefaction of the air has come because of our sins the remedies of the medical art are of little value, for only He who binds can unbind."[44] Prayers and other efforts seeking divine intervention, such as requesting the aid of the saints, were often a response to medical emergencies. People asked saints to intervene with God on their behalf for all manner of problems from lost animals, sick children, broken bones, and any sort of mysterious ailment. The Virgin was the quintessential saint for people seeking aid for their problems in medieval Europe. Although people often asked local saints for aid, requesting the Virgin's help was a standard procedure. The poet John Lydgate provides two examples of prayers to the Virgin asking her intercession to help prevent the plague that are typical in their simplicity and need.[45] In addition to the Virgin, people turned to the other saints for aid in preventing the plague and curing it.

Two saints, St. Sebastian and St. Roch, became known as plague saints in the late Middle Ages. Sebastian, who was martyred in the third century, was an established saint when the Second Plague Pandemic got underway. Roman authorities tried to kill Sebastian with a hail of arrows, which he survived only to be killed later. He became the patron saint of archers and the arrow motif came to be connected with plague arrows directed at a sinful world. People saw him as able to avert "plague arrows" and so requested his aid. In the fifteenth and sixteenth century, he came to be the subject of suffrages which were prayers directed toward individual saints. A York popular prayer found in a devotional work from 1536 is typical in requesting Sebastian's aid in warding off the plague.[46] Sebastian's martyrdom is somewhat tangential to the plague, but people made the connection as they sought to avert harm. St. Roch was born around 1350 and seemed to have contracted the plague which he survived. He was imprisoned in Montpellier in 1379, dying in prison while on a pilgrimage on which he cured victims of the plague. Roch at least had a connection to the plague. His and Sebastian's cults were stronger in southern Europe, but Roch, too, had a suffrage directed to him in the York devotional work.[47] Along with Mary, Roch's and Sebastian's aid was often sought although more commonly in southern than northern Europe. Although known as plague saints, both Sebastian and Roch may have had less impact in the Middle Ages than later.[48]

Many people in fourteenth- and fifteenth-century England probably had not heard of St. Roch although some may have known of St. Sebastian and of course the Virgin. People also turned to almost any saint for aid with their problems. When the miracle lists of "new" late medieval saints such as Henry VI are examined, a few plague miracles can be found. Henry's cult developed after his murder in 1485. Around the turn of the sixteenth century, a list of 182 miracles was compiled as part of an attempted canonization supported by Henry VII. Seventeen of Henry's reputed miracles were cures of the plague during outbreaks in the late fifteenth century.[49] In reality, 12 of the cures imputed to King Henry involved the prevention of the disease. Thomas Syman invoked Henry's protection for himself and 11 other inhabitants of his house in Farlington, Hampshire when a plague outbreak occurred. None of the households contracted the disease and so Syman visited Henry's tomb at Windsor to give thanks for their miraculous preservation from harm.[50] More established saints also had a mixed track record when it came to the plague. The shrine of St. Thomas Becket, which enjoyed an international reputation, displayed an increase in offerings in the mid-fourteenth century over the early fourteenth century.[51] The track record of other shrines is mixed. Saints came and went in fashion and this pattern seems to have persisted even if people were seeking relief from the plague. The fortunes of the shrine of St. Thomas Cantilupe are typical. Soon after Bishop Thomas Cantilupe of Hereford died in 1282, miracles began to be recorded at his tomb in Hereford and he would be canonized in 1320. The offerings at his tomb in 1290–91 were substantial, totaling £178 10s. 7d. Thomas's cult was essentially a local one and interest soon declined and even the challenges posed by the plague did not lead to a return of popular attention. By 1386–87, offerings at his tomb were only £1 6s. 8d.[52] Even though records are unavailable for the fourteenth-century plague years, it is unlikely that the tombs of local saints such as St. Thomas Cantilupe saw an increased influx of visitors. However, the translation of Thomas's remains to a new tomb in October 1349 was credited by some with a decline in plague cases around Hereford, although this was probably an act of self-aggrandizement by the custodians of the tomb as the plague was already waning by then.[53] Unlike some mysterious disease or a broken bone or wound that could heal on its own, a diagnosed case of the plague often led to death. People often invoked the aid of saints in the case of what appeared to be sudden death, but in many instances, the victim was simply stunned rather than dead. For example, return from the dead is the largest category of Henry VI's miracles with 24 cases while cure of wounds is second with 22 cases.[54] Although there is some difference between saints, a larger sample comprising 1,695 miracles of ten English saints from the eleventh through the fifteenth century indicates that the cure of continuing ailments and crippling was the most common form of miracle, with twenty-two percent of the total miracles, a likely result given the hazards of medieval life. Return to life was the next largest category comprising fifteen percent of the ten saints' miracles.[55] People may well have appealed to various saints, but the high mortality rate of the plague made it unlikely that they survived so no cures were reported at the saints' tombs. The evidence from saints' tombs and written proceedings is spotty, but it seems that many people considered saintly medicine no more effective than other forms of aid although the desperate family of a plague victim might well have tried invoking a saint's aid in addition to trying other remedies. The ineffectiveness of saintly medicine in regard to the plague did not, however, seem to have had much impact on popular veneration of the saints which remained strong throughout the fifteenth century.

The medical response to the plague was grounded in accepted doctrine that had a logic behind it. Popular remedies might also involve herb lore, but they too were traceable to remedies that may have been effective in other situations. The medicine of the saints was an accepted part of medieval life. The saints were credited with all sorts of cures and the authority of the Church stood behind the acceptance of miracles.[56] The devastation caused by the Black Death also generated fear in society. Later outbreaks of the disease generated less fear and by the fifteenth century, the disease had become almost a routine part of English life. The high death rates that were not always explainable by the usual means led to a fear of the unknown resulting from the 1347–50 outbreak that produced a variety of responses that were aimed at stopping the spread of the disease by looking to non-natural causes for it.

Because almost every one recognized that the ultimate origin of the Black Death was God, prayers to avert the plague were a natural response to the new threat. Even as the first cases of the *pestis* began to be reported Archbishop Zouche of York ordered on 28 July 1348 that "devout processions are to be held every Wednesday and Friday" in churches throughout the diocese as well as "a special prayer be said in every mass every day for allaying plague and pestilence."[57] Thereafter, the clergy regularly offered prayers to try to avoid ward off the pestilence. By late December of 1349, as the epidemic had wound its course through southern England Simon Islip, Archbishop of Canterbury wrote to the bishops of the southern province ordering a general rejoicing to commemorate the final passage of the disease.[58] Later outbreaks of the plague generally did not produce the same widespread response. Individual bishops continued to urge prayer and congregations and individuals continued still seek divine help to ward off the plague, but there were few national or regional responses.

Prayer was an acceptable response to many problems in the Middle Ages, one that people engaged in for a variety of issues. Beseeching divine help was one means of avoiding the wrath of God. At times, people saw the plague as divine punishment and while prayer could help to alleviate divine anger, removing the source of the anger could be another response. By the sixteenth century, a plague epidemic often led to calls for moral reform although some of these calls were caught up in the religious disputes of the Reformation and the changing religious dynamic in England. For example, in *Spirituall Preservatives against the Pestilence* (1593) Henry Holland described pestilent spirits that poisoned people's souls, indicating that a sound moral attitude was a defense against disease.[59]

Scapegoating and a turn to unconventional religious action provided a different means for alleviating the divine anger that had produced the pestis. In some parts of the continent, such as the Rhineland or Switzerland, people blamed the Jews for causing the plague usually by poisoning wells. Persecution of the Jewish population followed as some people thought to remove the threat. England engaged in no persecutions of the Jews during the fourteenth and fifteenth centuries because there was no Jewish population. Edward I had expelled the Jews from England in 1291 and so one potential scapegoat was removed. As the plague became increasingly concentrated in poorer sections of cities such as London by the early sixteenth century, some commentators focused calls for moral reform on the poor, in essence blaming them for being plague victims.

Another scapegoating response of a sort was the turn to unconventional religious practices that the Church often came to regard as heresy. In some parts of Italy, for example, flagellants abased themselves in efforts to assuage God's wrath that had led to the plague. At times, these flagellant groups turned on the clergy or engaged in theft or other threats to public order. Some flagellants went farther contending that the coming of the millennium was nigh.[60] What had started as displays of popular religious enthusiasm often went into such unconventional directions as to lead to prosecutions for heresy. Even though the island of Britain could not be sealed against the plague, royal authorities were more successful at keeping heresy out. People might turn to God for aid in dealing with the plague, but it was more an individual effort in England than a group effort.

Clerical mortality and the ensuing shortage of clergy were a direct consequence of the Black Death and the subsequent outbreaks. An example from the diocese of Bath and Wells is illustrative. There had been a total of 35 institutions to clerical livings in Somerset every year prior to the Black Death, but there were 32 for December 1348 after the plague hit. In the following year, 232 new livings were presented indicating a crisis with the number of the clergy.[61] Monasteries and cathedral chapters were also hard hit, often losing many of their members and often causing economic distress. However, some houses, such as Tavistock Abbey, were already in economic trouble before 1348.[62] The English church took several measures to deal with the clerical shortage such as decreasing the age of ordination and the founding of new colleges to train priests such as Corpus Christi at Cambridge (founded 1352) and New College, Oxford (founded 1378). In his wide-ranging essay on the impact of the plague in late medieval English religion, Christopher Harper-Bill argues that the pessimism found in some theological tracts of the late fourteenth century also found its way into popular religion. Two changes are important although we must be careful in attributing them solely to the impact of the plague. By the end of the fourteenth century, various writers were making a distinction between the deserving and the undeserving poor when it came to charity, in part spurred by the availability of employment. Nonetheless, the labor shortage that ensued from plague deaths seemed to have an impact on the moral outlook of some people. Harper-Bill also indicates that people were also becoming more concerned with questions of sexual morality than before even though official views did not change until the sixteenth century.[63] What came to be called Puritanism was coming early. Connecting the latter development directly to the impact of the plague is difficult as a variety of factors were at work.

Literature and art

The plague outbreaks of the fourteenth century had a cultural impact, but it is difficult to separate the impact of the plague and the evolution of a cultural ethos from each other. Dating from the early twentieth century, scholars such as Johan Huizinga saw a darker outlook in the late Middle Ages although they differed in the causes for this perspective. Huizinga, for example, was clear about the pessimistic spirit of the age: "At the close of the Middle Ages, a somber melancholy weighs on people's souls."[64] More recently, some scholars have questioned the concept of decline. The Second Pandemic played in role in shaping late medieval outlooks, but it is difficult to see a consistent, clear-cut impact arising from the plague. John B. Friedman indicates this lack of clarity in the concept of decline: "Perhaps the most striking feature of medieval art dealing with the plague is its indirection."[65] As Friedman indicates in his wide-ranging study, medieval wall paintings and manuscript miniatures rarely depicted the dead and dying, leaving these subjects to Renaissance artists who often depicted saints saving the dying through their intervention or saints caring for the afflicted. Instead, medieval depictions of the impact of the plague were often symbolic, focusing on the themes of the Dance of Death and the Three Dead and the Three Living. For example, in the north cloister of the Pardon Churchyard at St. Paul's Cathedral, there is a fresco of the dance of death done between 1430 and 1440.[66] Christine Boeckl indicates that these types of images originated before the middle of the fourteenth century although the plague provided a focusing mechanism that encouraged depictions of these subjects.[67] The Italian writer Giovani Boccaccio used the outbreak of the plague as the motive force that drove his storytellers into the country in *The Decaemeron*, which he probably began in the 1350s when the impact of the Black Death was still fresh in Italy. Even though he was not a medical man, Boccaccio provided one of the better lists of symptoms in providing background to why his storytellers fled Florence. Earlier Gabriele de Mussis, a lawyer from Piacenza, provided what has come to be the main account for the arrival of the plague in Europe in his *Historia de Morbo*.[68] Aside from chroniclers, English authors were slower to include the plague in their writings although they gradually came to use the plague to help shape the moral lessons they were trying to convey to their readers.

Born in 1332, William Langland entered the Church but took only minor orders. A young man when the Black Death struck, he often depicted the plague in his classic, *Piers Plowman* that appeared in three versions to symbolize the presence of sin, particularly pride, in society and the need for reform.[69] Langland likely composed the three texts between 1370 and the early 1390s so he was able to take into account the 1361 and 1369 outbreaks of plague as well as the social disorder that resulted from the plague. His theme is the search for truth in society, a theme he explores with feeling, faith, and satire. Later in *Piers Plowman*, in a chapter dealing with the coming of pestilence, Langland does explicitly describe the impact of death in society although in somewhat convoluted terms.[70] The image of society presented in *Piers Plowman* is essentially a conservative one that supports the social status quo even though Langland pokes fun at the pretensions of some elements of society. In sum, the plague appears in *Piers Plowman*, but only as a means for moving along Langland's critique of late fourteenth-century English society.

By the end of the fourteenth century, English authors were turning to the plague either directly or indirectly as they took the plague as a metaphor for death. Written sometime after 1400 John Lydgate's "A Dietary and a Doctrine for Pestilence," provided remedies and preventatives for the plague in 21 stanzas. He indicated that changing one's behavior, attitudes, and diet could help people avoid the plague.[71] His "Dietary" is an unoriginal cribbing from standard medical advice books of the time and contains little that is specifically directed against the plague although it does reflect current medical thinking.[72] Lydgate explored the theme of death using the plague as its agent in his "The Daunce of Machabree," which he translated from a French text sometime after 1426.[73] Lydgate used the

Dance of Death to show the inevitable progression of death through its agent, pestilence. Lydgate was well-read in the current medical advice books as noted in his "Dietary." The "Daunce of Machabree" captures the relationship of physicians and death, as physicians are depicted as essentially irrelevant in the battle against the plague.[74] Death comes for us all is Lydgate's theme and the learning of medical men avails us little in this inevitable battle. The moral lesson is clear: everyone is defenseless against the inevitability of Death and so we should prepare for it by repentance and atonement. Lydgate's Death does have a personality, which is revealed in some stanzas. At times, Death threatens those he encounters in savage fashion and at other times mocks their concerns for earthly life; there is little pity here. Only a few characters drawn from the lower reaches of society receive some pity as some welcome Death's embrace. Throughout the poem, Death deigns to respond to the complaints of those he encounters save for the Hermit who Death replies to saying "that is wel sayd … A better lesson there can no clerke expresse. Than til to-morrow is no man sure to abide."[75] The Dance Macabre was composed some 70 years after the plague first struck England so it cannot be labeled an immediate response to the fear created. It must be seen as both a response to the continued dislocations, particularly as the plague continued to affect England, and within a growing unease with the search for salvation, an unease that led others to emphasize the inevitability of death and the need to prepare for God's judgment.

Lydgate's near contemporary, Geoffrey Chaucer, had been a child when the plague struck for the first time. In the period from April to June 1349, two of John Chaucer's (Geoffrey's father) half-brothers died of the plague.[76] The young Geoffrey must have been struck by the inevitability of death coming to all for turned to the theme in the "Pardoner's Tale" when he composed the *Canterbury Tales*. The three blaspheming protagonists are drinking in a Flemish tavern when:

> … they heard a bell toll before a corpse which was being carried to its grave. [identified as a crony of the men] … and last night he was suddenly killed as he sat straight up on his bench completely drunk. A stealthy thief, whom men call death, who kills all the people in this country, came and cut his heart in two with a spear, and went away without a word. During this plague, he has slain a thousand.[77]

Chaucer's Death might be less obviously cruel than Lydgate's Death, but the result was the same and the agent of death—pestilence—was the same.

The literary impact of the plague was one embedded in overall attitudes toward salvation and death.[78] More often than not, writers used the plague as a vehicle for enunciating moral concerns. Even late medieval chroniclers, who often provided simply a dry recitation of events, emphasized the moral lessons to be learned from the attack of disease. From the early fifteenth century until the end of the sixteenth century, the plague and its impact might be in the background but it rarely figured overtly with the writers of the time. Near the end of the Second Plague Pandemic, Daniel Defoe drew on the outbreak in Marseille in 1720 for his *A Journal of the Plague Year*, a depiction of the final plague outbreak in England.

The Black Death inspired various other writers, especially science fiction authors who use the idea of a massive pandemic, although usually driven by some other disease, as the basis for their story of societal collapse. Two notable works deal specifically with the plague and how it affected social outlooks. Albert Camus told the story of a plague outbreak in the Algerian city of Oran in his novel *Le Peste* (*The Plague*) written in 1947. The existential novel shows how various inhabitants of Oran tried to cope with a plague outbreak although Camus based it on a cholera epidemic in Oran in 1849, not a plague outbreak. Ingmar Bergman used the Black Death in Sweden and how people reacted to it in his widely acclaimed film (1957) *The Seventh Seal*. The film ends with Death leading several of the main characters over the horizon in a Dance of Death.

Popular and artistic attitudes toward death in the fourteenth and fifteenth centuries were grounded in theology and the experiences of daily life.[79] Society made a distinction between natural death, which came to all in the course of time, and unnatural death that resulted from murder, accident, or disease. Embedded in both conceptions was the awareness that death could come at any time leading to the concepts of a good and a bad death. The person who died at home surrounded by family after making peace with God was considered to have died a good death. The body would then be prepared for interment often in a shroud for the less-well-off and usually in a coffin for the well-off. Once the body was prepared, a funeral, at times with appropriate ceremony and large groups of mourners, would be followed by burial in hallowed ground. The elite expected that they would be commemorated by an often substantial tomb although the poor might have to make due with a board, placed above their shallow graves, indicating who they were. People considered that the person taken by death unexpectedly with no chance for preparation had made a bad death. The medieval Church indicated that people should live every day as though it were their last in order to be prepared for death. Some people may have done this but death caught many by surprise. The onset of the plague gave at least some warning to its victims but it did not always allow for the usual rituals of death. Artists and writers often tried to capture the concepts of good and bad death and how life was fleeting. As Philippe Aries has indicated, care must be taken to separate the macabre depiction of death found in works of art and some writers with the popular conception of death as they were not always well-aligned.[80]

Starting with the publication of Millard Meiss's influential *Painting in Florence and Siena After the Black Death* in 1951, a variety of scholars have concluded that the shock to the system rendered by the Black Death created a watershed in which society turned increasingly to the macabre as a means for coping with the magnitude of the dead.[81] Although Meiss clearly limited his conclusions to the art of two cities in Italy, his approach was often seen as an explanation of art and literature elsewhere. As the examples from Lydgate and Chaucer illustrate, the macabre was present in the literature of the late Middle Ages, often represented by the Dance of Death. As Paul Binksi points out, such an interpretation is based on special pleading that over-emphasizes plague as an exogenous shock.[82] Focusing largely on art, Binski examines changes in the rituals of death that had already started to occur before the Black Death. The plague may have helped to push changes in the rituals of death, but it was, at most, a contributing factor, not the prime mover. Moreover, changes in religious practice such as the rise of the new Franciscan order and the Spiritual Franciscans who took some of Francis's teaching on poverty and salvation to a logical, if not acceptable, extreme also helped to increase a focus on the need to seek salvation as the day of judgment was coming. Some of the millennial movements of the later thirteenth and early fourteenth century emphasized the day of judgment was nigh, a time in which all would die no matter their standing in society. The plague could provide a convenient metaphor as the agent of death for writers such as Lydgate or Chaucer, but the seeds of what they described had been planted long before the Black Death and would be reinforced thereafter by continued disorder and in the fifteenth century by the threat that the Mongols posed to Christian Europe.

The same sort of shifting interpretation of the impact of the plague on artistic representation on the continent also occurred with the treatment of late medieval art in England. First, there was the acceptance of a large impact on artistic expression, followed by a reaction against this approach. Phillip Lindley indicates that for England and by extension the continent that the truth lies somewhere in between. Changes were already underway in the treatment of death before 1348, but the plague played a role and may have helped to accelerate the changing, more macabre, depiction of death. Undeniably, the plague did have an impact on architectural patronage, and, thus by extension, on construction. Churches were left unfinished not necessarily because of change in attitude, but because of contractions in clerical finances that made building projects impossible to continue.[83]

The visual arts captured the attitudinal changes toward death that were occurring in the late Middle Ages, even if not directed by the impact of the plague as Meiss claimed. It was understandable that people turned to the saints for aid, saints such as the Virgin, Lawrence, Christopher, or Barbara, or the two patron saints of the medical profession, Cosmos and Damian. As noted above, the cults of St. Sebastian and St. Roch also became popular in some areas and led to their artistic depiction. Artists depicted Sebastian at times as having a bubo-like growth in his groin, a characteristic of the plague. The Romans had reputedly martyred Sebastian in the third century by shooting him with arrows. Some commentators described the intense pain sometimes associated with the plague as almost coming from divine arrows. St. Roch had survived the plague and later comforted plague victims. The two most notable plague saints seem to have been more popular in Italy and southern France than in northern Europe. Beyond representations of plague saints, some artists of the fourteenth and fifteenth centuries tended to emphasize the coming Last Judgment awaiting mankind. By the sixteenth century, depictions of saints aiding the plague-stricken in some way became commonplace, especially in Italy. Tintoretto depicted St. Roch ministering to the poor in a 1549 painting with the implication that a miracle was soon to follow. Cardinal St. Charles Borromeo (1538–1589) became a common artistic subject, but the pictures drew on Counter-Reformation values rather than the earlier views express in pictures of St. Roch as they displayed a cardinal ministering to the poor, some of whom appeared to have the plague.[84] In England, from the time of Henry VIII onward such pictures of the saints were decidedly unwelcome although other artistic representations of the impact of the plague were still created. These representations often included an obviously pestilential figure as representing death. In some cases, the representation took on the form of the Dance of Death or the Three Living and Three Dead. Tomb architecture was also changing. An interred worthy might be depicted in lordly array on one level of the tomb, but the lower level of the tomb depicted a decomposing skeleton, the transi, the ultimate fate of mankind.[85] As Binski has noted, the Black Death was only part of a changing array of forces that led to these macabre depictions of the dead.

A personalized Death was central to the Dance of Death and even with the encounter of the three living men with the three corpses. Death, the fourth rider of the Apocalypse, could kill with any means available: pestilence, war, and famine. The advent of the plague in the mid-fourteenth century added to Death's power, but it was already considerable. The images of the three living and three dead tried to introduce a personal rapport with Death through conversation between the living and Death. Both themes, especially the Dance of Death, also introduced a leveling theme—all were equal before Death, no matter their social status. Kings, bishops, knights, priests, and peasants all joined in the line following Death. While the Dance of Death became a commonplace theme in continental art and literature, it found less of a place in England. John Aberth speculates, probably correctly, that themes of leveling would have been unpopular in certain circles after the Peasants' Revolt of 1381.[86] The continuing outbreaks of the plague emphasized that death was always present in society and so entered artistic and literary consciousness as well as the preaching of the day.

It is still difficult to see how much the presence of Death and the increased turn to the macabre affected popular life. For many people, life went on after a plague outbreak. They might be momentarily more aware of the omnipresence of death, but they had crops to be gotten in and children to raise. Bishops or members of the nobility might be more aware of the transience of life and so erect transi tombs, but the poor did not erect tombs. Other factors as well as the plague influenced popular consciousness and lead to a turn toward the macabre. Surviving the plague and other challenges could also lead in another direction contra-Huizinga, a relief at survival and an appreciation that opportunities could be seized from Death.

Plague and the late medieval economy

Some economists indicate that the pre-industrial world was locked into a situation in which population governed economic well-being. Derived from the arguments of the eighteenth-century parson, Thomas Malthus, this approach postulates what is known as a Malthusian trap, a world with a stationary population neither declining nor growing. Whenever population moved away from its natural equilibrium point, the tendency was for either birth or death rates to increase to bring it back into balance. With a stationary population, birth rates are equal to death rates. Birth rates are governed by social custom but generally rise, as the material living standard of the society increases. The death rate declines as living standards increase. Finally, the material living standard declines as the population increases.[87] This latter point is derived from the Law of Diminishing Returns that owes its origin to David Ricardo. The Law of Diminishing Returns indicates that production systems have a variety of inputs, most notably, land, labor, and capital. If one of the inputs is fixed, in this case, land by the mid-fourteenth century, using more of one of the other inputs will increase output, but by progressively smaller levels.

With a Malthusian model, it might be expected that the standard of living in England was on the verge of decline because of the growth in population through the end of the thirteenth century and the population was poised to return to an equilibrium lower than what it had been in the mid-fourteenth century. Population had been growing for some time as the death rate had remained constant but the birth rate had increased. Land, however, was in limited supply so little additional land could be put into cultivation. Under the Law of Diminishing Returns, the increases in population would lead to smaller positive impacts on the standard of living.

It is easy to fall into the trap of indicating that a decline in population **had to occur** in mid-century because the English population had so far exceeded its equilibrium. There are simply too many variables in place for such a deterministic argument to be successful. However, it is possible to argue that the standard of living might well have declined had population continued to grow unchecked. As Gregory Clark demonstrates, the standard of living was declining in the early fourteenth century, with a low point in the decade of 1310–19.[88]

The economic impact of the first outbreak of the *pestis* was quite severe, as we might expect. The Black Death was not the only shock to the English economy as the 1361 epidemic caused another drop in population numbers. There was a succession of severe winters between 1349 and 1352 and in 1363–64 that complicated the situation as did an abnormally hot summer in 1361 and another cattle plague in the 1360s.[89] Plague deaths meant that fewer workers were available to work the land. Agricultural laborers grasped this situation and tried to negotiate for higher wages and tenants also tried to negotiate better terms with their landlords. In urban areas, laborers also attempted to negotiate for higher wages. It appears that the disadvantaged made some gains as a result of the plague although grain prices also rose in the years after 1350 so that wage gains did not always lead to an improved standard of living. Many of the last vestiges of villeinage vanished by 1360 although serfdom continued to persist in some areas. Lords were no longer able to enforce required labor services and peasants refused to make the usual customary payments. A lord who tried to maintain the old regime soon found himself with no tenants. Free tenants negotiated for more land or better terms such as contractual tenure for leasing their holdings. Some of these changes did not happen overnight, but some appeared quite soon after an outbreak of the *pestis*.

The Black Death and continuing plague outbreaks provided a severe shock to the institution of serfdom.[90] The labor shortage gave peasants more bargaining ability and many were able to negotiate contractual tenancies rather than servile tenures in the 1350s and 1360s. This changing relationship is important in light of the participants and their stated goals in the Peasants' Revolt of 1381. R.H. Hilton makes the strongest argument for seeing serfdom as the major cause for the Revolt finding evidence in calls for abolition of serfdom by some of the participants.[91] The *Anonimalle Chronicle*, a contemporary account indicates that one of the rebel demands put forward at Mile End outside of London on 14 June was freedom "from all manner of serfdom."[92] Peasant grievances, including serfdom, were some of the goals of the Peasants Revolt, but not the only goals. Serfdom was already in decline in many places although for some it continued to be burdensome. However, many of the participants were free peasants and urban dwellers, people less concerned with servile tenure. Moreover, many of the individual targets of the rebels were not landlords but were political (and religious) figures, such as the Chancellor, Simon Sudbury Archbishop of Canterbury, or judges. The Peasants Revolt had its roots in the Black Death, but also in royal tax policy, innovations in royal justice, and an anti-Flemish immigrant attitude.

The changes disturbed lords or merchants who had benefited from the old regime but also anyone else who felt threatened by such rapid social change. William Langland, a minor cleric and author of *Piers Plowman*, was one such person. To Langland, it seemed that the social order was in danger of collapse as peasants tried to rise above themselves. Piers the Plowman, the central character in the work is depicted as a frugal, honest, diligent, loyal, and godly peasant who knew his station in life. He was devoted to the cultivation of his half-acre of land and to achieving salvation but did not aspire to more. In his contract with a knight, he promises to work for the knight's benefit as long as the knight provides law and order. In essence, Langland described an ideal world of mutual obligation of the three orders (those who prayed, those who fought, and those who worked) in contrast to what he saw going on around him. Langland also describes a fourth-order comprised of wage workers, beggars, and criminals. Piers tried to put some of these people to work on his land, but they soon deserted him for better conditions elsewhere. Harshly, Langland argues that it was the threat of hunger that kept the idle at work a point he elaborates on elsewhere with his criticism of the greed of laborers.[93] To someone such as Langland, the demands of tenants for better conditions or of workers for higher wages violated the tacit social contract. There is certainly much more in *Piers Plowman*, but Langland's critique of the economic impact of the plague must have resonated with many as the work was the equivalent of a best seller with numerous manuscript copies made. Langland was not alone in his criticism of those who were coming to be regarded as the idle poor. Henry Knighton, a canon of St. Mary's Abbey in Leicester displayed a similar view indicating that: "Nevertheless the workmen were so puffed up and contrary-mined that they did not heed the king's decree [concerning returning wages to pre-Black Death levels], and if anyone wanted to hire them then he had to pay what they asked: either his fruit and crops rotted or he had to give in to the workmen's arrogant and greedy demands."[94] A moralism, tinged with self-interest, influenced how some people viewed poverty and charity as distinctions were coming to be made between the deserving and the undeserving poor who would not work or who demanded more for their labor. This trend of distinguishing between the deserving and the undeserving poor intensified by the sixteenth century. Commentators continued to urge charity for those who deserved it, but became increasingly harsh in their condemnation of many of the poor.

The criticisms of workers and tenants also had an impact on the English government. The major landowners, merchants, and wealthy townspeople who sat in the Lords or who were elected to the Commons quickly took action. In 1349, Parliament passed the Ordinance of Labourers and followed it up with the Statue of Labourers in 1351.[95] The intent was to set the clock back to pre-1348. Laborers were forbidden to demand wages higher than those that prevailed before the Black Death or to refuse to work or break a labor contract before the end of the term of employment. Landowners or merchants were forbidden to pay more as well but the thrust of the legislation was directed toward those people who were seen as profiting from the labor shortage. The Ordinance went further and prohibited giving charity to those capable of work "so they may be compelled to labour."[96] The Statute also mandated fixed prices so that merchants could not benefit from the dearth that resulted from the labor shortage. The demand for higher wages continued, however, and in 1388, the Statute of Cambridge further addressed the fear of social decay. It particularly addressed efforts to control those people who wandered about in search of work and prohibited beggars from leaving their place of origin.[97] The powerful enforced these laws first with the Justices of Labourers in the 1350s and later through local Justices of the Peace.

The legislation at first glance seemed to be a reasonable effort at coping with unreasonable times; something that was fair to all. When the impact is examined, the result was anything but that. The price of food was regulated after all as well as wages, and anyone who offered higher wages was subject to prosecution. The reality was something different. The nobility and the gentry controlled the courts, not the peasantry. Even when peasants brought actions under the Statute, it was likely to be peasants with substantial holdings who wanted to hire laborers at low wages. As Christopher Dyer illustrates, the system was biased against those at the bottom of the social and economic pyramid. In the June 1378 session of the court in Hinckford Hundred in Essex, several laborers were fined for taking high wages including a group of 26 ploughmen, roofers, and a disabled carpenter. No lords of the manor, gentry, or bailiffs were fined for paying these wages. The fines collected under the Statute of Labourers also tended to indirectly benefit the well-off more so than the poor. In 1352, the village of Beauchamp St. Paul in Essex owed a subsidy of 75s. to the crown. It had collected 60s. in fines for violating the Statute so only 15s. more was needed to make up the difference. The well-to-do peasants, who would typically have paid the bulk of the subsidy, had their taxes effectively reduced by the impact of the Statute of Labourers.[98] Both directly and indirectly, the Ordinance of Labourers and the Statute of Labourers did little for the poor, nor were they intended to do so.

Parliament's efforts to control wages had some impact, but the demand for labor forced wages up. Interestingly, prices did not seem to increase as rapidly so the standard of living for those people at the bottom of society improved. The initial increase in wages was staggering, a hundred and one percent increase from 1349 to 1350. Parliament's actions did have some impact as wages declined by fourteen percent from 1351, when the Statute of Labourer's was passed, to 1352. After this setback, wages and their purchasing power continued to rise until the middle of the fifteenth century, especially after the price of grain declined in the 1370s. The impact of epidemic disease continued to be felt, holding down population and providing opportunities for laborers to negotiate for better conditions. By the 1380s, laborers' purchasing power had risen above that of what it would only reach in the decade of 1860–69 and remained above the 1860–69 level until the first decade of the sixteenth century.[99] These changes had gotten well underway and continued to develop over time for the rest of the century. Mark Bailey points out that the idea that a new economic equilibrium existed from 1375 to 1400 may be a stretch and he argues that the economy did not reach a post-plague equilibrium until the 1390s.[100]

In spite of efforts at maintaining low wages, the standard of living for the poor crept upward as the Malthusian model predicts. Higher wages meant higher purchasing power and some wage earners or agricultural laborers began to make purchases that might be labeled luxury goods. The effrontery of such actions seems to have been too much for some powerful people. The Sumptuary Law of 1363 attempted to address this situation although there seems to be no evidence of its enforcement and it was soon repealed. The Sumptuary Law prohibited "excessive apparel" and set maximums on what could be spent for cloth and accessories by the poor. Part of the motivation for the law seems to have been a concern with prices for goods being driven up by demand. Part of the motivation also came from a concern with the poor trying to rise above their proper social position.

The return of the plague as well as other diseases throughout the fifteenth century helped continue the labor shortage and the concomitant improvement in the standard of living for the poor. Without the impact of epidemic disease, the higher fertility rate would have been likely to drive down wages once again. If indeed some epidemics of the *pestis*, such as that of 1361, took the young who were the future producers of children, this further contributed to maintaining a low population growth rate for a time. In addition, the plague (and other health problems) seemed to claim more men than women as victims so that there was a shortage of men by the fifteenth century.[101] Although it would be unwise to speak of a golden age for English peasants and working men and women in the late Middle Ages, it does appear that the standard of living for those who survived the continued bouts of disease improved, only to drop in the sixteenth century when population began to grow once again.

The only fly in the ointment regarding this positive interpretation of the impact of the *pestis* is the impact of food shortages caused by a lack of producers. In some localities, this situation seems to have existed. Individual families or villages suffered for a time when too few laborers were available to produce adequate food. When this situation was coupled with inclement weather, increased prices and famine were the results. It was local rather than national famine, but famine nonetheless. Prices appear to have gone up considerably in the years immediately after the Black Death in response to the labor shortage. However, by the mid-1370s, the inflated prices for grain began to drop rapidly falling by forty to fifty percent by October 1372, well below the average of the 1360s.[102]

Once the death rate declined by the end of the fifteenth century, population grew until it produced a declining standard of living. As Clark indicates, this situation eventually overcame England in the sixteenth century and the overall standard of living declined.[103] It would not be until improvements in technology in the late eighteenth and early nineteenth centuries led to an upward shift of the population curve that the standard of living would grow in a permanent fashion.

Epidemic disease alone could not produce the changes necessary to propel England forward into sustainable economic growth. For that to happen, structural changes to the economy were necessary. The *pestis* and other diseases did, however, have a short-term positive impact on the economy. Overall, the positive economic impact of the plague improved the lot of those at the bottom of the social pyramid more than those at the top. The abandonment of serfdom was caused by a variety of factors, but the labor shortage resulting from disease played a major role. When population equilibrium returned it was too late to re-impose serfdom on English society.

The economic impact of the first outbreak of the *pestis* also had affected the political structure of England. Until the mid-fourteenth century, the crown had rarely interfered in the economic aspects of the kingdom. English monarchs obtained taxes, imposed tariffs, coined and at times debased money, and borrowed money with little thought to the economic impact these actions would have. They did not otherwise interfere in the economic activities of their subjects. The *pestis* changed this. With the Ordinance and Statute of Labourers, the Sumptuary Law, and the Statute of Cambridge, the English government attempted to legislate economic and social conditions. It was a conservative approach designed to return the changing situation to a pre-1348 situation and was designed to ensure the welfare of the well-to-do rather than the poor. Undoubtedly, the nation's elite welcomed, nay even demanded the actions. These laws were seen as maintaining good government, an expectation of kings, by maintaining the status quo. Nonetheless, it was an expansion of the power of government even if Edward III or Richard II or their ministers saw their actions only as affecting the economy.

The infrastructure of society and its institutions

The large number of plague deaths coupled with the fear generated by the disease had a tangible effect on how English society was organized. The impact of the labor shortage on agricultural production is obvious. The manpower shortage coupled with times to a capital shortage curtailed many building projects. In the sixteenth century, there were several parish churches that looked unbalanced because they stood incomplete with one section obviously larger than the rest of the church or a truncated steeple. Perhaps, a patron had started an elaborate addition to the church in the years immediately before the Black Death, but as labor and capital vanished, the building scheme fell victim to circumstances. In villages with declining populations and/or changing economic fortunes of the patron, the addition might never be completed. Colin Platt provides numerous examples of village churches throughout England with elaborate construction projects started before the mid-fourteenth century never to be completed such as an abandoned church in the deserted village of Wharram Percy, Yorkshire, or the church at Kersey in Suffolk.[104] Building might continue in places such as London, driven by royal will, but not always in the countryside. In some places, the population never returned to pre-Black Death levels so there were some communities with large churches that served small congregations. People moved away from other places in search of economic opportunity in the late fourteenth and fifteenth centuries. The landscape of sixteenth-century England was much different in some places than it had been before 1348.

Many of the parish clergies gave their lives serving their parishioners during plague outbreaks. Some, however, left their churches driven at times by fear and at times by a desire to move on to better livings. While bishops struggled to find clergy to fill benefices, they did not always meet with success. Without a local priest, a person facing death faced it unshriven. One response was to allow the laity to hear confessions in an emergency as the Bishop of Bath and Wells directed in January 1349.[105] Although the Church leadership took stringent measures to recruit more clergy, a clerical shortage, often coupled to declining population led to amalgamations of parishes as the Bishop of Hereford did with Great and Little Collington in Herefordshire in April 1351.[106] Monastic communities also suffered from the loss of monks during plague outbreaks and a declining sense of vocation that did not refresh the number of monks. By the end of the fifteenth century, some houses were down to only a few monks, something that

Thomas Cromwell latched on to in the sixteenth century as he sought to confiscate monastic foundations to buttress the coffers of Henry VIII. The Church remained an important part of English society in the fifteenth century and some aspects of devotion, such as pilgrimage, may have even increased. The visible institutions of the Church did suffer a blow.

The Black Death: A turning point?

At one time, many historians indicated that the Black Death produced a turning point in medieval society. Some indicated that the impact of the plague helped to produce a more pessimistic attitude in the fifteenth century. The great French historian Fernand Braudel called the Black Death and the accompanying recession of the mid-fourteenth century "a spectacle of this disintegration, this headlong tumble into darkness—the greatest drama ever registered in European history."[107] Others have maintained that the economic changes wrought by the Black Death helped to produce a modern outlook that enabled northern Europe to progress beyond southern Europe and ultimately for Europe to become a dominant force by the nineteenth century—the Little Divergence and the Great Divergence. Most recently scholars have become more cautious in their estimation of the impact of the Black Death. Recent accounts are more nuanced than earlier ones as they take many factors into account and trace the development of change over longer periods of time. The historian Colin Platt, for example, maintains that the massive number of deaths caused by the Black Death precipitated social and economic change in England, but grants that many of the developments that ensued after 1348 had earlier precedents.[108] Many scholars now look to other factors in addition to the plague as precipitating change and see the changes as having earlier roots and taking longer to occur. Some also point to the plague as having a devastating impact on some regions, but not others, rather than seeing a uniformly negative impact everywhere.

The continued plague outbreaks helped produce economic changes favorable to people on the bottom rungs of society in England, most notably enhancing their economic and social mobility. Others who could take advantage of the changes affecting society, such as some of the gentry also benefited. Some of these changes such as the abandonment of villeinage were permanent. Others, such as increased wages and an improved standard of living, did not last. Wages for both agricultural and urban workers began to decline in the sixteenth century and remained low until the nineteenth century.[109] Long-distance trade began to expand long before the first outbreak of the plague in 1347. It appears that in spite of fear of the disease that little was done to curtail trade. Individual villages might keep outsiders out, but overall trade went on especially in large cities such as London.

The situation of the nobility and wealthy merchants is harder to gauge. In some cases, mortality was high among these groups but they probably had a better chance of surviving any outbreak of epidemic disease than did the poor. In some cases, opportune deaths even provided opportunities for advancement in the royal service. Yet, noble fathers who died with no surviving sons had their line die out and the estates were dispersed or taken by the crown. The plague alone did not cause this situation but it furthered an existing process. Some land-lords suffered when they were forced to negotiate higher wages or lower service requirements with their tenants. Masters who raised the wages of skilled crafts-men also suffered the economic consequences of the plague if they were unable to raise the prices of their goods. In reality, the situation was not always bleak for the upper echelons of society. Merchants benefited from increased demand for their products. In addition, the impact of the Hundred Years War in the reigns of Edward III and Henry V appears to have been positive for many members of the nobility as well as some merchants. The collection of ransoms from French captives benefited some military leaders, as well as war profiteering which added to the coffers of military leaders and merchants who supplied the royal armies.

Even before the arrival of the plague in 1348, English towns were often unhealthy places to live. Diseases such as dysentery often took a toll on urban life. At least in London, the crown and the London city government made efforts at improving sanitation. For example, Edward III ordered the London city government to put a stop to the blood and offal that was dropped on the streets when it was transported from butcher shops to a dumping place along the bank of the Thames.[110] The crown generally respected the prerogatives of the City of London but had to continually remind the City of health hazards. In February 1377, King Edward threatened the City with a fine of 100 marks because of "the accumulation of refuse, filth and other fetid matter on Tower Hill, whereby the air was foully corrupted and vitiated and the lives of those dwelling or passing there are endangered."[111] As early as 1309, the Common Council ordered that householders should not dump their chamber pots in the streets, and seems to have, at least sporadically, enforced the ordinance was when it fined Richard Baker, a brewer 2s. in February 1372 for casting dung into the streets.[112] No wonder that London remained unhealthy with various diseases originating from filth in addition to visitations by the plague. Towns continued to grow in spite of public health problems and epidemic disease, except during severe outbreaks of disease such as that of 1348–49, but the growth was often spurred by in-migration. Until the nineteenth century, death rates exceeded birth rates in English cities.[113] Epidemics of the plague helped to slow the growth of urban population, but the upward trend continued. In spite of improving conditions on the land, after the Black Death, places such as London or Norwich still seemed to offer more opportunities for advancement and so people continued to flock to some towns. A.R. Bridbury, an historian who sees economic life of the late Middle Ages in a positive light, has argued that towns continued to prosper in the late Middle Ages based on trade and supplying goods not available in the countryside.[114]

The Second Pandemic helped to spur governmental efforts to improve public health. Local governments had already begun to focus on removing waste from the streets before the Black Death. Driven by the miasma theory, governments redoubled efforts at dealing with air and water quality. The Plague Orders of the sixteenth century were another effort by government to enhance the health of the population. Although motivated by public health concerns, both efforts also led to an expansion in the role of government.

The continuing magnitude of the impact of the plague also forced the medical community to reassess how it viewed disease. Galenic medicine came under stress in the sixteenth century from a variety of sources. The inability to cope with plague was one important focal point. Medical practitioners began to focus on the plague as a unique entity that had to be described. At first, this approach was directed at the plague, but its adoption opened the way to a new approach to disease.

Public health movements tended to be urban-based and designed to improve the health and reputation of communities. Not all towns prospered, however, from the fifteenth century onward. A combination of epidemic disease, changing trade patterns, and out-migration left some towns with little reason for existence. Already before the plague struck, some towns were in decline in the early fourteenth century.[115] Boston, a Lincolnshire port, was a growing town prospering from the coastal trade in the early fourteenth century. The ravages of disease decreased its population by half and the decline of its trading position helped ensure that few people would move to Boston seeking opportunities in the fifteenth century.[116] Boston was not alone in suffering decline; Colchester, Grimsby, and Winchester also lost population, not to regain their earlier numbers and prosperity (never for Grimsby) until the sixteenth century. In some cases, plague helped reinforce a trend already underway, in other cases, it precipitated decline. Some small villages that were particularly hard hit vanished entirely as the few remaining inhabitants moved away in search of a better life elsewhere.

Overall, the impact of the plague on the economic life of England seems to have been uneven. There was an immediate discernable positive impact on wages and the standard of living for the working poor. This impact diminished over time. For many people, even if not the country as a whole, England remained caught in a Malthusian system until the nineteenth century.[117] There does not appear to have been a shift to technology as a replacement for workers. Some towns suffered decline that the continued reoccurrences of the plague helped cause or reinforce.

While we can measure wages or economic growth, social attitudes are always harder to explain. On one level, it might be expected that massive numbers of deaths and the continued reoccurrence of disease would have a negative impact with a spirit of decline, perhaps even a preoccupation with death. Yet even Johan Huizinga, often credited with seeing a decline in the fifteenth century, did not view the plague as a major contributor to this spirit. To be sure, the plague provided a framework for Boccaccio's *Decameron* in Italy, but the disease did not really figure in the work except at the beginning. In England, the disease was reported in the chronicles and its impact on wages figured in *Piers Plowman*.

The shortness of life was a theme in some sermons, but other factors had long emphasized the frailty of human existence; the plague provided a fillip to add to this trend. The continued impact of disease may have helped to precipitate the emphasis on death, but even that is hard to gauge.

Constructing an accurate appraisal of the *mentalité* of medieval people is often difficult as the views of most people are not represented in chronicles and other documents. Without a time machine, in which to visit the fourteenth century and interview people we can only try to approximate popular views from the remaining accounts. One such was written by John Clyn, a Franciscan located in Kilkenny, Ireland and writing at Lent in 1349. His account is worth quoting at length:

> And in case things which should be remembered perish with time and van-
> ish from the memory of those who are to come after us, I seeing so many
> evils and the whole world, as it were, placed within the grasp of the evil
> one, being myself as if among the dead, waiting for death to visit me, have
> put into writing truthfully all the things that I have heard. And, lest the
> writing should perish with the writer and the work fail with the labourer,
> I leave parchment to continue this work, if perchance any man survive and
> any of the race of Adam escape his pestilence and carry on the work which
> I have begun.[118]

The chronicle breaks off at this point although another hand wrote at a later date: "Here it seems the author died."

It is hard not to be moved by John Clyn's account, but life went on. The historian Alfred Crosby tried to explain why the Great Influenza of 1918–19, which killed more people worldwide than who died in combat in World War I, was soon forgotten by the 1920s. He concluded that in the United States some people saw the flu as an outgrowth of the Great War while others, even those with relatives who died from influenza, wanted to forget it. Dying on the field of battle in France was heroic, dying of the flu was not.[119] Crosby's line of reasoning can be of use in examining why the plague did not always appear to have a large impact on the *mentalité* of the people. People were certainly afraid of the disease, especially in major epidemics, but there was also an awareness that everyday life had to go on. As time passed and the outbreaks in the fifteenth century, and thereafter came at longer intervals, there was more time to focus on the mun-dane. Plague became almost routine in the fifteenth century with moments of sheer terror during major outbreaks such as 1563.

The plague had varied impacts on English society that was not the same in 1500 as it had been in 1300. As Chris Dyer shows, the world of 1500 was much different than that of 1350, but the changes came gradually, were caused by many factors, and were already starting to affect English society even before 1300 and were still occurring in the early sixteenth century.[120] Although he ended his title *An Age of Transition?* with a question mark, Dyer intended that his readers would accept the period from 1300 to 1500 as an age of transition.

In *The Great Transition,* Bruce M.S. Campbell indicates that the Black Death ushered in a period of change for European and especially English society that started in the early fourteenth century and was largely complete by the end of the fifteenth century that served as a precursor to what some have labeled the Great Divergence in which Europe came to dominate the world.[121] Campbell focuses largely on the related impacts of climate change and disease in his densely reasoned account. He does note other factors that affected outlooks and helped to precipitate change such as the fall of Acre, the last of the crusader states, in 1291 and the beginning of the Hundred Years War. Along the way, he addresses the importance of commercial expansion and how it was related to the developments that led to economic recovery and expansion. Campbell wisely does not address other factors that helped to shape the transition although he alludes to issues such as political fragmentation and war which helped to hold the European economy back.[122] The succeeding plague epidemics that comprised the Second Pandemic had a demographic impact that then produced economic impacts when coupled to other factors. As noted above, the plague also affected European culture and attitudes.

Focusing on England and the Netherlands, other historians label the period that started in the crisis of the fourteenth century and ended by the early seventeenth century as the Little Divergence.[123] They use a number of variables to show that the changes wrought by the plague help pushed English and Dutch economic development ahead of that of the rest of Europe. While the plague had caused GDP per capita and real wages to rise in the fourteenth and fifteenth centuries, real wages had declined for much of Europe by the sixteenth century but not the Netherlands and England. Several scholars have labeled this growing disparity the Little Divergence.[124] There is overall agreement that England and the Netherlands had moved ahead of northeastern Europe by the sixteenth century; the debate has centered on what variables caused this to happen. One variable sometimes cited is the change in the European Marriage Pattern (EMP) with the average age of women at first marriage to be late and many women not marrying. Such a situation would tend to decrease family size and translate into higher per capita outputs producing higher income.[125] There are several other variables that were more likely to produce the Little Divergence such as agricultural changes leading to greater productivity, investment in labor-saving and capital-intensive goods, a change to a more materialistic cultural outlook, a rise in representative government.[126]

The Black Death and the succeeding outbreaks of plague that came in the fourteenth century helped to precipitate the changes that led to the Little Divergence. Economists Daron Acemoglu and James A. Robinson argue that the Black Death was a critical juncture that disrupted the economic balance of society. Once such an event happens, small continuing events will help to create a feedback loop that furthers the change in direction.[127] With their argument, we return to the argument of institutional economists that the institutions in which developments happen matter. Different institutions give different weights to different variables.[128] The Second Plague Pandemic helped precipitate economic changes, but the institutional constraints present in various countries also influenced the overall impact.

The changes affecting English society in the late Middle Ages are striking. Some of these changes can directly be traced to the Second Plague Pandemic, while other changes were generated by other forces or a synergy of several forces operating at once. But all was not changed. People mourned lost relatives and may have had to adapt to changing economic circumstances. Once the mourning was over, they still needed to tend their crops and their families. The king and barons played out their disputes with each other and with other countries. Life went on. The overall impact of the Second Plague Pandemic was great, greater than any other disease episode, but its impact on individual lives is often hard to trace and may have seemed transitory to even those affected

Plague and climate change may have been major drivers of change, but so too were war, the growing impact of representative institutions (i.e., Parliament) in some countries, the intellectual changes found in the Renaissance already underway in Italy, and the Mongol invasion of Eastern Europe. These forces helped to lead Europe to look outward in the latter part of the fifteenth century. A strengthening economy enabled Europe to take advantage of the discovery of the New World, but the discovery itself and everything it opened up also helped to further change Europe in the sixteenth century. The development of the printing press in the latter part of the fifteenth century made it possible to publicize knowledge of the Americas as well as giving medical treatises wider circulation and provided the venue for Luther and the other religious reformers of the sixteenth century to plead their cause. The late medieval climate change roller coaster that produced first warmer then colder conditions helped to set the table for change. The wider-ranging demographic impact arising for the Second Plague Pandemic furthered the changes. And finally, there were a large number of other forces at work that amplified or retarded change. Disease, even something of the magnitude of the Second Plague Pandemic, does not work alone.

The Second Plague Pandemic clearly produced major changes in English society. It was not the only infectious disease to affect premodern England. In addition to everyday ailments, such as diarrhea, other infectious diseases, such as the English Sweat, smallpox, typhus, and syphilis produced major outbreaks, perhaps even epidemics, in premodern England. Their impact will be examined and contrasted with the impact of the plague in succeeding chapters.

Notes

1 James Tait, ed. *Chronica Johannis de Reading et Anonymi Cantaurienis 1346–1367* (Manchester: Manchester University Press, 1914), 109.
2 G. H. Martin, ed. and trans., *Knighton's Chronicle, 1337–1396* (Oxford: Clarendon Press, 1995), 84–85.

3 John Aberth, *From the Brink of the Apocalypse* (New York: Routledge, 2001), 124. At one point inquisitions post mortem were the primary source of information for British medieval population patterns as was the case with the pioneering study by Josiah Cox Russell, *British Medieval Population* (Albuquerque: University of New Mexico Press, 1948).
4 Aberth, *From the Brink of the Apocalypse*, 125. Aberth summarizes the data reported in various local studies, 264, 272–74.
5 Aberth, *From the Brink of the Apocalypse*, 127.
6 E.A. Bond, ed., *Chronicon Monasterii de Melsa*, 3 vols. (Rolls Series, 43, 1866–69), 3: 37.
7 Gregory Clark, "The Long March of History: Farm Wages, Population and Economic Growth, England 1209–1869," *EconHistRev,* 60 (2007), 120.
8 Mark Bailey, *After the Black Death* (Oxford: Oxford University Press, 2021), 4.
9 Bailey, *After the Black Death*, 137.
10 Jon Arrizabalaga provides a telling discussion of Avicenna's views on the airborne causes of fevers. "Facing the Black Death: Perceptions and Reactions of University Medical Practitioners," in Luis García-Ballester, Roger French, Jon Arrizabalaga, and Andrew Cunningham, eds., *Practical Medicine from Salerno to the Black Death* (Cambridge: Cambridge University Press, 1994), 251–52.
11 Jacme d'Agramont, "Regiment de preservacio a epidimia o pestilencia e mortaldats," M.L. Duran-Reynals and C.E.A. Winslow, trans., *BHM,* 23 (1949), 57–89.
12 d'Agramont, "Regiment de preservacio a epidemia o pestilencia e mortaldats, 76–78.
13 An excellent account the continuity with pre-plague medicine found in the medical treatises is Arrizabalaga, "Facing the Black Death," 237–88.
14 Ann G. Carmichael addresses the problem posed by physicians' need to explain the cause of what appeared to be considered a universal disease in "Universal and Particular: The Language of Plague, 1348–1500," *Medical History* 52, S27 (2008): 17–52.
15 *Compendium de epidemia per Collegium Facultatis Medicorum Parisius.* Printed in Rosemary Horrox, ed. and trans., *The Black Death* (Manchester: Manchester University Press, 1994), 159–60. Two pioneering works that examine the early plague tracts are: Dorthea W. Singer, "Some Plague Tractates (Fourteenth and Fifteenth Centuries)" *Proceedings of the Royal Society of Medicine* 9 (1916), 159–214 and Anna Montgomery Campbell, *The Black Death and Men of Learning* (New York: Columbia University Press, 1931).
16 Horrox, *Black Death.*, p. 160–61.
17 Horrox, *Black Death,* p. 163.
18 Anonymous, German, c. 1360s, Horrox, *Black Death,* pp. 177–82.
19 Joseph P. Pickett, trans., "A Translation of the 'Canutus' Plague Treatise," in Lister M. Matheson, ed. *Popular and Practical Science of Medieval England* (East Lansing: Colleagues Press, 1994), 263–82.
20 E. M. Thompson, ed., *Chronica Galfridi le Baker de Swynebroke* (Oxford: Oxford University Press, 1899), pp. 98–99.
21 E.M. Thompson, *Adae Murimuth continuatio chronicarum; Robert de Avesbury de gestis mirabilibus reis Edwardi Tertii* (Rolls Series, 93, 1889), 406–07.
22 Guy de Chauliac, *The Cyrurgie of Guy de Chauliac,* Margaret S. Ogden, ed. (London: E.E.T.S., 265, 1971), 155.
23 Giovania Boccaccio, *The Decameron,* G.H. McWilliams, trans. (Harmondsworth: Penguin, 1972), 50–51.
24 Nancy G. Siraisi, *Medieval and Early Renaissance Medicine* (Chicago, 1990), p. 128.
25 Karl Sudhoff, "Pestschriften aus den ersten 150 Jahren nach der Epidemie des 'schwartzen Todes' 1348, II," *Archiv für Geschichte der Medizin,* 4 (1910–11), 405–6.
26 John of Burgundy, *Treatise on Epidemic Sickness,* Printed in Karl Sudhoff, "Pestschriften aus den ersten 150 Jahren nach der Epidemie des 'schwartzen Todes' 1348, III," *Archiv für Geschichte der Medizin,* 5 (1911–12), p. 62.
27 John of Burgundy, 69.

28 A modern edition of Moulton's *Glass of Health* is found in Rebecca Totaro, ed., *The Plague in Print* (Pittsburgh: Duquesne University Press, 2010), 5–15.

29 Chauliac, *Cyrurgie of Guy de Chauliac*, 155–57. The question of medical ethics in a time of pestilence is examined in Darrel W. Amundsen, *Medicine, Society, and Faith in the Ancient and Medieval Worlds* (Baltimore: Johns Hopkins University press, 1996), 289–309.

30 Philip Zeigler, *The Black Death* (New York: Harper, 1969), 75.

31 Darrel W. Amundsen, *Medicine, Society, and Faith in the Ancient and Medieval Worlds* (Baltimore: Johns Hopkins University Press, 1996), 303.

32 Slack provides a discussion of this early effort at trying to control the spread of the disease (*Impact of Plague*, 201–03) as well as discussing the implementation of plague orders later in the century.

33 Ann G. Carmichael, "Contagion Theory and Contagion Practice in Fifteenth-Century Milan," *Renaissance Quarterly*, 44 (1991), 213–256.

34 Slack (*Impact of Plague*, 207–13) discusses the background to the Plague Orders. A version in modern English is found in Totaro, *Plague in Print*, 180–96.

35 Moulton, "Glass of Health," in Totaro, *Plague in Print*, 6–7.

36 Slack, *Impact of Plague*, 23.

37 Margaret Healy, *Fictions of Disease in Early Modern England* (New York: Palgrave, 2001), 70. An interpretation that places more emphasis on Bullein, the physician can be found in Andrew Wear, *Knowledge and Practice in English Medicine, 1550–1680* (Cambridge: Cambridge University Press, 2000).

38 Bullein's *Dialogue* is reprinted in modern English in Totaro, *Plague in Print* (52–177). All references are to this edition.

39 Bullein, *Dialogue*, 98, 93.

40 Bullein, *Dialogue*, 92, 87, 90.

41 Bullein, *Dialogue*, 94–96.

42 Bullein, *Dialogue,* 164.

43 Ákos Tussay makes a strong argument, perhaps too strong, that the Plague Orders were elitist designed to control the poor rather than provide for their well-being. "Plague Discourse, Quarantine and Plague Control in Early Modern England: 1578–1625," *Hungarian Journal of Legal Studies*, (2020).

44 D'Agramont, *Regiment de preservacio a epidemiia o pestilencia e Mortaldats*, 78.

45 H.N. MacCracken, ed., *The Minor Poems of John Lydgate*, Part 1 (EETS, 107, 1907), 291. Lydgate "O Heavenly Star, Most Comfortable of Light," in Carleton Brown, ed., *Religious Lyrics of the XVth Century* (Oxford: Oxford University Press, 1967), no. 135, p. 206, lines 15–18. See also Lydgate, "*Stella Celi Extirpavit* in Brown, no. 136, p. 209, line 32, where Lydgate begs God to "save all thy servants from the stroke of pestilence." Spelling modernized.

46 Christopher Wordsworth, ed., *Horae Eboracenses* (Surtees Society, 132, 1920), 129.

47 Wordsworth, *Horae Eboracenses*, 131.

48 Heinrich Dormeier, "Saints as Protectors against Plague: Problems of Definition and Economic and Social Implications," in Lars Bisgaard and Leif Søndergaard, ed., *Living with the Black Death* (Odense: University Press of Southern Denmark, 2009), 163–86.

49 J.M. Theilmann, "The Miracles of King Henry VI of England," *The Historian*, 42 (1980): 465. The miracles are compiled in Ronald Knox and Shane Leslie, eds., *The Miracles of King Henry VI* (Cambridge: Cambridge Univesity Press, 1923).

50 Paul Grosjean, ed. *Henrici VI Angliae regis mircula postuma* (Brussels: Bollandist Society, 1935): 24–25.

51 Ben Nilson, *Cathedral Shrines of Medieval England* (Woodbridge: Boydell Press, 1998), 211–15, 234.

52 W. Nigel Yates, "The Fabric Rolls of Hereford Cathedral, 1290/1 and 1386/7" *National Library of Wales Journal* 18 (1973), 79. Penelope E. Morgan, "The Effect of the Pilgrim Cult of St. Thomas Cantilupe on Hereford Cathedral," in *St. Thomas of Cantilupe, Bishop of Hereford*, Meryl Jancey, ed. (Hereford: Friends of Hereford Cathedral, 1982), 145–52.

53 Ronald C. Finucane, *Miracles and Pilgrims* (Totowa: Rowman and Littlefield, 1977), 179.
54 Theilmann, "Miracles of Henry VI," p. 465.
55 John Theilmann, "On the Road to Health: Pilgrimage in Medieval England," in Gabriel R. Ricci, ed., *Travel, Discovery, Transformation* (New Brunswick: Transaction Publishers, 2014), 177–97. These numbers might be compared to the types of cures reported for the eleventh and twelfth centuries in France in Pierre-André Sigal, *L'homme et le miracle dans la France médiévale* (Paris: Les Éditions du Cerf, 2007) or modern miracles in Jacalyn Duffin, *Medical Miracles* (New York: Oxford University Press, 2009).
56 The most comprehensive account of medieval saints and their impact on society is Robert Bartlett, *Why Can the Dead Do Such Great Things* (Princeton: Princeton University Press, 2013). Also useful, especially for the Late Middle Ages is André Vauchez, *Sainthood in the Late Middle Ages*, Jean Birrell, trans. (Cambridge: Cambridge University Press, 1997). For pilgrimage in England: Diana Webb, *Pilgrimage in Medieval England* (London: Hambledon and London, 2000), Colin Morris and Peter Roberts, eds., *Pilgrimage: The English Experience from Becket to Bunyan* (Cambridge: Cambridge University Press, 2002), and Theilmann, "On the Road to Health." For shrines: Nilson, *Cathedral Shrines of Medieval England*, and John Crook, *English Medieval Shrines* (Woodbridge: Boydell Press, 2011).
57 James Raine, ed., *Historical Papers and Letters from Northern Registers* (Rolls Series, 61, 1873), pp. 395–7.
58 David Wilkins, *Concilia Magnae Britanniae et Hiberniae, A.D. 446–1718,* 4 vols. (London, 1737), 2: 752.
59 Healy, *Fictions of Disease,* 42.
60 There are numerous accounts of heresy in the late Middle Ages. Good starting points are Gordon Leff, *Heresy in the Later Middle Ages* (Manchester: Manchester University Press, 1967), Norman Cohn, *The Pursuit of the Millennium*, rev. ed. (New York: Oxford University Press, 1970), R.I. Moore, *The War on Heresy* (Cambridge: Harvard University Press, 2012).
61 Christopher Harper-Bill, "The English Church and English Religion after the Black Death," in Mark Ormrod and Phillip Lindley, eds., *The Black Death in England* (Donington: Shaun Tyas, 2003 [1996]), 85.
62 Harper-Bill, "English Church after the Black Death," 99.
63 Harper-Bill, "English Church after the Black Death," 115, 117.
64 Johan Huizinga, *The Waning of the Middle Ages* (Garden City: Anchor Books, 1954 [1924]), 31. The most recent translators of this work argue that it was not as pessimistic as it seemed because of mistranslations. *The Autumn of the Middle Ages*, R.J. Payton and U. Mammitizsch, trans. (Chicago: University of Chicago Press, 1997).
65 John B. Friedman, "'He Hath a Thousand Slayn this Pestilence': The Iconography of the Plague in the Late Middle Ages," in Francis X. Newman, ed., *Social Unrest in the Late Middle Ages* (Binghamton: Medieval and Renaissance Texts and Studies, 1986), 75. While Friedman ranges across Europe in his study of art, he focuses more closely on England in his examination of literature (75–112).
66 John Aberth, *The Black Death* (Oxford: Oxford University Press, 2021), 137.
67 Christine M. Boeckl, *Images of Plague and Pestilence, Sixteenth Century Essays and Studies* 53 (Kirksville, MO: Sixteenth Century Essays and Studies, 53, 2000), 69.
68 The excerpt published in translated form in Horrox, *Black Death*, 14–26, gives a good idea of the detail that de Mussis provided.
69 Bryon Lee Grigsby sums up the impact of plague in *Piers Plowman* in *Pestilence in Medieval and Early Modern English Literature* (New York: Routledge, 2004), 103–05.
70 William Langland, *Piers the Plowman*, J.F. Goodridge, trans. (Harmondsworth: Penguin, 1959), 125.
71 Grigsby, *Pestilence in English Literature*, 132.
72 MacCracken, *Minor Poems of John Lydgate*, 702–7.

73 Henry Bergin, ed., "The Daunce of Machabree," in *Lydgate's Fall of Princes* 4 vols. (EETS, extra ser., 121–24, 1923–7), 123: 1025–44. A good discussion of the themes raised in this work is Karen Smyth, "Pestilence and Poetry: John Lydgate's Danse Macabre," in Linda Clark and Carole Rawcliffe, eds., *The Fifteenth Century, XII: Society in an Age of Plague* (Woodbridge: Boydell Press, 2013), 39–55.
74 "Daunce of Machabree," 123: 1037, lines 417–24.
75 "Daunce of Machabree," 123: 1042, lines 625, 631–2.
76 Barney Sloane, *The Black Death in London* (Stroud: The History Press, 2011), 60.
77 Geoffrey Chaucer, *The Canterbury Tales of Geoffrey Chaucer*, R.M. Lumiansky, trans. (New York: Washington Square Press, 1948), 293–94.
78 The starting point for questions of the representation of death in the late Middle Ages is Paul Binski, *Medieval Death* (Ithaca: Cornell University Press, 1996).
79 Two chapters in Peter C. Jupp and Clare Gittings, eds., *Death in England* (Manchester: Manchester University Press, 1999) provide a concise overview of attitudes toward death and how it was portrayed in the late Middle Ages: Rosemary Horrox, "Purgatory, Prayer and Plague: 1150–1380" (90–118) and Philip Morgan, "Of Worms and War: 1380–1558" (119–46).
80 Philippe Aries, *The Hour of Our Death*, Helen Weaver trans. (New York: Alfred A. Knopf, 1981), 126.
81 Millard Meiss, *Painting in Florence and Siena after the Black Death* (Princeton: Princeton University Press, 1951).
82 Paul Binski, *Medieval Death: Ritual and Representation* (Ithaca: Cornell University Press, 1996), 127–30.
83 Phillip Lindley, "The Black Death and English Art. A Debate and Some Assumptions," in Ormrod and Lindley, *Black Death in England*, 125–46. See also Colin Platt, *King Death* (Toronto: University of Toronto Press, 1997), 137–75.
84 Boeckl, *Images of Plague and Pestilence*, 58–60.
85 Aberth provides a helpful discussion of changing fashions in late medieval architecture. *From the Brink of the Apocalypse*, 182–257.
86 Aberth, *From the Brink of the Apocalypse*, 214.
87 Gregory Clark provides a good discussion of the Malthusian model in *A Farewell to Alms* (Princeton: Princeton University Press, 2007), p. 20–29. A critique of the Malthusian model as well as other models intended to explain economic growth in the Middle Ages can be found in John Hatcher and Mark Bailey, *Modelling the Middle Ages* (Oxford: Oxford University Press, 2001).
88 Clark, *Farewell to Alms*, 41. Gregory Clark, "The Condition of the Working-Class in England, 1209–2004," *Journal of Political Economy* 113 (2005), 1307–40; Clark, "Long March of History," 99.
89 Mark Bailey, *After the Black Death* (Oxford: Oxford University Press, 2021), 168.
90 Bailey (*After the Black Death*, 83–109) provides a good overview of the impact of plague on the institution of serfdom as he argues that it helped to weaken the institution. Various perspectives on the Peasants' Revolt are found in R.H. Hilton and T.H. Aston, eds., *The English Rising of 1381* (Cambridge: Cambridge University Press, 1984). A work that places the Peasants' Revolt in the context of urban risings throughout the fourteenth century is Samuel K. Cohn, Jr., *Popular Protest in Late Medieval English Towns* (Cambridge: Cambridge University Press, 2013).
91 Rodney Hilton, *Bond Men Made Free* (New York: Viking, 1973), e.g., pp. 137–40.
92 V.H. Galbraith, ed., *The Anonimalle Chronicle, 1333 to 1381* (Manchester: Manchester University Press, 1927), 149.
93 *Piers Plowman*, 87–90.
94 G.H. Martin, ed. and trans. *Knighton's Chronicle 1337–1396* (Oxford: Clarendon Press, 1995), 102–03.
95 Ordinance of Labourers: in A. Luders, et al., *Statutes of the Realm 1101–1713*, 11 vols. (Record Commission, 1810–28), 1: 307–08; Statute of Labourers: 1: 311–13.
96 *Statutes of the Realm*, 2: 311–13.

97 Statute of Cambridge: *Statutes of the Realm*, 2: 59–60.

98 Christopher Dyer, *Making a Living in the Middle Ages* (New Haven: Yale University Press, 2002), 283.

99 Clark, "Long March of History," 116–17, 100.

100 Bailey, *After the Black Death*, 234–70.

101 Jim Bolton, "'The World Upside Down'. Plague as an Agent of Economic and Social Change," in Ormrod and Lindley, *Black Death in England*, 37. Bolton provides a helpful, well-referenced discussion of the state of the economy in the late Middle Ages.

102 John Hatcher, "England in the Aftermath of the Black Death," *Past & Present*, 144 (1994), 34.

103 Clark, *Farewell to Alms*, 47.

104 Platt, *King Death*, 137–49.

105 Wilkins, *Concilia Magnae Britanniae et Hiberniae*, 2: 745–6.

106 J.H. Parry, ed., *Registrum Johannis de Trillek* (Canterbury and York Society, 1912), 7: 174–76.

107 Fernand Braudel, *Civilization and* Capitalism, Siân Reynolds, trans., 3 vols. (New York: Harper and Row, 1984), 3: 314–15. David Levine echoes this view calling the new mortality regime produced by re-occurring epidemics "the specter haunting Europe." *At the Dawn of Modernity* (Berkeley: University of California Press, 2001), p. 333.

108 Platt, *King Death*, 177.

109 Clark, "Long March of History," 99–100.

110 A.H. Thomas, ed., *Calendar of Plea and memoranda Rolls; A.D. 1364–1381* (Cambridge: Cambridge University Press, 1929), p. 93.

111 *Plea and Memoranda Rolls, A.D. 1364–1381*, p. 140. The mayor and aldermen followed up with an inquest that revealed that John Gardiner alone had dumped one hundred carts of rubbish on Tower Hill, Ibid., pp. 140–41.

112 Riley, *Memorials of London*, 67–8. *Plea and Memoranda Rolls, A.D. 1364–1381*, p. 135. A wide-ranging discussion of public health issues in late medieval England, particularly London, can be found in Rawcliffe, *Urban* Bodies, and J.M. Theilmann, "The Regulation of Public Health in Late Medieval England," in J.L. Gillespie, ed., *The Age of Richard II* (New York: St. Martin's, 1997), c. 10.

113 An extensive account of English population history from the mid-sixteenth century to the mid-nineteenth century is E.A. Wrigley and R.S. Schofield, *The Population History of England, 1541–1871* (Cambridge: Cambridge University Press, 1989), especially 136–42.

114 A.R. Bridbury, *Economic Growth: England in the Late Middle Ages* (London: Allen and Unwin, 1962), 70–82.

115 Richard Britnell, "The Black Death in English Towns," *Urban History*, 21, pt. 2 (1994): 196.

116 Platt, *King Death*, 19–20.

117 Clark provides an interesting assessment of the interaction of the interaction of fertility and social mobility in a Darwinian system. *Farewell to Alms*, 112–32.

118 John Clyn, *Annalium Hiberniae Chronicon*, R. Butler, ed. (Dublin: Irish Archaeological Society, 1849), 37. Philip Zeigler treats Clyn's mental state in sympathetic fashion indicating his chronicle was "a memorial to the terror and grief of those who were still alive." *Black Death*, 195.

119 Alfred W. Crosby, *America's Forgotten Pandemic* (Cambridge: Cambridge University Press, 1989), 311–25.

120 Christopher Dyer, *An Age of Transition?* (Oxford: Clarendon Press, 2005), 244.

121 Bruce M. S. Campbell, *The Great Transition* (Cambridge: Cambridge University Press, 2016).

122 Campbell goes so far as to condemn climate determinists such as David Zhang et al., who argue that climate change was the ultimate driver for the human crises of pre-industrial Europe (p. 395). Aware of the risks of producing an overly long book by including other factors such as war Campbell wisely focused on climate

change and disease and the changes they produced. David D. Zhang, et al., "The Causality Analysis of Climate Change and Large-Scale Human Crisis," *PNAS* 108 (2011): 17296–301.

123 The impact of the Black Death on several of the economic variables that contributed to the Little Divergence is detailed in Remi Jedwab, Noel D. Johnson, and Mark Koyama, "The Economic Impact of the Black Death," *Journal of Economic Literature* (2021).

124 Bailey (*After the Black Death*) provides a good summary of the impact of the variables used to measure the Little Divergence, 283–325.

125 Nico Voigtländer and Hans-Joachim Voth make the argument for the impact of the EMP in connection with other demographic variables. "The Three Horsemen of Riches: Plague, War, and Urbanization in Early Modern Europe," *Review of Economic Studies*, 80 (2013), 774–811. Changes in fertility regimes arising in part from age of marriage are also part of Mattia Fochesato's explanation for the Little Divergence although he also emphasizes changes in rural and urban labor organization. "Origins of Europe's North-South Divide: Population Changes, Real Wages and the 'Little Divergence' in Early Modern Europe," *Explorations in Economic History*, 70 (2018), 91–131.

126 Bailey (*After the Black Death*, 283–325) stresses these variables, among others, over change in marriage patterns. Alexandra M. De Pleijt and Jan Luiten van Zanden give some credence to demographic variables, but emphasize the rise of representative institutions. "Accounting for the 'Little Divergence': What Drove Economic Growth in Pre-Industrial Europe, 1300–1800," *European Review of Economic History*, 20 (2016), 387–409. Stephen Broadberry emphasizes the impact of the Black Death, but also the opening of new trade routes as he first details the Little Divergence and then the Great Divergence. "Accounting for the Great Divergence," London School of Economics and Political Science, Department of Economic History Working Papers, No. 184 (2013).

127 Daron Acemoglu and James A. Robinson, *Why Nations Fail* (New York: Crown, 2012), 101, 107.

128 A good introduction of the impact of medieval institutions on economic life is Avner Greif, *Institutions and the Path to the Modern Economy* (Cambridge: Cambridge University Press, 2006), 14–53, 350–57.

7

NEW DISEASES AT THE TURN OF THE SIXTEENTH CENTURY: THE MYSTERY OF THE ENGLISH SWEAT

On August 22, 1485, Henry Tudor, Earl of Richmond, gained the English throne by defeating Richard III at the Battle of Bosworth. Soon afterward, a new, mysterious, and deadly disease struck the land, killing readily and quickly. Writing in 1513, when memories of the disease were still fresh the chronicler Polydore Vergil described the new disease:

> "it was a baleful affliction and one which no previous age had experienced. A sudden deadly sweating attacked the body and at the same time head and stomach were in pain from the violence of the fever. When seized by the disease, some were unable to bear the heat and (if in bed) removed the bed-clothes or (if clothed) undressed themselves; others slaked their thirst with cold drinks; yet others endured the heat and the stench (for the perspiration stank foully) and by adding more bedclothes provoked more sweating. But all died alike, either as soon as the fever began or not long after, so that of all the persons infected scarcely one in a hundred escaped death. And those who survived twenty-four hours after the sweating ended (for this was the period when the fever raged) were not then free of it, since they continually relapsed and many thereafter perished.[1]

What Polydore Vergil described was the advent of a disease previously unknown in England that came to be known as *Sudor Anglicus*, or the English Sweat, although some contemporaries also called it Stup-Gallant, Stoupe Knave and know thy Master, and the New Acquaintance. After its first appearance in 1485, the English Sweat reappeared in 1508, 1517, 1528, and 1551 and then disappeared from sight not to be seen again. Later outbreaks were not as well recorded as the first one although John Caius, the Padua trained physician of Edward VI, Mary, and Elizabeth I, described the medical aspects of the 1551 outbreak in some detail in two treatises.

DOI: 10.4324/9781003215219-8

The English Sweat was not the only disease to appear for the first time in the late fifteenth century. Syphilis (described in the next chapter) made its appearance in 1494 in Italy and then spread throughout Europe including England. Syphilis did not come and go in epidemic patterns; it struck people at any time in the year, and in the first 20 years with ferocity and with a large number of victims. The two diseases illustrate historian Charles Rosenberg's point that a disease does not exist until it has been named.[2] Naming the English Sweat proved to be an easy proposition as it was found almost exclusively in England and an obvious symptom was copious sweating. Naming syphilis proved to be more challenging as it became a disease that people wanted to blame someone else for starting (see the discussion in the next chapter).

Syphilis and *Sudor Anglicus* are classic examples of "new" diseases. They appeared suddenly, had a large impact on society, and medical thought tried to incorporate them into the existing structure of medical explanation, in this case, the Galenic approach to medicine. The plague in the fourteenth century had also been a "new" disease, but by the late fifteenth century, it had become almost routine save epidemics that still produced death rates as high as ten percent or so. The three diseases all posed challenges to Galenic medicine. Medical men tried to fit the symptoms of these diseases into the existing Galenic framework and succeeded to some degree with the plague. The other two diseases, however, stretched the existing approach to medicine although medical men did their best to fit their symptoms, purported causes, and cures into the framework of humor theory and Galenic treatment regimens.

The Sweat posed a different set of problems than syphilis. It was an epidemic disease with five clear outbreaks although the likelihood exists that a few cases occurred between the epidemics. Commentators mostly agreed upon its symptoms, but did not always agree on treatment, displaying some differences concerning how they fit it into humor theory. The Sweat also appeared to be more of a disease of only England although an epidemic occurred in Germany in 1529 that many contemporaries regarded as the Sweat. Mysteriously *Sudor Anglicus* did not reappear after the 1551 epidemic leading the medical community to lose interest although not late twentieth-century commentators who tried to construct a retrospective diagnosis of *Sudor Anglicus*.

The importance of *Sudor Anglicus* is less in the number of deaths that it caused, but in seeing how people viewed a "new" disease, one that struck all levels of society, and how it affected society, and how the medical community reacted to it. Examining the Sweat also enables us to gain some knowledge concerning unknown diseases in the past that enables a comparison of the impact of diseases over time.

The arrival of the English sweat

The plague was omnipresent in fifteenth-century England, so much so that only major outbreaks, such as that of 1479–80, received much attention. Almost as if the disease had a life of its own and could sense the upcoming political turmoil resulting from the death of Edward IV in 1483 and the usurpation of the throne by his brother as Richard III, there were no major outbreaks of the plague during the 1480s. By 1485, Englishmen could describe the symptoms of the plague and how it progressed. The plague had come to provide a reference point for describing the symptoms and impact of other diseases. When the disease described by Polydore Vergil as the sweating sickness appeared, people recognized it as something new, something different than the plague although seemingly almost as lethal.

Although it is possible that cases of what came to be described as the English Sweat had occurred before 1485, it was not until September 1485 that the disease came to have an impact on English society. Thereafter, it reappeared periodically although it never seemed to reach the intensity of the first outbreak. Whenever people described the Sweat, they were quite clear that whatever it was, it was not the plague. Even the plague had warned of its coming as chroniclers noted outbreaks elsewhere long before the disease arrived in England. The sudden arrival of the English Sweat almost out of the blue helped to contribute to its fearsome reputation and left people scrambling for remedies and preventatives.

Henry Tudor's invasion force landed at Milford Haven in the west of England on August 7, 1485, after leaving France on the first. Their line of march took them across the western counties toward London. Henry's forces defeated those of King Richard III on the twenty-second at the battle of Bosworth and thereafter, his march was more a triumphal progress than an invasion although some mopping up of Richard's supporters remained to be done. The first reported cases of the English Sweat occurred on September 19. Writing in 1490, shortly after the first outbreak of the disease, the French physician Thomas Forrestier, who had been resident in England at the time, indicated that the Sweat started in London and spread to the countryside. The Sweat certainly was present in London in September 1485. Two lord mayors of London, Sir William Stoker and Thomas Hall succumbed to the disease within eight days of each other, as did six aldermen, and Forrestier reports that 15,000 people died from the disease in 1485 although he is unclear as to whether this was in the whole country or London alone.[3] The first mayoral death occurred on 23 September just as the disease broke out in London, weakening the ability of the City government to cope with it.[4] The suddenness of the onset of the Sweat was matched by its quick departure from London. The late sixteenth-century chronicler Raphael Holinshed reported that it had passed by the end of October.[5] Forrestier may have overestimated the number of deaths, but Henry VII's reign was off to a bad start nonetheless. Writing from the perspective of the late sixteenth century, Holinshed noted that "this disease coming in the first yeare of king Henries reigne, was iudged (of some) to be a token and signe of a troublous reigne of the same king, as the proofe partlie afterwards shewed it selfe."[6] Polydore Vergil, who arrived in England in 1501, provided a subtler interpretation than Holinshed, as he indicated that Henry had to work to maintain his rule as he was continually beset by treachery, in essence, he had to "reign in the sweat of his brow."[7] Both authors had the advantage of hindsight in viewing Henry's turbulent reign when they wrote their accounts of the 1485 epidemic. Writing closer in time to the epidemic, Thomas Forrestier read no political implications into the outbreak. As might be expected, the deaths in London received the attention of chroniclers writing in London, but the disease may not have originated there and cases appeared throughout southern England. Instead, the Sweat may have first appeared in the rural western counties that Henry's army marched through on their way to London. Deaths there would have been unlikely to have been reported, being ascribed to the hardships of campaign.

Scholars John Wylie and Leslie Collier, on the other hand, find no evidence for either a London or west country origin for the English Sweat as they argue for the appearance of cases in the north of England earlier in 1485.[8] Before Henry Tudor landed at Milford Haven Thomas, Lord Stanley indicated that he would be unable to join King Richard's forces because he feared that he was infected with the sweating sickness.[9] Because this is a rather vague reference, we must be careful of inferring too much from it. Another piece of evidence for an earlier northern origin is an entry in the York civic records that a shoemaker was releasing his apprentice from his indenture "for fere of the plage of pestilence that reigned."[10] Whatever the disease was, it continued throughout the summer as the local council ordered an alderman, who had fled York during the summer, to return on 16 August 1485 to help deal with "the plage that reigneth."[11] Pestilence, however, was a generic term that often referred to plague but could refer to any sort of epidemic disease. Wylie and Collier as well as Paul Heyman, Leopold Simon, and Christel Cochez build their cases for a northern origin of the Sweat on what is a rather flimsy piece of evidence.[12] As Paul Slack points out, plague was present in York in 1485–86 so the disease noted in the York records was likely that.[13] The origin of the English Sweat outbreak in 1485 remains a mystery. Possibly, it came to England on a disease vector such as a tick that one of Henry's mercenaries carried on board ship. The French origin might help to explain a continental outbreak in 1529. On the other hand, it may have already been in the country in 1485, perhaps in the rural western counties or even London. Examination of the geography of the disease, in 1485 and later, creates as many questions as it answers.

Several characteristics of later outbreaks of the English Sweat appeared in the accounts of the first epidemic. First, there was the copious sweating that resulted from a high fever. Second, was the sudden onset of the disease and the quick death it often produced. Third, the disease often reappeared in its victims after the first episode so there seemed to be no lasting immunity. Fourth, people seemed to learn from observing the course of the disease. Polydore Vergil and Richard Grafton, two commentators on the 1485 outbreak, reported a means of fighting the disease. Once a person felt the onset of the disease, he should retire to bed for 24 hours, remain tightly covered, and drink only minimally.[14] Taking in only a little fluid may have done more harm than good when it came to fighting a fever, but the other two remedies couldn't have hurt and may have helped in fighting the Sweat although they may have also made the fever worse. A fifth point also emerges as it was apparent with the deaths of the London mayors and aldermen that the English Sweat seemed to be no respecter of persons. Some commentators have gone so far as to indicate members of the aristocracy were often likely victims, although numbers, as well as specific instances, do not seem to support this argument.[15] If Forrestier's high mortality figures are at all likely, most of the victims had to come from the bottom rungs of society, not just the aristocracy.

If the English Sweat had disappeared after the 1485 epidemic, later writers such as Polydore Vergil, Richard Grafton, or Raphael Holinshed might have accorded it less notice in their chronicles in spite of a substantial number of deaths. The Sweat reappeared four more times, helping to keep it in the public's consciousness although later outbreaks did not receive nearly as much attention as did the first one. This point is consistent with accounts of the plague that were quite fulsome regarding the first outbreak and much less so on later occasions. Once a disease began to occur on almost regular intervals, it became almost routine and commentators noted its presence briefly, but did not comment extensively on the disease. Moreover, if the Sweat was a virgin soil epidemic in which the first outbreak is far more lethal than subsequent ones is accepted, the later outbreaks of the English Sweat would have had much less of an impact than did the first one as some people developed immunity to the disease.

After the first outbreak, the English Sweat returned four more times before vanishing from sight. In 1508, it struck again although its impact this time is hard to gauge. Polydore Vergil argued that it had a diminished impact because people had learned to cope with it during the first outbreak.[16] He maintained that its coming presaged the death of Henry VII in 1509 as Henry had won the country by "the sweat of his brow." Contemporaries did not adopt Polydore Vergil's view, nor did they mention the Sweat in discussing the death of the King. Sir Thomas More is reported mentioning to Cardinal Wolsey an outbreak of the sweating sickness among the students of Oxford and Cambridge in 1509.[17] Certainly, if there was an outbreak in England, students arriving from various parts of the country, especially London, would have been likely to spread the disease, particularly if it was passed from one person to another. There are references to an outbreak of an unknown disease in Chester ascribed to *Sudor Anglicus* that killed less than one hundred people in a three-day period but they are sketchy at best.[18] From the lack of attention, it seems that the Sweat may have had little impact in 1508 and that largely in London.

Following a lapse of several years, the Sweat returned again in 1517. Holinshed's description of the symptoms and course of the disease mirrors that of Polydore Vergil for the 1485 epidemic.[19] Reporting to the Venetian government, the Venetian ambassador noted the large number of deaths and the rapid progress of the disease in August, indicating that many victims died in as little as four or five hours after contracting the disease and almost all of the deaths occurring 24 hours after the onset of the Sweat.[20] Edward Hall indicates that many in the King's court fell victim to the Sweat including Lord Clinton and Lord Gray of Wilton. He indicates that as the disease progressed many people died "and in one town half of the people died, and in another a third perished," but gives no specifics.[21] Hall's numbers are probably an exaggeration, an exaggeration driven in part by the fear that the epidemic generated. Even Cardinal Wolsey, Henry's chief minister contracted the disease and retired to his county house where he recovered, but only after suffering through four attacks of the Sweat.[22] The epidemic lasted from July to December and led to the abandonment of the Michaelmas setting of the law courts and a "solemn Christmas" for the royal court as Henry VIII was afraid to have a large number of people around him.[23] Again, cases were reported at the universities of Oxford and Cambridge. In a letter of August 6, Francesco Chieregato, papal nuncio to England noted that "such was the universal dread of the disease, that very few were those who did not fear for their lives, whilst some were so terrified by it that they suffered more from fear than others did from the sweat itself."[24] Most probably, the 1517 outbreak involved a larger region than the 1508 outbreak, but it is impossible to know how widespread or how deadly the epidemic was without further information.

The English Sweat seemed to be following an almost ten-year cycle and a fourth epidemic is reported in 1528. London again seemed to be a focal point for the disease as Hall indicated the epidemic began in May in London and then affected the rest of the country.[25] Already in early June, Sir Brian Tuke, royal treasurer, wrote to Cuthbert Tunstall, Bishop of London indicating there was a case of the Sweat in his household. In early June, Cardinal Wolsey's household was afflicted and he fled to his palace at Hampton Count to avoid the disease, where he received a letter from Anne Boleyn, with a postscript from Henry VII, inquiring as to his health.[26] The household of William Warham, Archbishop of Canterbury, also reported several cases, as did the London Charterhouse. Anne Boleyn herself developed a case of the sweating sickness in mid-June causing King Henry to flee to Waltham in Essex after sending his beloved to her father in Kent. Henry, still in the blush of new romance, wrote her a heartfelt letter on the sixteenth,

> There came to me in the night the most afflicting news possible. I have to grieve for three reasons: first, to hear of my mistress's sickness, whose health I desire as my own, and would willingly bear the half of yours to cure you; secondly, because I fear to suffer yet longer that absence which has already given me so much pain—God deliver me from such an importunate rebel! Thirdly, because the physician I trust most is at present absent when he could do me the greatest pleasure. However, in his absence I send you the second, praying God he may soon make you well.[27]

A few days later, he further tried to console her indicating that few women contracted the disease and so far, no one in the royal court had died from it. She and her father, who was also infected, survived their bout with the Sweat and Anne had returned to the royal court later in the summer.[28] However, four members of the court came down with the Sweat there leading Henry to flee once again, this time to Hunston in Hertfortshire. The French ambassador reported on the thirtieth of June that 40,000 people had contracted the disease in London and 2,000 people had died with some people dropping dead in the streets.[29] His figures may be accurate regarding total deaths, but they may also have been driven by fear. In some ways, government came to a halt as both Henry VIII and Cardinal Wolsey, his chief minister, isolated themselves. The situation seemed to be improving by early July when Anne Boleyn returned to court. Cases continued to be reported among members of the royal court who remained in London throughout the month, but they were usually infections, not deaths.[30] Brian Tuke, whose wife suffered through an attack of the Sweat, was somewhat suspicious of the predisposition of many victims to assume that they were infected by the Sweat, as he indicated that children who did not know of the disease did not suffer from it and indicated that he did "not think that every man who sweats is infected."[31] The 1528 epidemic appears to have been more widespread than the second and third outbreaks with cases in London, Cambridge, Kent, Wiltshire, and Yorkshire.[32] *Sudor Anglicus* was essentially a summer ailment in 1528 with cases first reported in June and the last cases in September.

Up to this point, cases of the sweating sickness had been confined to England, hence the name the English Sweat. In 1529, the disease seems to have spread to the continent with cases reported in Germany in July. Martin Luther, for example, spoke of cases of the English Sweat in a letter to his wife, written from Marburg on 4 October 1529.[33] The disease spread across southern Germany and into Switzerland during the summer and was nearly over by October although deaths from the Sweat continued to occur until January 1530.[34] The first cases seem to have occurred in the port of Hamburg as Hansa merchants may have brought the disease from England and it served as a transmittal point to other ports such as Danzig and Novgorod and along inland trade routes to cities such as Cologne.[35] As had been the case in many places in England, the Sweat infected Hamburg for only two weeks, but chroniclers reported that 1,100 died during the first week (in 1500, the population of Hamburg was 15,000) producing the usual sudden spike in deaths associated with the Sweat.[36] The disease also spread around the Baltic with nearly simultaneous outbreaks in Lübeck, Bremen, and Copenhagen where some of the Danish royal family fell victim to the disease.[37] Most contemporaries seem to have regarded the continental disease as the same one that had been afflicting England and believed that the epidemic originated from England. Writing in the nineteenth century, Hecker thought that the continental epidemic was independent of the English outbreak of 1528, but this seems unlikely because of the extensive contacts between England and Hansa merchants of the Baltic cities in the sixteenth century.[38] Unlike in England, several continental commentators prepared treatises describing the disease in much the same fashion as Forrestier and Caius, and described several cures.[39] Even Girolomo Francastoro took note of the Sweat in his comprehensive work on disease, published in 1546, as he traces its cause to a miasma in the air.[40] Although there may have been some cases in Calais in 1519, the 1529 outbreak appears to be the first time that the disease visited the continent. The reported cases in Calais in 1519 may well have been people who contracted the disease in England and brought it to the city that was a military outpost for England. The disease did not seem to spread in 1519 as it did in 1529 with a full-scale epidemic in Germany.

The sweating sickness made a fifth and final appearance in England in 1551. The fifth epidemic was better documented than previous outbreaks of the Sweat with two new sources in addition to the chroniclers and letter writers who described the earlier outbreaks. The first are two treatises in English and Latin on the sweating sickness written by the physician John Caius, while the second comes from the parish registers that had started being compiled by the mid-sixteenth century. These new sources help in describing the symptoms of the disease, its geographic impact, as well as providing a more accurate appraisal of the mortality rate of the Sweat.

The chronicle accounts and letters concerning the earlier sweating sickness epidemics often made it seem as if London bore the brunt of the disease. This may have been so but it may also have been an artifact of the chroniclers' focus on London. The 1551 epidemic appeared to cover much of the country and did not seem to have originated in the capital. The chronicler Charles Wriothesley was quite certain that the epidemic originated in Shrewsbury in the west of England. John Stow, writing in the 1590s, concurred, saying that the first case was reported in Shrewsbury on 15 April and spread from there to London with cases beginning to be reported on the seventh or ninth of July and continuing throughout the month.[41] John Caius reports that cases in 1551 occurred in Wales before the disease spread to Coventry, Oxford, and then southward to London.[42] As was the case with earlier epidemics, the aristocracy were not spared in 1551. The teenage Duke of Suffolk, Henry Brandon and his younger brother Charles both fell victim to the Sweat.[43] As had occurred with earlier epidemics of the Sweat, panic seems to have set in London, at least according to the Venetian ambassador. He reported that shops were closed and many people fled the city.[44] Writing at the end of the sixteenth century, John Stow confirmed this judgment calling it "a terrible time."[45] Examination of parish registers reveals that the disease was present in almost all counties of England with a concentration from Shropshire east to London and another wide swath from Cheshire across Lancashire to Yorkshire and the North Sea. Only Northumberland along the border with Scotland seems to have been spared.[46]

The accounts of deaths found in the parish registers reaffirm much of what earlier chroniclers said about the sweating sickness. Most early accounts spoke of how the disease seemed to appear almost overnight, quickly killed a number of people, and then vanished as if by magic. The burial notices from several parishes in 1551 confirm this appraisal. In the parish of Thaxted, Essex eleven corpses attributed to the Sweat were buried during a four-day period in July while in the parish of East Down in Devon twelve burials occurred from the fifteenth to the twenty-second of August with five on the seventeenth. Data are present from twenty-eight of the London city parishes and these data indicate that ninety per-cent of the deaths attributed to the Sweat in 1551 were reported from the tenth to the twentieth of July.[47] Most parishes were fairly small in the sixteenth century so the concentration of burials is explainable. Even in the parish of Halifax, in the West Riding of Yorkshire in which 42 of 44 deaths noted as being caused by the Sweat, were recorded from the second to the thirtieth of August. This parish was quite large, covering 118 square miles, and even there the deaths were grouped chronologically in regions of the parish.[48]

The various narrative accounts as well as the parish registers record a large number of deaths although nothing of the order of magnitude caused by some of the earlier plague epidemics. Unlike the plague deaths, however, those from the Sweat occurred over an extremely short period. John Caius reported that 903 people died in London in 1551, not counting those who died in the first two days of the epidemic while John Stow, writing later in the century, set the figure at 800.[49] The contemporary chronicler Robert Fabyn, who may have been the source of Stow's information, indicated that 800 people died during the week the disease was present in London.[50] None of these figures is particularly large and Caius's number is approximately 1.25% of the population of London that Wrigley and Schofield calculated as about 80,000 in 1560.[51] Using data available from twenty-four London parishes, Alan Dyer confirms this mortality rate indi-cating a 1.2% death rate. His estimates from provincial parish data are somewhat higher with a mean mortality rate of 2.2% derived from 69 parishes in 12 coun-ties.[52] In many parishes, of course, no deaths were recorded while in others the death rate was higher. Overall, Dyer calculates that between 15,000 and 20,000 people died from the sweating sickness in 1551 out of a population of more than three million.[53] When compared to the impact of the influenza epidemic of 1557–59 or the plague epidemic of 1563, the sweating sickness epidemic of 1551 barely registers.[54] Its impact derived from the short period of time in which the death occurred and the disease clusters of several family members or neighbors dying at once.

The numbers of deaths in London and elsewhere both in absolute numbers and as measured by the mortality rate do not seem to confirm Stow's judgment that the summer of 1551 was "a terrible time." Numbers alone do not tell the whole story in this case. First, unlike plague epidemics that tended to last sev-eral months or influenza epidemics that lasted even longer in some cases, the sweating sickness epidemics lasted a month at most, and often most of the deaths in one parish occurred in the space of a week. The sudden mortality peaks that occurred almost out of nowhere emphasized the suddenness of death as well as its unexpected nature that helped to generate fear out of proportion to the actual demographic impact. A large number of deaths in such a short period could influence local patterns of life just as significantly as did a larger number of deaths over a longer period. Second, both the plague and influenza killed both men and women without respect to gender although some chroniclers indicated some-what of a gender bias with the 1361 outbreak of the plague. The victims of the sweating sickness, on the other hand, were more likely to be male than female except in 1551 when larger numbers of women also fell victim to the disease.[55] Contemporaries made enough of this point to indicate that they considered it significant that men rather than women died from the Sweat. Third, the sweat-ing sickness was no respecter of social status. It did not kill just mayors or noble-men although not too much should be made of the reported deaths among the upper levels of society as this may have been celebrity bias, but the very fact that it killed members of the aristocracy was considered noteworthy at the time. The plague at its worst was no respecter of personage but later outbreaks took most of their victims from the poor, and someone who received better care during an illness, most likely the better off, was more likely to survive influenza. Fourth, the symptoms of the sweating sickness themselves were likely to engender fear in a way that influenza could not. The plague could produce such fear, but it had also become familiar by the sixteenth century with continued outbreaks so that its arrival generated less fear.

John Caius and the Sweat

Writing in response to the 1551 epidemic, the physician John Caius provided a fulsome account of the symptoms, progression, prevention, and treatment of the sweating sickness in two treatises. Educated at Cambridge and the University of Padua, which possessed one of Europe's leading medical schools, Caius had a distinguished career. He served as royal personal physician for a time, served as the long-serving president of the College of Physicians, and was the sec-ond founder and sixteenth master of what came to be known as Gonville and Caius College at Cambridge University. He could also be autocratic and petty and excluded the blind, the deaf, the halt, the lame, sufferers from incurable diseases, and Welshmen from his refounded College.[56] He published the *Boke or Counseill against the Disease Commonly Called the Sweate or Sweatyng Sickness* in 1552, basing it on the 1551 epidemic. The *Counseill against the Sweate,* was intended for a wide audience rather than simply medical practitioners. Caius wrote his account in English, not Latin, although he also produced a Latin work dealing with the Sweat, *De Ephemera Britannica*, at the same time that enabled him to display his learning with numerous phrases in Greek. In the first part of sixteenth century, medical men were expected to show their eru-dition by publishing in Latin, not the vernacular. Even though Caius produced the Latin *De Ephemera Britannica*, he was defensive about writing in English. He took pains in the first pages of the *Counseill against the Sweate* to defend writing it in English arguing that he was "compelled I am to use this our Englishe tongue as best to be understande and moste needful to whom it most foloweth."[57] Following the style of the time, Caius described the causes and symptoms of the Sweat and then provided a full list of largely dietary remedies for the Sweat that anyone, at least anyone with enough wealth to afford the ingredients, could follow. His approach, as befitting a Padua trained physician, was Galenic in origin and so there are limitations to both his diagnosis and approach to combating the disease.

Caius studied medicine at the University of Padua from 1539 to 1541 when he received his M.D. degree and imbibed deeply from the well of Galenic medicine there. The leading Galenist physician at Padua was the influential Gianbaptiste de Monte. Andreas Vesalius whose *De humani corporis fabrica* ("On the Fabric of the Human Body"), published in 1543 became one of the leading anatomy texts of the day, was another professor at Padua. Vesalius revered Galen, even helping to produce a new edition of his works, and placed his own work squarely in the Galenic tradition. Although Vesalius acknowledged the errors in Galen, he still upheld the Galenic approach and organized *De fabrica* according to the principles of Galenic philosophical anatomy.[58] Like other humanists, Vesalius placed a great deal of emphasis on recovering ancient texts (in this case Galen) and presenting them as accurately as possible. While this approach had a good deal of merit, it also ran the risk of locking in the ancients' ideas in a way that could be stultifying. Vesalius rarely attempted to question the basis of Galenic physiology and presented it as the accepted approach although he did emphasize the value of empirical knowledge. John Caius drew on this approach to physiology and became such an ardent Galenist that he devoted part of his intellectual life to providing an edition of the master's works.[59] No innovator, Caius tried to put the sweating sickness into the context of the existing Galenic medical fabric.

Others had reported the symptoms of the sweating sickness before and Caius's account was consistent with them although he added a few points. The rapidity of the progression of the Sweat clearly influenced Caius as it had earlier commentators as he noted: "But that immediately killed some in opening theire windowes, some in plaieing with children in their street dores, some in one hour, many in two it destroyed & at the longest, to these that merilye dine it gaue a soroful Supper."[60] He went on to provide a comprehensive list of symptoms that included the sudden onset of sweating that produced a foul stench, a high fever, headache, nausea and vomiting, and pains in the back and extremities. The disease produced what Caius (and Thomas Forrestier before him) called a passion of the heart which was probably tachycardia or heart palpitations as well as leading to massive organ failure (such as the liver), or insanity.[61] This was quite a list although headaches, nausea, or organ failure could all be the product of a very high fever.

Fever is a double-edged sword in the body's defense mechanism. Fevers can suppress some pathogens, but some pathogens, such as those with metabolic processes that speed up with higher body temperatures, can even benefit from a high fever. Suppressing a fever (e.g., with drugs such as aspirin) can have either positive or negative impact depending on the pathogen. High fevers can also have other negative impacts on the body such as leading to the organ failure noted above.

Good physician that he was, Caius tried to distinguish the sweating sickness from the plague as well as describing the causes for the disease and some possible remedies. Caius took a Galenic approach to describe the two causes of the Sweat as infection and corruption produced by an imbalance in the humors. This situation could be caused by many factors, but Caius indicated it likely came from an imbalance between the planets Mars and Venus.[62] Because summer was hot and moist under a Galenic regime, it was an appropriate time for the sweating sickness to occur. The sun drew "cruel" mists from the ground producing many deaths as had occurred with the Greeks in the siege of Troy. The miasma was coupled in 1551 to an unfortunate conjunction of the constellations to create an ideal moment for the Sweat. The corruption produced what Caius called "unstirred" air that came from graves and old wells with the miasma often released by earthquakes helping to produce a predisposition to illness. Caius was consistent with miasma theory with this point although miasma theory would be in decline by the end of the sixteenth century. Dietary habits, in particular, helped to produce the imbalance in the humors that led a person to be vulnerable to diseases such as the Sweat. Climatic conditions as well as the diet of Englishmen made them more susceptible to diseases of this sort than say people in Scotland where the Sweat did not penetrate.[63]

The Galenic explanation described above could apply to men or women, or rich or poor almost equally. Caius went on to explain why men and men of a certain type were likely to fall victim to the Sweat. The likely victims of the Sweat

> were either men of welthe, ease, & welfare, or of the poorer sorte such as wer idle persones, good ale drinkers, and Tauerne haunters. For these, by ye great welfare of the one sorte, and large drinkyng of thither, heped vp in their bodies moche euill matter; by their ease and idleness, could not waste and consume it.[64]

Caius's moralism mixed with his Galenism in this explanation for there is a degree of moralistic criticism of idleness and potential debauchery combined with the argument to keep the humors in balance. The latter aspect of good health Caius addressed with several dietary recommendations of specific foods as well as overall moderation in diet designed to maintain the body in balance. He went on to advocate exercise in moderation.[65] All of this advice also was found in other medical treatises of the time designed to ward off illness of almost any sort. In trying to prevent the onset of the sweating sickness, Caius advocated the standard Galenic remedies (with perhaps a touch of moralistic asperity) intended to ward off sickness in general rather than speaking to the specific symptoms of *Sudor Anglicus*.

John Caius was too good a physician, however, to believe that even if the path to avoiding harmful diseases was the same for most diseases, then fighting them once people contracted the Sweat was likewise similar. He wisely advocated prevention but went on to describe means for fighting the sweating sickness once a person contracted it. Because of the progression of the disease, the first 12 to 14 hours after it appeared were crucial to returning to health. As Polydore Vergil had done, Caius advocated bed rest and quiet once the Sweat was diagnosed. In an age in which many people slept more than one person to a bed, he indicated that only the sick person should be in a bed, no one else, probably from fear of contagion. He further advocated no food for 24 hours and no drink for the first five hours of the illness and then only a little clarified ale.[66] This latter recommendation had the potential to do a good deal of harm as the afflicted suffered from a high fever and were likely to become dehydrated, particularly if they were also vomiting. Caius believed that the act of sweating was itself something that aided in fighting the disease and advocated the encouragement of copious sweating through various means. Once the victims were on the mend, they should receive a bland diet seasoned with herbs such as fennel, rosemary, and mace. Caius saw these herbs as encouraging sweating as a means of voiding the system of harmful contaminants.[67] Sleep, Caius maintained, was harmful to afflicted people because the "venom" produced by the disease ran toward the heart during sleep. He advocated that those people attending those afflicted by the Sweat should go so far as to pull their ears or nose in order to keep them awake.[68] Confident of the value of his remedies Caius indicated that they were likely to produce a return to good health although they might have to be repeated in cases in which they did not immediately produce a cure or in those in which a relapse occurred.[69] Unlike the other accounts of the sweating sickness, Caius provided a full-scale treatment, one in keeping with the traditions of sixteenth-century medicine.

Because he provided the only full-scale treatise on the Sweat in English, many observers have celebrated John Caius. In many ways, the *Counseill against the Sweate* is an old-fashioned work, exhibiting the strengths and weaknesses of the Galenic medicine that was beginning to be challenged in the sixteenth century. He tells his readers little new about the Sweat and his preventative measures and treatments could just as easily have been applied to many other diseases. He does not go beyond superficial symptoms in attempting to diagnose the Sweat. If there had been epidemics subsequent to the 1551 outbreak, other commentators might have entered the lists, but interest died away when the disease did not return.

Diagnosing the English Sweat

John Caius, as well as other observers, regarded the sweating sickness as something new, outside the known diseases even though their remedies did not reflect this situation. None of the commentators on the sweating sickness confused it with the plague that was a clearly known disease, nor, it seems, did they regard it as influenza, which produced high mortalities on occasion. During the nineteenth century, the first efforts were made to reconcile the Sweat with a known disease, efforts that continued throughout the twentieth century. The historian Jon Arrizabalaga has argued that retrospective diagnosis is doomed to failure; diseases should be regarded as social constructions by people of the time.[70]

Such an approach begs the question of "new diseases" and their impacts as something that needs to be consistently described. Developing a diagnosis for a disease in past time enables us to understand how the disease affected society and how human society interacted with the disease. Without understanding the biology of a disease and how it may have evolved over time, scholars adopt an anthropocentric viewpoint that distorts the past. We should do retrospective diagnosis with care, but attempting such a diagnosis provides a more fulsome picture of the past than an anthropocentric approach gives. In this case, it helps to give us some insights into aspects of the sweating sickness such as who was infected, how the disease was spread, and its lethality.

At first, it seems that it should be easy to provide a diagnosis for the sweating sickness. Caius and others provided a wealth of symptoms to work with. Unfortunately, for the goal of achieving a concrete diagnosis, many of these symptoms are also those of other diseases so it is possible to call almost any potential diagnosis related to a "modern" disease into question. Near the turn of the twentieth century, the physician Charles Creighton tried to relate the sweating sickness to a known disease. He acknowledged that the Sweat cannot be reconciled exactly with another disease, but concluded that it must have been some form of influenza.[71] Some of the symptoms such as a high fever and the resulting sweating could be those of influenza, and Creighton's diagnosis remained plausible and R.S. Roberts echoed it when he refuted a view that food poisoning caused the Sweat.[72] Two problems exist with an influenza diagnosis, however. First, it does not take into account the vomiting and bleeding described by some contemporary observers. Second, contemporaries, who had experienced influenza, and would do so again in 1557–58, did not diagnose the Sweat as influenza, regarding it as something different. Typhus, too, has many of the same symptoms as the Sweat, but like influenza, it tends to produce epidemics in winter and spring not in summer as was the case with the Sweat.

Often identified as a potential health threat today, hemorrhagic viruses exhibit many of the symptoms of the sweating sickness. Some viruses that cause hemorrhagic fevers are arboviruses, bunyaviruses, or filoviruses. The hemorrhagic viruses include some of the most lethal diseases presently known such as Ebola as well as some that generally do not present a major health risk. Today hemorrhagic viruses are found on all continents and vary widely in their clinical symptoms and pathogenicity. The means of transmission also varies (unknown vector in the case of filoviruses) with some having an arthropod vector that might help to explain the possible rural origin for the Sweat and others transmitted from one person to another.

A possible diagnosis is to regard the sweating sickness as viral in nature. John A.H. Wylie and Leslie H. Collier forwarded an arbovirus diagnosis arguing for an insect vector of transmission.[73] Some arboviruses such as encephalitis do have many of the same symptoms as the English Sweat but there are also some important differences. Insect vectors can transmit two bunyaviruses, Hantavirus and Crimean-Congo Hemorrhagic Fever, and can be quite lethal to humans. Three arboviruses, Lassa, Marburg, Ebola, cause hemorrhagic fevers and can be transmitted through human-to-human contact as well as by a disease vector such as ticks. Some arboviruses seem to infect the young and the elderly, not the middle-aged people often described as victims of the Sweat. Arthropod borne arboviruses cause human illness through insect bites rather than human-to-human transmittal. This is certainly a possibility, but if so, an insect vector needs to be identified. There are several questions concerning an arbovirus diagnosis but it has the possibility to be a diagnosis for the sweating sickness

We can appreciate the challenges in retrospective diagnosis when we examine the three candidates for diagnosis as the Sweat. Table 7.1 highlights the epidemiological aspects of the three diseases as well as the Sweat. Table 7.2 provides a listing of the symptoms of *Sudor Anglicus* in a comparative framework with three diagnostic candidates. The three diagnostic candidates are two viruses of the *Bunyaviridae* family: Crimean-Congo Hemorrhagic Fever (CCHF) and Hantavirus, as well as meningococcal disease caused by the bacteria *Neisseria meningitidis*. CCHF may have been described in Tajikistan in the twelfth century and was first identified in the Crimea in 1944 and later in parts of Asia, Africa, and the Balkans.[74] Hantavirus has four serotypes that primarily cause hemorrhagic fever with renal syndrome and another type found in the Americas that causes an acute pulmonary syndrome. Hantavirus has its advocates in spite of a

TABLE 7.1 Symptoms Comparison

English sweat	Crimean-Congo Hemorrhagic Fever	Hantavirus	Meningococcal disease
High fever	X	X	X
Pain in back & neck	X	X	X
Pain in extremities		X	X
Vomiting	X		X
Sub-cutaneous bleeding/black blotches	X	X	X
Organ failure	X	X	X
Passion of the heart/heart failure	X	X	X

TABLE 7.2 Conditions Comparison

English sweat	Crimean-Congo Hemorrhagic Fever	Hantavirus	Meningococcal disease
Sudden onset		X	X
Rapid progression	X		X
High death rate	X	X	X
Infection does not confer later immunity			X
Summer/early autumn	X	X	?
Present in England		?	X

telling criticism.[75] Meningococcal disease can lead to a variety of medical problems including some that are not serious, but when meningococcemia develops, it can be fatal. Meningococcal disease was first diagnosed in 1806 but there is some evidence that the disease, or something much like it, was present in the sixteenth century.[76]

One essential aspect of disease diagnosis is identifying how a disease spreads. Contemporary commentators seemed to be unsure how *Sudor Anglicus* spread. Unlike a disease, such as syphilis in which people came to understand the means of transmission, the Sweat was less forthcoming as to how it spread. Crimean-Congo Hemorrhagic Fever spreads by bites from infected ticks. Today sporadic outbreaks occur across parts of Asia, the Balkans, and Africa usually in rural areas where people would be likely to encounter ticks.[77] Hantavirus spreads by contact with the bodily fluids of rats and voles, particularly saliva from bites and inhalation of viral particles from aerosols from urine and feces. Meningococcal disease is spread through human-to-human transfer from respiratory secretions through coughing, kissing, or prolonged contact. Although contagious, meningococcal disease is not as contagious as influenza or the common cold. However, crowded living conditions such as those of poor households, student housing at university, and even some noble households could serve as a major factor for the spread of the disease.[78]

By 1551, the availability of parish death records helped give a clearer conception of the spatial and temporal distribution of the Sweat. The Sweat seemed to come and go in an area in quick fashion, but during its stay often produced several deaths, often in one household or neighborhood. Rats and voles, the carriers of Hantavirus, were omnipresent in the early modern world making it somewhat unlikely that an outbreak would fall neatly into a one-week period although it is possible that everyone in a household could have become infected. Ticks, the vector for CCHF were unlikely to vanish suddenly from an area reducing the threat of disease overnight. Today, CCHF often produces a few cases at a time, not the clustering that the Sweat seemed to exhibit. Meningitidis outbreaks today can occur in schools or households where people are crowded together and oral discharges readily spread. In such cases, disease clusters often develop as everyone around the initial carrier becomes infected.

Geography is also a factor in the spread of a disease. The Sweat was a disease of London with cases reported in all five epidemics but it also appears to have been a disease of the countryside. The disease also visited other town such as Chester and the university towns of Oxford and Cambridge in 1508 and 1517 but it was also a disease of small hamlets.[79] In 1528 and 1551, these urban areas were the same focus with cases also reported in Kent, Wiltshire, and a band running from Chester across to the North Sea in 1551.[80] A hierarchal diffusion model for the spread of disease indicates that diseases spread from large population centers, such as London, to smaller ones via human contact. The Sweat cases were always reported in London but often nearly simultaneously in small villages as well. This situation suggests that Sweat epidemics, except for perhaps the first one, originated in London and spread outward. Parish death records from 1551 enable a more precise plotting of the deaths that occurred throughout England than is possible for the earlier epidemics. This pattern is perplexing, as the Sweat seemed to be a disease of both crowded urban centers and small villages.

The disease remained almost an exclusive English phenomenon although this may reflect poor reporting from Scotland or Wales. Only in 1529 did the disease appear to spread to the continent with cases first appearing in the Hansa cities of the Baltic and then the disease appeared farther south in Germany. There was extensive trade between England and the Hansa cities in the early sixteenth century so it is possible that a vector-borne disease or one spread by infected people could have spread to the continent. The question is why not on other occasions. However, closer examination indicates outbreaks with symptoms similar to the Sweat, most notably the copious sweating, in Ireland, especially Cork in 1591–92, Antwerp and Flanders in 1517 and 1529, Calais in the 1520s.[81] Some contemporaries indicated the Sweat may have arrived in England in 1485 from the continent with the mercenaries of Henry of Richmond, soon to be Henry VII, but this is more hearsay than something based on evidence.

Timing is often an important key to disease diagnosis. Some diseases can occur at any time while others are seasonal in nature. The Sweat was primarily a disease of summer and early autumn. The epidemics lasted for only one season, either because of growing immunity in the population, a lack of susceptibles, or a collapse in the vector pathway. The first outbreak of the Sweat was in August 1485 and it had disappeared by November. Contemporaries noted later outbreaks in May or June and lasted through September with occasional cases during the winter. Such timing occurs with diseases that have arthropod vectors such as fleas, ticks, or lice. While ticks can live through the winter in protected surroundings, they flourish in summer, helping to provide the vector for transmitting a disease such as CCHF. A disease that required human-to-human transmission, such as Meningitidis, is more common in winter when people are more likely to be crowded together indoors although there are exceptions such as 1918 when the influenza epidemic made a second appearance late in the summer. Rats and voles, the secondary vectors for Hantavirus, can flourish at almost any time.

The biological aspects of the English Sweat, especially its infectability are also important in arriving at a diagnosis. In order to spread a pathogen's basic reproductive number, R_0 should exceed one, where R_0 is the average number of secondary infections arising from one infected individual in a completely susceptible population in order for an epidemic to sustain itself. Pathogens with an $R_0 < 1$ are unable to sustain an infection in a given population. The Sweat was able to sustain itself for a time with each outbreak but soon died out raising the question of its R_0 value. Recent research indicates that in some cases that the basic reproductive number may decline in three to five generations, helping to limit the spread of a disease.[82] Areas with small populations, and this was most of England, tend not to experience cycling during an epidemic as all susceptibles are infected and either die or recover. This situation would produce disease-free periods until the area was re-infected from the outside. However, it is possible that as the R_0 approached 1, a disease might be evolving in such a way as to make an epidemic more likely.[83] If the R_0 hovered around 1, it might have been possible for the disease to turn into small-scale outbreaks. Often this can occur when individuals known as superspreaders are present. These infected people may have numerous contacts and be highly contagious enabling a disease to spread rapidly at least in a small-scale setting. Such an occurrence can then produce disease "hotspots" such as the royal court that are centers of contagion enabling a disease to spread. A superspreader event in a small village could turn it into a hotspot that might serve to spread the disease to nearby villages. If conditions changed enough so that Sweat could not evolve enough to produce an $R_0 > 1$ but instead an $R_0 < 1$ after 1551, it is plausible that so few new cases were generated as to lead the disease to slip out of public notice.

The ease of transmission of a disease is related to its case fatality rate although not in all instances. Measles, for example, has an R_0 of between 16 and 18, indicating that the disease spreads readily but it also has a low mortality rate except in some virgin soil epidemics. Ebola has an R_0 between 1 and 2 indicating that it is difficult to transmit the disease and somewhat difficult to sustain epidemics, but it has a case fatality rate of approximately sixty percent indicating that most people who are infected die. Plague, on the other hand, has an R_0 of approximately 3, which when coupled to a high mortality rate helps to explain the impact of the Black Death. Hantavirus, which is usually spread by indirect contact with rats or voles, usually has an R_0 between 1 and 2.[84] A basic reproductive number in this range often indicates that it is difficult to sustain an epidemic as the R_0 may drop below one and epidemic stalls out, something that the Sweat outbreaks tended to exhibit. CCHF also has a low R_0 of slightly higher than 1 in European settings, indicating that it is difficult for CCHF epidemics to sustain themselves.[85] Meningococcal disease also exhibits this same pattern with an R_0 of 1.36.[86] The transmission rate of all three candidates fits the pattern described for *Sudor Anglicus* outbreaks and helps to explain why the outbreaks were sudden but lasted for short periods.

The case fatality rate of a disease also affects its impact. As earlier chapters indicated, plague has a high case fatality rate (CFR) and an overall mortality rate that was close to sixty percent on occasion that helped to produce the dramatic population decrease of the fourteenth century. Because we do not know the incidence rate of the sweating sickness, it is not possible to determine a CFR so instead an overall mortality rate must be used. If the letters of 1528 are an indication, it seems that the Sweat infected many people in June and July, but not many died. This situation argues for a lower rather than higher case fatality rate for *Sudor Anglicus*. None of the three diagnostic candidates has a CFR that are as high as the plague, but they still had the ability to produce a substantial number of deaths. Today, Hantavirus renal syndrome can produce a CFR between five percent and fifteen percent and Hantavirus pulmonary syndrome can produce a CFR from thirty percent to fifty percent while CCHF has a CFR of up to thirty percent and meningococcemia can have a CFR of forty percent.[87] In a society with limited treatment options, the CFR could have been even higher. These CFRs appear to be consistent with the descriptions of the death rate for the Sweat.

Symptoms are an important diagnostic tool at any time and arriving at a list of symptoms for past diseases is both easy and complex. The terms used for describing symptoms in the sixteenth century are often the same as those of today but may have different meanings. In some cases, they are so vague or commonplace, such as a fever, as to be almost meaningless. They do have the advantage of reflecting a common medical and popular conception of disease. There are several accounts of the Sweat with lists of symptoms that are roughly the same throughout the period. The two most fulsome accounts are the works of the physicians Thomas Forrestier in 1490 and John Caius in 1552. Forrestier and Caius are in near agreement concerning symptoms providing continuity of description from the first outbreak to the last although Forrestier devotes a bit more attention to pulmonary symptoms.

A defining characteristic of *Sudor Anglicus*, common with other diseases, was a high fever that produced a copious amount of perspiration. Polydore Vergil reported the onset of the disease in 1485: "it was a baleful affliction and one which no previous age had experienced. A sudden deadly sweating attacked the body and at the same time head and stomach were in pain from the violence of the fever."[88] The course of the disease ranged from three to 14 days and those who survived the initial onslaught were likely to survive. As the list of symptoms in Table 7.2 indicates, many of the symptoms are associated with a high fever such as delirium or headaches, and are present for all three of our diagnostic candidates. John Caius's list of symptoms reflected the impact of a high fever although he indicated pain in the back and extremities and organ failure (e.g., the liver), both of which could also be produced by a high fever. Caius and Forrestier before him also noted "a passion of the heart," a symptom that was used in a variety of ways by medieval medical writers, but that appears to be tachycardia, or heart palpitations, which would significantly increase the likelihood of stroke or sudden cardiac arrest and death. Forrestier and Caius also reported black blotches on the skin that were probably caused by subcutaneous bleeding.[89]

Three other characteristics of the Sweat were that surviving the disease conveyed no immunity as it could return, and victims often died before many symptoms were manifest, as Caius noted that from onset to death was often less than 24 hours something that could have resulted from tachycardia.[90] Information concerning the 1528 and 1551 outbreaks indicate that cases often occurred in household clusters with several people ill at the same time.[91]

Surviving an attack of Hantavirus or Crimean-Congo Hemorrhagic Fever generally confers immunity from further attacks that is fortunate today as there are currently no vaccines for the diseases and treatment is largely supportive. Meningococcal disease, on the other hand, may reoccur at later date. Today, it is largely preventable as there is a vaccine available. As several accounts, such as the letter describing Wolsey's four attacks in 1517, indicate the Sweat was capable of returning to attack a victim on more than one occasion although these may have indicated relapses rather than recovery and reinfection.

Neither CCHF nor Hantavirus usually leads to death as rapidly as six-teenth-century commentators indicated although meningococcal disease is another matter. Hantavirus pulmonary syndrome usually starts with a few days of non-specific symptoms that lead to coughing, shortness of breath, and heart palpitations. Death from cardiovascular shock may occur rapidly after that, but the overall progression of the disease is not as rapid as indicated for the Sweat. Hantavirus renal syndrome usually proceeds through five distinct phases. The febrile (first) stage lasts three to seven days with victims exhibiting headaches, backaches, nausea, vomiting, and abdominal pains. Many of the deaths that occur during the second, hypotensive stage, that may last from several hours up to two days.[92] CCHF does exhibit a more rapid course with a one-to-three-day incubation period after a tick bite, often followed by flu-like symptoms during the prodomal phase. With some victims, signs of bleeding may appear within three to five days of the onset of the disease. In severe cases, kidney failure, liver failure (Forrestier's yellow complexion?), and acute respiratory distress may occur. When death occurs, it is usually during the second week of the illness. Although not always fatal, CCHF can lead to death six to eight days after onset, often terminating in cardiac arrest, a sudden resolution that corresponds with that attributed to the Sweat.[93] Death may occur for up to thirty percent of the victims by the end of the second week of the illness. CCHF often produces a hemorrhaging that leaves a black tinge on the skin, something listed as a symp-tom by Forrestier and Caius.[94] Crimean-Congo Hemorrhagic Fever symptoms are rarely fully apparent when an infection first occurs, a situation likely to have been the case with the Sweat, so the brief progression of the disease is somewhat comparable.

Both Hantavirus Pulmonary Syndrome and Renal Syndrome have the poten-tial, even today, to be a deadly companions. There is currently no treatment save supportive care and the diseases have a mortality rate between five percent and fifty percent depending on circumstances. About ten days after generalized symptoms such as fever and headaches appear, the late symptoms of the disease appear which include coughing, shortness of breath, and cardiovascular shock leading to death. Although people might not have noticed all of the early symp-toms in the sixteenth century, Hantavirus progressed at a slower rate than was indicated for the Sweat.

Meningococcemia, the most serious form of meningitis, generally starts with fever, nausea, chills, and general malaise. In severe cases, the disease progresses to produce acute respiratory distress and multiple organ failures. One sign at this stage is a purple rash resulting from blood leakage that may cover large parts of the body. The resulting sepsis often leads to death.[95] Before the 1920s, mortal-ity rates could approach seventy percent. Even today with antibiotic treatment, Meningococcemia may kill ten percent of its victims and have a permanent impact on the central nervous system. Meningococcemia may run a course from initial presentation of symptoms to death within a 24-hour period.

Some accounts indicate that the disease tended to affect men more than women as Henry VIII reminded Anne Boleyn in 1528. Meningococcal disease today tends to claim more women than men as victims so the gender bias of the victims may be important. Children and young adults were victims of the Sweat, but middle-aged people were the more likely victims. Today meningo-coccal disease tends to affect children and young adults in industrialized coun-tries although it has a wider age dispersion in Africa, and indeed today more cases occur in the 23 to 64 years old group worldwide than any other segment of the population.[96] It might be expected that meningococcal disease would have readily affected all age groups in England if it had been present.

A comparison of the symptoms and characteristics listed in Tables 7.1 and 7.2 indicates that any of the three diseases could have plausibly been the English Sweat. Meningococcal disease aligns with many characteristics of the Sweat save that it tends not to be a disease of summer. James Carlson and Peter Hammond, the leading advocates of Crimean-Congo Hemorrhagic Fever as the diagnosis for the Sweat admit that it is not a perfect match, as do the advocates of Hantavirus, Paul Heyman, Leopold Simons, and Christel Cochez.[97] None of the three diagnostic candidates is a perfect match for the Sweat based on symptoms and characteristics, but all three are more plausible than other candidates espe-cially if the disease evolved over time.

There is one other characteristic of the three diseases that must be taken into account: presence in England in the fifteenth and sixteenth centuries. All three of our candidates were identified by the nineteenth century, but evidence for their existence as recognized disease entities before then is sparse. If we can indeed identify the Sweat as one of the three, then we would have evidence for its existence at an earlier time. Geography is another factor in locating our candidates in England. Today, meningococcal disease is present in England. Scientists have identified Hantavirus pulmonary syndrome in the Americas but not Europe. Hantavirus renal syndrome is found in Europe, but its symptoms do not match those of the Sweat as well as the pulmonary syndrome variant. There have never been any cases of CCHF identified in England. Both CCHF and Hantavirus could have been present in England in the past but it is troubling that there is no trace of them today.

Perhaps the most perplexing issue regarding the Sweat is why there were no more cases after 1551. It is possible to explain the appearance of the disease in 1485 as arising from a zoonotic disease that crossed species and began to infect humans. Why it did not continue to affect humans after 1551 is more difficult to explain. There may have been a smattering of cases after 1551, but the disease did not reach epidemic proportions again. There does not seem to be a major climate shift, population shift or sudden immunity introduced by say a change in diet to warrant the disappearance of the disease. The development of immunity to the Sweat is a possibility but difficult to countenance with five outbreaks over a 65-year period. Possibly, the Sweat evolved to a more benign form after 1551, but this sort of rapid evolution is difficult to countenance and should still have led to a smattering of cases after 1551. One possibility is the Picardy Sweat, a milder disease with many of the same symptoms that appeared in France in 1718 and continued into the early nineteenth century.[98] Explaining why there were no more cases reported after 1551 is an important aspect of identification of the Sweat and explaining its impact. None of our three candidates appears to help solve this final conundrum. Perhaps the mid-twentieth century virologist Hans Zinsser had the best answer, when he asserted that the English Sweat was a virus that had been present on the continent for some time before it arrived in England where it relapsed back to this benign form without trying to identify the virus.[99]

Another approach, related to Zinsser's, is to diagnose the sweating sickness as its own disease. The high fever that is an important characteristic of the sweating sickness may have been caused by a manipulation by the disease pathogen rather than a response to it. If the former and the disease evolved in a more benign direction in the sixteenth century, the high fever that came to identify the sweating sickness would have been less noticeable, potentially leading to fewer sweating sickness diagnoses. Such an approach avoids the difficulty of matching symptoms but it still raises the question of why and how the Sweat appeared and disappeared in England. It also does not answer the question of why the disease appeared to be present in only England with the exception of the 1529 continental outbreak. In many ways, we are no farther along in diagnosing the sweating sickness than John Caius was in 1552.

In spite of being unable to arrive at a definitive diagnosis for *Sudor Anglicus*, this close examination of the characteristics and symptoms of the disease helps to expand our knowledge of the Sweat. We now have a better idea of why the disease produced clusters of infection and why it came and went so quickly. There is some indication that the Sweat did have a high morbidity rate across various sectors of society, but it did not produce an overall high mortality rate, unlike the plague. Addressing these questions helps to explain the fear that the Sweat generated beyond its mortality rate. Questions of the gender and class of the victims are more problematic but do help to explain why the Sweat had such an impact on public opinion. The examination also helps to explain why the Sweat presented such a challenge to the received medical opinions of the time. One final reason for trying to diagnose the English Sweat is that whatever the causal agent, it may still be present awaiting a triggering factor to re-emerge.[100]

The impact of *Sudor Anglicus*

The impact of the plague, with the Black Death of the fourteenth century and later outbreaks is easy to trace. The disease changed the demographic profile of England for nearly two hundred years. The demographic changes led to economic impacts as well. The five outbreaks of the English Sweat clearly did not have the same impact as did the plague. Here and there, parishes or even whole villages might have suffered a dramatic population downturn for a generation. The Sweat affected cities such as London less in spite of the inflated number of deaths that some commentators reported. Because the Sweat appeared in episodic fashion rather than being a continual presence, it didn't produce a substantial drop in population. Even in years in which the Sweat contributed to an increase in the number of deaths, the plague was also active.[101] Without a large demographic impact, it is hard to detect a concomitant economic impact. Unlike the dramatic population decline and accompanying labor shortage caused by the Black Death in the mid-fourteenth century, there was no Sweat created labor shortage in the early sixteenth century. A labor surplus did not yet exist, but population was on the increase again. Even the series of epidemics arising from various diseases in the years from 1556 to 1560 that led to a six percent drop in population did not stem the overall trend toward an increasing population.[102]

At times, it seemed that an outbreak of the Sweat might cripple the English government. Henry VIII's flights from London, the sickness of Cardinal Wolsey and other courtiers, and the failure to hold sessions of law courts probably had a negative impact on the smooth functioning of government. So too, the death of a large number of local officials such as the deaths of two London mayors and several aldermen in short order in London in 1485. These were only minor blips in the functioning of government. The Venetian ambassador might note the absence of the king or a royal official but the business of government went on as usual.

The sweating sickness had some influence on the medical thinking of the time. Physicians such as Thomas Forrestier and John Caius struggled with how to treat the disease. It appeared to be a new disease that was not contained in the Galenic corpus. The medical elite's authority-based approach to medicine indicated that the ancients had defined all diseases so a new disease was a challenging anomaly. Caius unsuccessfully tried to force the Sweat into the existing Galenic structure. The nature of *Sudor Anglicus* may have led to a further questioning of the accepted medical tenets by the medical elite. Unfortunately, no commentaries by empirics survive so we cannot tell if they accepted the novelty of the Sweat. It seems that some commentators at least followed this approach in indicating that the Sweat was a new and frightening disease.

The Sweat produced fear more than anything else. Its symptoms were horrifying as was the sudden death of its victims, if, indeed it killed within a day. The randomness of the Sweat both in when and where it occurred must have been troubling. So too, did the clusters of victims in the same family or neighborhood especially as the Sweat seemed to appear and sicken its victims and then be gone in a matter of days although sometimes to reappear a week or ten days later. By the end of the fifteenth century, many people had come to expect that epidemic disease affected the lower orders of society more than the aristocracy. The Sweat was no respecter of class and contemporaries noted with dismay its aristocratic victims, a situation that may have helped to further a climate of fear concerning the disease. The plague produced fear aplenty even before it reached

the island. Dating from the first outbreak in 1485, the Sweat also alarmed people. Not all outbreaks were of the same magnitude but the sudden, short epidemics coupled to symptoms and all-encompassing nature of the social class of
its victims led people to fear the Sweat. Fear, however, is often transitory; once
the episode generating fear is over people tend to forget although some tried
to indict outbreaks of other diseases in the late 1550s as the Sweat although the
evidence is scant.

The English Sweat did leave a fictional legacy, at least from the reign of
Henry VIII. Philippa Gregory describes Anne Boleyn's bout with the Sweat in
The Other Boleyn Girl (based on the 2008 film of the same name) with Anne's
sister Mary as the protagonist. Her depiction is accurate as both Anne and Mary's
husband William Carey were afflicted with the disease. Gregory captures the
suddenness of the onset of the Sweat and the fear it generated: "The sweat had
come to court with a vengeance. Half a dozen people who had been dancing
were in their chambers. One girl had already died."[103] Hilary Mantel also makes
use of the Sweat in *Wolf Hall,* her novel (and PBS TV series) about Thomas
Cromwell. She has Cromwell's wife become ill with the Sweat, something that
did not happen, but it provided a good plot twist.[104] The Sweat also makes an
appearance in the HBO series concerning the Tudors with Anne Boleyn and
Cardinal Wolsey both falling ill and surviving, as they did. Some of the Sweat's
characteristics make it highly serviceable for film and fictional treatment.

The true legacy of *Sudor Anglicus* may be its mysterious nature. It first arose
suddenly in 1485 and apparently vanished after 1551. There did not seem to be the
astrological portents of impending doom with the Sweat as sometimes preceded
plague outbreaks. The suddenness of the outbreaks and their short duration even
though with the ability to generate high mortalities in limited areas also contributed to the mystery of the Sweat. In some ways, it is the ultimate mystery disease
that may in part help to explain the various efforts at retrospective diagnosis for
fear that it presages something similar today.

Notes

1 Polydore Vergil, *The Anglica Historia,* Denys Hay ed. and trans. (Camden Society, 74, 1950), 6–9.
2 Charles Rosenberg, *Explaining Epidemics and Other Studies in the History of Medicine* (Cambridge: Cambridge University press, 1998), 306.
3 John Stow, *The Annales of England* (London, 1608), 788. Raphael Holinshed, *Chron-icle of England, Scotland, and Ireland,* 6 vols. (London: J. Johnson and F.C. and J. Rivington, 1808), 3: 482. Thomas Forrestier, *Tractus contra pestilential thenasomen et disserterium* (Rouen, 1490), c. 7, not paginated.
4 A.H. Thomas and I.D. Thornley, eds., *The Great Chronicle of London* (Gloucester: Alan Sutton, 1983 [1938]), 239, 438.
5 Holinshed, *Chronicle,* 3: 482.
6 Holinshed, *Chronicle,* 3: 482.
7 Vergil, *Anglia Historia,* 8–9.
8 John A.H. Wylie and Leslie H. Collier, "The English Sweating Sickness (*Sudor Anglicus*): A Reappraisal," *Journal of the History of Medicine,* 36 (1981): 444.

9 Wylie and Collier, "English Sweating Sickness," 428.
10 Angelo Raine, ed., *York Civic Records*, vol 1, (Yorkshire Archaeological Society Record Series, 98, 1938), 117.
11 *York Civic Records*, 118.
12 Wylie and Collier, "English Sweating Sickness," 428. Paul Heyman, Leopold Simons and Christel Cochez," "Were the English Sweating Sickness and the Picardy Sweat Caused by Hantaviruses?" *Viruses*, 6 (2014),152. Paul Heyman, Christel Cochez, Mirsada Hukić, "The English Sweating Sickness: Out of Sight, Out of Mind,' *Acta Medica Academica*, 47 (2018), 102.
13 Slack, *Impact of Plague*, 61.
14 Vergil, *Historia Anglicana*, 8–9. Richard Grafton, "Continuation" of *The Chronicle of John Hardyng*, Henry Ellis, ed. (London: F.C. and J. Rivington, 1812), 550–51.
15 In their detailed analysis of the etiology of the English Sweat, James R. Carlson and Peter W. Hammond take pains to explain why the aristocracy may have been victims of the disease. "The English Sweating Sickness (1485–c. 1551): A New Perspective on Disease Etiology," *Journal of the History of Medicine and Allied Sciences*, 54 (1999), 23–54.
16 Vergil, *Anglia Historia*, 142–43. Grafton, "Continuation," 589. Grafton does not discuss the portents ascribed to the Sweat but otherwise his and Polydore Vergil's accounts are nearly word for word.
17 Wylie and Collier, "English Sweating Sickness," 430.
18 M.B. Shaw, "A Short History of the Sweating Sickness," *Annals of Medical History*, 5 (1933): 252
19 Holinshed, *Chronicle*, 3: 626.
20 *Letters and Papers, Foreign and Domestic of the Reign of Henry VIII*, 22 vols. (London, 1862–1932), 2: 3558.
21 Edward Hall, *Hall's Chronicle; Containing the History of England during the Reign of Henry the Fourth and the Succeeding Monarchs, to the End of the Reign of Henry the Eighth*, Henry Ellis, ed. (London: J. Johnson, F.C. and J. Rivington, 1809), 592. Spelling modernized.
22 *Letters and Papers*, 2: 3638.
23 Hall, *Chronicle*, 592.
24 *Calendar of State Papers Relating to English Affairs in the Archives of Venice*, 2: *1509–1519*, Rawdon Brown, ed. (London, 1867), 945.
25 Hall, "*Chronicle*," 750.
26 *Letters and Papers*, 4: 1903, 4332, 4360.
27 *Letters and Papers*, 4: 4382.
28 *Letters and Papers*, 4: 4403, 4542.
29 *Letters and Papers*, 4: 4391.
30 *Letters and Papers*, 4: 4453, 4440, 4489, 4510, 4560.
31 *Letters and Papers*, 4: 4510.
32 Shaw, "Sweating Sickness," 255. Creighton, *Epidemics*, 1: 250–55.
33 John L. Flood, "'Safer on the Battlefield than in the City': England, the 'Sweating Sickness', and the Continent," *Renaissance Studies*, 17 (2003): 155.
34 Flood, "Safer on the Battlefield," 157.
35 Flood, "Safer on the Battlefield," 158–9; Wylie and Collier, "English Sweating Sickness," 434.
36 John Christiansen, "The English Sweat in Lübeck and North Germany, 1529," *Medical History*, 53 (2009), 415–24.
37 Wylie and Collier, "English Sweating Sickness," 433.
38 J.F.C. Hecker, *Epidemics of the Middle Ages*, trans. B.G. Babington (London, 1844), 246–54. For a discussion of England's trade with the Hansa see E.M. Carus-Wilson and O. Coleman, *English Export Trade 1275–1547* (Oxford: Clarendon Press, 1963).
39 Flood, "Safer on the Battlefield," 165–73.
40 Fracastoro, *Contagion*, 96–99.

41 Charles Wriothesley, *A Chronicle of England during the Reigns of the Tudors*, W.D. Hamilton, ed. (Camden Society, O.S., 11, 1875), 49–50. Stow, *Annales of England*, 1021.
42 John Caius, "A Boke or Counseill against the Disease Commonly Called the Sweate or Sweating Sickness," in E.S. Roberts, ed., *The Works of John Caius, M.D.* (Cambridge: Cambridge University Press, 1912), 11.
43 Wriothesley, *Chronicle of England*, 50.
44 *Calendar of State Papers Relating to English Affairs in the Archives of Venice*, 5: *1534–1554*, Rawdon Brown, ed. (London, 1873), 934.
45 Stow, *Annales of England*, 1021.
46 Alan Dyer, "The English Sweating Sickness of 1551: An Epidemic Anatomized," *Medical History*, 41 (1997): 368–69.
47 Dyer, "English Sweating Sickness of 1551," 365.
48 Dyer, "English Sweating Sickness of 1551," 366.
49 Caius, "Counseill against the Swete," 11; Stow, *Annales of England*, 1021.
50 Robert Fabyn, *The New Chronicles of England and France in Two Parts*, Henry Ellis, ed. (London: F.C. and J. Rivington, 1811), 711.
51 A.L. Beier and R. Findlay, *London 1500–1700: The Making of the Metropolis* (London: Longman, 1986), 45.
52 Dyer, "English Sweating Sickness of 1551," 379.
53 Dyer, "English Sweating Sickness of 1551," 380.
54 E.A. Wrigley and R.S. Schofield, *The Population History of England, 1541–1871* (Cambridge: Cambridge University Press, 1989), 496. Paul Slack labels the demographic impact of the sweating sickness in 1551 as "not impressive." *Impact of Plague*, 70.
55 Dyer, "Sweating Sickness of 1551," 375–6.
56 Vivian Nutton, "John Caius and the Linacre Tradition," *Medical History*, 23 (1979), 373.
57 Caius, *Counseill against the Sweate*, 8.
58 Peter Dear, *Revolutionizing the Sciences* (Princeton: Princeton University Press, 2001), 38.
59 Marie Boas, *The Scientific Renaissance, 1450–1630* (New York: Harper, 1962), 136.
60 Caius, *Counseill against the Sweate*, 9.
61 Caius, *Counseill against the Sweate*, 9. 13.
62 Caius, *Counseill against the Sweate*, 7.
63 Caius, *Counseill against the Sweate*, 14–17.
64 Caius, *Counseill against the Sweate*, 19.
65 Caius, *Counseill against the Sweate*, 20–24, 27–28.
66 Caius, *Counseill against the Sweate*, 30.
67 Caius, *Counseill against the Sweate*, 32.
68 Caius, *Counseill against the Sweate*, 33.
69 Caius, *Counseill against the Sweate*, 33–34.
70 Jon Arrizabalaga, "Problematizing Retrospective Diagnosis in the History of Disease," *Asclepio*, 54 (2002): 62–67.
71 Creighton, *Epidemics*, 1: 280.
72 R.S. Roberts, "A Consideration of the Nature of the English Sweating Sickness," *Medical History*, 9 (1965): 385. Roberts wrote in rebuttal to Adam Patrick who argued food poisoning caused that the Sweat. "A Consideration of the Nature of the English Sweating Sickness," *Medical History*, 9 (1965): 272–79.
73 Wylie and Collier, "English Sweating Sickness," 444.
74 Sara Shayan, Mohammad Bokaean, Mona Ranjvar Shahrivar, and Sadegh Chinkar, "Crimean-Congo Hemorrhagic Fever," *Laboratory Medicine*, 46 (2015), 180–9.
75 Martin Zeier, Michaela Handermann, Udo Bahr, Baldur Rensch, et al., "New Ecological Aspects of Hantavirus Infection: A Change of a Paradigm and a Challenge of Prevention—A Review," *Virus Genes*, 20 (2005), 157–80. Guy Thwaites, Mark Taviner, Vanya Gant, "The English Sweating Sickness 1485–1551," *New England*

Journal of Medicine, 336 (1997), 580–2. Taviner, Thwaites, and Gant, "The English Sweating Sickness, 1485–1551: A Viral Pulmonary Disease," *Medical History*, 42 (1998), 96–8. Eric Bridson, "The English 'Sweate' (*Sudor Anglicus*) and Hantavirus Pulmonary Syndrome," *British Journal of Biomedical Science*, 58 (2001), 1–6; Heyman, et al., "English Sweating Sickness and the Picardy Sweat," 151–71; Heyman, Cochez, and Mirsada Hukić, "The English Sweating Sickness," 102–16.

76 Nancy E. Rosenstein, Bradley A. Perkins, David S. Stephens, Tanja Popovic, and James M. Hughes, "Meningococcal Disease," *New England Journal of Medicine*, 344 (2001), 1378–88.

77 Harry Hoogstraal, "The Epidemiology of Tick-Borne Crimean-Congo Hemorrhagic Fever in Asia, Europe, and Africa," *Journal of Medical Entomology*, 15 (1979), 307–417. Chris A. Whitehouse, "Crimean-Congo Hemorrhagic Fever," *Antiviral Research*, 64 (2004), 145–60. Dennis A. Bente, Naomi L. Forrester, Douglas M. Watts, Alexander J. McAuley, Chris A. Whitehouse, et al., "Crimean-Congo Hemorrhagic Fever: History, Epidemiology, Pathogenesis, Clinical Syndrome, and Genetic Diversity," *Antiviral Research*, 100 (2013), 159–89.

78 Michael Baker, Anne McNicholas, Nicholas Garrett, Nicholas Jones, Joanna Stewart, et al., "Household Crowding a Major Risk Factor for Meningococcal Disease in Auckland Children," *Pediatric Infectious Disease Journal*, 19 (2000), 983–90.

79 Wylie and Collier, "English Sweating Sickness," Grafton, *Continuation of Hardyng*, 551, Dyer, "English Sweating Sickness of 1551."

80 Dyer, "English Sweating Sickness of 1551."

81 Flood, "Safer on the Battlefield," 147–76; Christiansen, "English Sweat in Lübeck," 415–24; R.S. Roberts, "The Use of Literary and Documentary Evidence in the History of Medicine," in E. Clarke, ed., *Modern Methods in the History of Medicine* (London: Athlone Press, 1971), 36–56.

82 Cécile Viboud, Lone Simonsen, and Gerardo Chowell, "A Generalized-Growth Model to Characterize the Early Ascending Phase of Infectious Disease Outbreaks," *Epidemics*, 15 (2016), 27–37; Gerado Chowell, Cécile Viboud, Lone Simonsen, and Seyed M. Moghadas, "Characterizing the Reproduction Number of Epidemics with Early Subexponential Growth Dynamics," *Journal of the Royal Society Interface*, 13 (2016), 20160659.

83 R. Antia, R.R. Regoes, J.C. Koella, C.T. Bergstrom, "The Role of Evolution in the Emergence of Infectious Diseases," *Nature*, 426 (2003), 658–61.

84 Thomáš Gedeon, Clara Bodelón, and Amy Kuenzi, "Hantavirus Transmission in Sylvan and Peridomestic Environments," *Bulletin of Mathematical Biology*, 72 (2010), 541–64.

85 A. Estrada-Peña, F. Ruiz-Fons, P. Acevedo, C. Gortazar, J. de le Fuente, "Factors Driving the Circulation and Possible Expansion of Crimean-Congo Hemorrhagic Fever Virus in the Western Paleartic," *Journal of Applied Microbiology*, 114 (2012), 278–86.

86 Caroline L. Trotter, Nigel J. Gay, and W. John Edmunds, "Dynamic Models of Meningococcal Carriage, Disease, and the Impact of Serogroup C Conjugate Vaccination," *American Journal of Epidemiology*, 162 (2005), 89–100. This study used data gathered from England and Wales in the current day.

87 T. Avšič-Županc, A. Saksida, and M. Korva, "Hantavirus Infections," *Clinical Microbiology and Infection*, 21 (2019), e10–e11. Whitehouse, "Crimean-Congo Hemorrhagic Fever," Anna Papa, Ali Mirazimi, Iftihar Köksal, Augustin Estrada-Pena, and Heinz Feldmann, "Recent Advances in Research on Crimean-Congo Hemorrhagic Fever," *Journal of Clinical Virology*, 64 (2015), 137–43. Rosenstein et al., "Meningococcal Disease."

88 Polydore Vergil, *Historia Anglicana*, 7.

89 Caius, *Counseill against the Swete*, 12–14, Forrestier, *Tractus contra pestilential thenasomen et dissenterium*, c. 7.

90 Forrestier, *Tractus contra pestilential thenasomen et dissenterium*, c. 7., Caius, *Counseill against the Swete*, 10.

91 Hall, *Chronicle*, 592; *Letters and Papers, Henry VIII*, 4: 4440, 4453, 4489, 4542; Dyer, "English Sweating Sickness of 1551," 365–66.

92 Avšič-Županc, et al., "Hantavirus Infections," e10.

93 Onder Ergonul, "Clinical and Pathologic Features of Crimean-Congo-Hemorrhagic Fever," in Onder Ergonul and Chris A. Whitehouse, eds., *Crimean-Congo-Hemorrhagic Fever* (Dordrecht: Springer, 2007), 209–10, and Mike Bray, "Comparative Pathogenesis of Crimean-Congo Hemorrhagic Fever and Ebola Hemorrhagic Fever," in Orgonul and Whitehouse, 223. Hoogstraal, "Epidemiology of Tick-Borne Crimean-Congo Hemorrhagic Fever," 380.

94 Chris A. Whitehouse, "Crimean-Congo Hemorrhagic Fever," *Antiviral Research*, 64 (2004): 152; Önder Ergönül, "Crimean-Congo Haemorrhagic Fever," *Lancet: Infectious Diseases*, 6 (2006): 208; Forrestier, *Tractus contra pestilential thenasomen et dissenterium*, c. 7. John Caius also mentions "partes with a blackeness," which may have been evidence of the cutaneous ecchymosis that is characteristic of CCHF. "Counseill against the Sweate, 34.

95 David S. Stephens, Brian Greenwood, and Peter Brandtzaeg, "Epidemic meningitis, meningococcaemia, and *Neisseria meningitidis*," *Lancet*, 369 (2007), 2196–2210.

96 Caroline L. Trotter and Martin C.J. Maiden, "Carriage and Transmission of *Neisseria Meningitidis*," in Ian Feavers, Andrew J. Pollard, and Manish Sadarangani, eds., *Handbook of Meningococcal Disease Management* (Adis, 2016), 19; Rosenstein, et al., "Meningociccal Disease," 1378.

97 Carlson and Hammond, "English Sweating Sickness (1485–c.1551), 23–54; Heyman Simons and Cochez, "Were the English Sweating Sickness and the Picardy Sweat Caused by Hantavirus?" 151–71. Both articles tend to draw their evidence from Caius and chronicle accounts and neglect the contemporary evidence from observers of the 1517 and 1528 epidemics.

98 Heyman, et al., "English Sweating Sickness and the Picardy Sweat."

99 Hans Zinsser, *Rats, Lice and History* (Boston: Little Brown, 1935), 100.

100 Heyman, Cochez, Hukić, "English Sweating Sickness," 104.

101 Slack, *Impact of Plague*, 57, 61, 71.

102 Slack, *Impact of Plague*, 7.

103 Philippa Gregory, *The Other Boleyn Girl* (New York: Touchstone, 2008), 300.

104 Hilary Mantel, *Wolf Hall* (New York: Picador, 2009), 92.

8

NEW DISEASES AT THE TURN OF THE SIXTEENTH CENTURY: THE CERTAINTY OF SYPHILIS, THE GREAT POX

The disease known as *Sudor Anglicus* first struck England in 1485. A few years later, another disease also struck the country, but unlike the Sweat it affected all of Europe.[1] The Italian physician Girolomo Fracastoro coined the term syphilis in his poem written in 1530, but contemporaries referred to it in a number of ways. The term the French disease (*morbus gallicus*) was often used in England and elsewhere, but the French referred to it as the Neapolitan disease and later as *Lues Venerea* and it was also known as the Polish Disease, the German Disease, and syphilis as well as other names reflecting the antipathy the writer had for a neighboring country. Some authors referred to it as the great pox in order to contrast one of its symptoms with smallpox, a known disease that produced much smaller pustules on its victims. Contemporaries did not achieve a consensus in naming the new disease. Although the authors of one account of the new disease use the term French disease throughout their work as they refuse to connect the sixteenth-century disease with the modern disease, their approach as Mary Healy indicates is a bit too rigid in denying continuities (and change) in nature in favor of social construction.[2] An understanding of syphilis in the sixteenth century is fraught with problems concerning its origin, how critics treated the disease and its victims, as well as the questions it posed to the Galenic consensus.

Although there is some dispute regarding its first appearance in Europe, a new disease first appeared among the troops of King Charles VIII of France during the siege of Naples in 1494/95. Soon reports appeared of a horrible disease that disfigured and killed many of the troops in often painful fashion. Largely a mercenary force, the dispersal of the army after the campaign meant that the troops often took home more than their wages and plunder. The disease rapidly spread throughout Europe and reached England before the turn of the fifteenth century. During the first 20 years of its presence in Europe, the new disease killed rapidly and often; thereafter either the disease evolved or its victims developed

DOI: 10.4324/9781003215219-9

some resistance for the disease took longer to kill and many of its victims survived the first attack albeit with scarring. Most likely, the disease mutated into a less virulent form as selection favored the milder strain that more opportunities to spread to other victims.[3] The approaches that various commentators took regarding the disease also evolved. First, commentators attempted to place it in a Galenic framework often displaying their misogyny at the same time as they often blamed women for the transmission of what was apparently a sexually transmitted disease. Medical writers never abandoned the Galenic approach when it came to looking for the root causes of the disease. However, many commentators adopted an increasingly moralistic approach that blamed sufferers of the disease for their own misfortune so that by the end of the sixteenth century, the English barber-surgeon William Clowes refused to discuss preventative measures in his discussion of the Pox saying that to do so would only encourage further immorality. Most sixteenth-century authors fit syphilis into the existing framework of disease to some degree. Unlike the English Sweat, which vanished after 1551, the Pox remained a problem that medical practitioners still needed to address.

Origins

Over time, explanations for the origins of syphilis, the new disease, have coalesced into three hypotheses. The Columbian hypothesis, proposed by the historian Alfred Crosby in 1969 and developed by scholars from a variety of disciplines is that Columbus's men acquired the disease in the West Indies and brought it to Europe upon their return.[4] The second hypothesis indicated that venereal syphilis was already present in Europe at the time of Columbus's voyage, having originated in East Africa, although early practitioners did not distinguish it from leprosy.[5] Examinations of skeletal remains from high medieval England have provided some evidence that treponemal disease was present in England in the Middle Ages although they do not provide conclusive evidence that it was venereal syphilis.[6] As might be expected, a third approach indicates that the disease was present on both sides of the Atlantic in four forms, pinta, yaws, endemic (nonvenereal) syphilis, and venereal syphilis all caused by *Treponema pallidum* which evolved simultaneously with humans.[7] Proponents of all three hypotheses agreed that various forms of treponemal disease were present in the New World at the time of Columbus's voyages. Some proponents of the second and third hypotheses indicate that treponemal disease was already present in Europe when Columbus's sailors returned.

Part of the disagreement revolves around the role of evolution. How has treponemal disease evolved and did the venereal syphilis present in Europe by the early sixteenth century evolve from American or European origins? Historians Jon Arrizabalaga, John Henderson, and Roger French argue that syphilis could not have been the disease that infected Europe in the early sixteenth century—it was something else so they use the terms "The Great Pox" or the "French

Disease" to refer to the disease.[8] Fortunately, paleopathology and now phyloge-
netics enables a nuanced answer that partakes in some ways of the third origin
hypothesis. In essence, the evidence indicates that a non-sexually transmitted
sub-species was present in Europe before Columbus. Columbus's sailors brought
a sexually transmitted species back to Europe. This sexually transmitted disease
probably interacted with the European sub-species to produce venereal syphilis.[9]
Currently, it appears that the Columbian voyages contributed to what became
the disease of syphilis, but several evolutionary links need to be explored in order
to understand how the disease evolved from a highly virulent to less virulent
form in the first third of the sixteenth century.

A class of bacteria known as spirochetes transmit the various treponemal
diseases. Although three kinds of spirochetes have become invasive parasites of
humans, the group known as Treponema are true parasites transmitted from
human to human. Syphilis belongs to *Treponema pallidum* as do yaws, pinta, and
endemic or nonvenereal syphilis. Pinta and yaws are both tropical diseases, with
pinta primarily affecting children. Neither is particularly deadly although both
can produce unpleasant symptoms. Nonvenereal or endemic, syphilis is largely
a childhood disease, and most adults in an area affected by the disease developed
a tolerance or immunity resulting from childhood exposure. Venereal syphilis is
another matter entirely and often led to death in the past (antibiotics such as penicillin make it possible to cure venereal syphilis today). It usually infects adults
although women who contract venereal syphilis can transmit it to their unborn
infants. Early transmission of syphilis often results in miscarriage or stillbirth.
Women who acquire the disease at a later stage in their pregnancies may give
birth to children with congenital syphilis.

Today, syphilis infections usually develop in three stages often with an interval between stages in which the infected person is symptom-free. Once infected,
usually through sexual contact, the person develops a lesion, a chancre, most
often on a genital organ between two and four weeks after being infected. The
secondary stage begins six to ten weeks later. During this stage, the person suffers
from a generalized infection with fever, rash, pain in the bones, headaches, and
inflammation of the eyes. Many early modern commentators emphasized the
bone aches and headaches, often at night, as characteristic of the disease. More
obvious symptoms may also appear during this stage such as external ulcers and
pustules and hair loss. After this progression of woe, the disease often goes into
remission, not to reappear for as much as five to 45 years. Someone who acquires
the disease later in life is more likely to die of something else rather than syphilis.
The third stage often leads to death but not before producing chronic ulcers on
the face, the gumma (large pustules), heart disease, tabor dorsalis (severe leg and
spinal pain) that can lead to deformity, arthritis, and dementia (not identified
until the nineteenth century). For someone infected with syphilis today and who
remains untreated, the progression is slow but often ultimately fatal. The progression of the disease is affected by the overall health of the person. During the
first 20 or so years that the new disease affected Europe, the disease progressed

rapidly from the second to the third stage and killed the afflicted person in speedy fashion. There were, however, some notable survivors who suffered from the disease with a longer period of remission than that enjoyed by many of their contemporaries.

The initial response to the new disease

Venereal disease was not unknown in late fifteenth-century Europe. Gonorrhea had been present for some time.[10] The physician Andrew Boorde noted both the Pox and what he called the "burning sickness," in his *Breviary of Health,* first published in 1547, and reprinted numerous times thereafter. He made a clear distinction between what he called the French pox and the "burning of an harlot."[11] Although Boorde blamed "unclean" women for transmitting the disease, he did indicate that unclean men could transmit it to women. He even provided a treatment: bathing the afflicted member in white wine and if this did not work then a surgeon should be consulted but said nothing about using mercury (a standard treatment for syphilis) for treating this problem. Gonorrhea coexisted with syphilis and generally, observers made a distinction between the two. In his discussion of Essex archdeacons' court cases in the latter third of the sixteenth century, W.G. Emmison indicates that only one of 32 cases involving venereal disease was described as the Pox, the others involved the "burning" of one or both parties.[12] The combination of its "newness" and more severe symptoms than those of gonorrhea, meant that most commentators focused on syphilis rather than the older disease.

Physicians confronted with the new disease turned to the teachings of Galenic medicine in order to explain it. Contemporaries usually maintained that the primary cause, of course, for any disease was divine punishment, but medical men advanced more immediate causes as well. They searched for an imbalance in the humors, which could be brought on by outside intervention. Joseph Grünpeck, one of the first to respond to the new disease, published a brief treatise in German and Latin in 1496. He devoted most of the work to astrology, rather than the disease or how to cure it. In keeping with this perspective, Grünpeck explained the coming of the disease by the conjunction of Saturn, Jupiter, and Mars.[13] Commentators such as Grünpeck indicated that people with melancholic or choleric temperaments were likely to be affected by the Pox as the influence of Saturn helped to produce melancholy and Mars produced a choleric temperament so the conjunction of the two helped to produce the black pustules on and around the genitals.[14] Grünpeck neglected the sexual aspects of the disease, but almost immediately other commentators indicated the sexual transmission of the disease as the proximate cause while continuing to acknowledge God's will and often the influence of the planets.

Italian medical practitioners were especially active in describing the new disease, which many labeled the French disease, as well as in prescribing cures. Because of the nearly epidemic proportions of the disease in Italy at the turn of the sixteenth century, this situation is not unsurprising. In spite of the variety of names for the disease and even an awareness that it may have originated in the New World, contemporaries did not seem to have engaged in the scapegoating of foreigners. Anna Foa and William Eamon have argued that the framing of the disease through its naming tended to focus on "others" who were not Christians. Jews and native Americans were not Christian and so could be blamed for the spread of the new disease and Eamon goes farther and adds lepers to this list.[15] Their arguments, especially concerning Native Americans and Jews, are plausible in the context of the time. However, these arguments fall apart when they are closely examined using the original sources. Jews and lepers are rarely mentioned in connection with the disease and no blame is attached to either group. Some commentators indicated that the disease originated in the Americas, with some Spaniards recognizing its origin with the term "mal de la ysla Espanola." Blame did not seem to be attached to any of these out groups as Samuel Cohn indicates in his insightful work dealing with how epidemic diseases have been treated by society.[16] The naming of the disease did not result in blame and by the end of the sixteenth century, many commentators had retreated to less loaded terms such as the Great Pox or *lues venera*. As the term indicates, contemporaries recognized the Pox as a venereal disease, but with different symptoms than the "burning disease" (gonorrhea) that had been present in the Middle Ages.

Perhaps because of the sexual transmission of syphilis, it may have been inevitable that women came to be seen as the immediate cause of the disease. Commentators, especially those who accepted the contagion approach to the spread of disease, viewed prostitutes and wet nurses as the means by which syphilis was transmitted. Such a perspective ignored how women acquired the disease in the first place although it recognized that syphilis was transmitted by coitus. Wet nurses were unlikely to transmit the disease to the children they nursed but class bias made it easier to accuse them of transmitting the disease to children who developed congenital syphilis rather than indicating it was acquired from a parent. For the most part, they did not call for wholesale action against women. By the latter half of the sixteenth century, some commentators more readily blamed "loose" women and those men who frequented them for the spread of the pox

The sexual transmission of syphilis as well as some of its symptoms such as skin lesions linked it back to leprosy for some. Leprosy had a declining medical impact by the early fifteenth century, but the moral repugnance regarding lepers remained. In 1500, jurors in Yarmouth indicted the notorious brothel-keeper Alice Dymock as a leper, suggesting that some people made a connection between leprosy and sexual deviance. Although given the similar symptoms at certain stages of the disease, she may have been instead the first person to suffer from syphilis in Yarmouth.[17] Because many commentators indicated that leprosy was transmitted through sexual contact, even though this was inaccurate, any disease that shared this means of transmittal was morally suspect. Syphilis gradually came to replace leprosy as a morally evil disease, a distinction that AIDS acquired in the latter third of the twentieth century.

Explaining the origin of the new disease and describing its symptoms was only part of the role of the early commentators. They also needed to provide a cure. While they operated within the framework of Galenic medicine, the early commentators responded as medical men had done with earlier diseases by describing approaches to treating the symptoms of syphilis that revolved around returning the humors to balance. Because physicians often avoided treating the disease, various other practitioners including surgeons, and various sorts of quacks often took on the treatment of the pox. Medical men had long advocated purging and bloodletting as a means of returning the humors to balance and these approaches became part of the treatment regimen for syphilis as well. Unfortunately, these treatments provided no relief and, as was often the case, even made the situation worse. Quicksilver, as mercury was known in the sixteenth century, had long been used for treating skin ailments so medical writers advocated various concoctions of mercury with wine, water, herbs, and other additives. Most often, the practitioner applied a paste-like substance containing mercury to the afflicted person who was then bundled up in blankets, sometimes in front of raging fire, to sweat the disease out. Other advocates of mercury combined it with ingredients such as wine for internal consumption. Some people turned to mercury cures to avoid the embarrassment of acknowledging the disease when symptoms became apparent. Mercury cures may have provided some relief but they produced their own symptoms such as a grey pallor and loose teeth, symptoms that indicated what the person was being treated for syphilis. Over-use of mercury may have avoided the full panoply of syphilis symptoms as mercury is a poison and too liberal application could kill the patient before he underwent the tortures of the late stages of syphilis.

Mercury cures had many supporters during the sixteenth century in spite of their unpleasant side effects. The Swiss physician Paracelsus was probably the most notable advocate of mercury and it did have some effectiveness against syphilis. Mercury was strongly sporicidal l and so was effective in dealing with secondary syphilis where large numbers of active spirochetes were present. It was less effective in dealing with primary infections as fewer spirochetes were present. Until the development of Salvarsan in the early twentieth century, mercury retained its place as the most effective cure for syphilis and continued to be used in limited circumstances until the highly effective remedy penicillin was discovered in the mid-twentieth century.[18]

Given the problems with the mercury cure, it is no wonder that contemporaries continued to search for other remedies. The bark of a West Indian tree, boiled down and then used in a fumigant environment promised some relief. A ready market developed for Guaiacum bark and wood imported into Europe and various empirics provided concoctions to treat the victims of syphilis. Writing in 1519, Ulrich von Hutten, Protestant reformer, humanist, and syphilis sufferer, defended the use of guaiacum in *De Guaiaci Medicina et Morbo Gallico*. This work was widely reprinted and translated with Thomas Paynel, a canon of Merton Abbey, providing an English translation in 1533.[19] Because of its expense, the guaiacum remedy was initially limited to only the wealthy, but it gradually came into wider use. Guaiacum produced a heavy sweat that many thought therapeutic, but in reality, it had no effect on the pox although it may have lined the pockets of the Fuggers who controlled the importation of guaiacum to Europe.

The usual means of preparation for guaiacum was to grind bark or wood from the guaiacum tree into a powder and then boil it in water. The practitioner then administered the remaining liquid orally to the patient. Often it was mixed with other ingredients to make it more palatable. The patient was usually swaddled in blankets in a warm room while this was done to induce sweating and was put on a strict diet. Patients usually had to follow this regimen for 30 days. Some medical men even combined guaiacum and quicksilver treatments, and if one proved ineffective would follow it with the other.

Fracastoro: Syphilis and contagion

Numerous medical men and laymen in Italy and Germany described the causes and symptoms of the new disease during its early years and often provided cures. In 1530, a physician of Verona, Girolamo Fracastoro coined the term syphilis to describe the new disease in his poetic commentary, *Syphilis sive morbus gallicus*. The work would be reprinted widely, converted to prose, and widely translated as it became a contemporary bestseller. Fracastoro described the disease as originating in classical Greece among idyllic shepherds. He went on to describe cures, favoring the guaiacum cure over mercury. In some ways, *Syphilis sive morbus gallicus* served to sum up knowledge concerning the new disease and its treatment at the end of the first generation of the disease. By 1530, the pox had already evolved into a less virulent disease than it had been at the turn of the century albeit a disease that now promised to afflict sufferers over a long period. Fracastoro's explanation was set in humanistic learning that emphasized the humor theory. Although it reflected an existing male bias in society, *Syphilis* was not overly moralistic or misogynistic in its approach.

Fracastoro returned to a consideration of syphilis in his treatise concerning what he considered to be contagious diseases, *De Contagione, Contagiosis Morbis et eorum Curatione*, published in 1546. Unlike *Syphilis* this work did not receive wide notice although it ultimately merited Fracastoro credit as one of the creators of the germ theory of contagion even though this was not his intent or how he saw his seeds of disease-causing infection.[20] As a university-trained physician with an intended audience of other educated practitioners, Fracastoro wrote *Contagion* in Latin not Italian. In *Contagion,* Fracastoro followed the traditional three-part approach to medical writing. In the first part, he provided a general definition of contagion, describes how it occurs, and the signs of contagion. The second part contains descriptions of various forms of contagious disease such as fevers, measles, plague, typhus, rabies, leprosy, phitis, and syphilis. Following conventional form, the third part described the treatments for each of the contagious diseases. Overall, it is a secular work with little moralism as Fracastoro described the disease in a matter-of-fact fashion. He betrays the Galenic origin of his thought as he indicates planetary influences on disease and the implication of his treatments is the need to restore humorial balance.

Fracastoro expanded upon his earlier treatment of syphilis which he referred to alternately as syphilis or the French sickness in *Contagion*. He described the progression of the disease through the development of its symptoms in straight forward fashion starting with lassitude, paleness, and small ulcers on the face, proceeding to large ulcers that might eat away the skin, irritability, catarrh which eroded the palate, gummata, and finally death.[21] He described most persons as becoming infected through sexual intercourse with some children being infected by nursing. Once he had described the symptoms of syphilis, Fracastoro followed up with a discussion of the causes of the disease. After discussing the possible American origins of the disease, Fracastoro questions this argument even going so far as to say that the medieval Arabic physician Avicenna may have described the disease. He then goes on to indicate that a probable conjunction of Saturn, Mars, and Jupiter was responsible for the disease. In further discussing the disease, Fracastoro places its immediate cause within his contagion theory which he uses to explain the latency period of the disease as well as some of its symptoms.[22] With *De Contagione* syphilis had finally arrived. It was a new disease, as Fracastoro indicated, but one that could be described within an existing framework encompassing other diseases.[23] In some ways, *De Contagione* reduced syphilis to yet another disease that could be described and treated rather than an unknown ailment that generated fear as it appeared in some earlier tracts such as Hutton's.

Once he had described the disease, Fracastoro did his duty as a physician and worked his way through the various treatment options available in the third section of the book. Wisely, Fracastoro indicates that the physician should be clear about what symptoms are present for this indicates the stage of the disease and what treatments are to be applied. He first described the environment necessary to lead to healing such as avoiding "impure" air as well as the proper diet for the patient. Fracastoro indicated that the patient should be active, he should "run, dance, hunt, play ball, wrestle, and fence," for this will help to "liquefy the sluggish substance, make it thinner, and drive it out, and along with it the germs of the contagion."[24] In conventional, Galenic fashion, Fracastoro started his treatment regimen with purging although he indicated this remedy was likely to be successful only in the early stages of the ailment. Aware that diet and purging were often unlikely to be successful, Fracastoro moved on to stronger remedies. He first turned to guaiacum and provided a fulsome discussion of the preparation of the various compounds as well as how it was to be administered and the pitfalls to avoid. Finally, he turned to the remedy that he indicates was once the first remedy of choice, quicksilver. Fracastoro detailed the various means of administering the mercury cure from inunction to fumigation and even ingestion as well as preparing the compounds to be used. He further described the less drastic use of mercury as topical creams to be applied to the ulcers. Unlike some empirics,

Fracastoro was well aware that mercury treatments could have very unpleasant side effects, which may preclude their use. In particular, he indicated that practitioners should use guaiacum rather than mercury for young sufferers.[25] All in all, Fracastoro reflects the class biases of the day. His patients were not likely to be poor or even middling sorts so milder rather than harsher remedies were to be preferred even though they may be more expensive. Although he rarely made it explicit, Fracastoro grounded his treatments in the tenets of educated, Galenic medicine. Especially in his poem *Syphilis sive Morbus Gallicus,* but also in *De Contagione,* he based his views on humanistic thought and he makes no moral judgments concerning the sufferers of the disease.

The pox in England

From reading the various accounts of the new disease that appeared until around 1530, it appears that the Pox was a major medical problem. Authors implied a high death rate and even those who did not die suffered greatly from the pox itself, or one of the prescribed cures, especially mercury. Obtaining numbers to confirm the impact of syphilis is another matter. Although commentators did not always consider the disease to be venereal during the first 30 years of its presence, in Europe, they came to see it as such by 1530. This sexual means of transmission may have made some sufferers unwilling to report its presence for fear of censure although others such as the aristocratic Ulrich von Hutten seemed to regard infection as a usual consequence of an aristocratic lifestyle. Unlike the plague or even *Sudor Angilicus,* reliable numbers of deaths for syphilis are nearly impossible to find. Commentators indicated that many people were infected and many of those died, but provided no concrete evidence. Part of the difficulty in deriving a mortality rate for the disease is that after the first years when the great pox quickly killed many of its victims, it had become a chronic disease so that people died each year from it but not necessarily in large numbers at any one time and place as could occur with outbreaks of the plague or the Sweat. The new disease was a major health problem during its first 30 years, but the fear arising from its symptoms generated some of the contemporary discussion. Nonetheless, it can probably be assumed that syphilis was present in epidemic proportions during its first 30 years even though it did not generate the mortality rate of a plague outbreak.

As Fracastoro and others indicated, the impact of syphilis was changing. The disease may have evolved into a less virulent form by 1530 decreasing mortality rates although not necessarily morbidity rates that remained high. The European population, or at least significant parts of it, may have evolved some degree to immunity to the disease that also helped to lower mortality rates. It seems that syphilis remained a major health problem for the rest of the century, but was often a chronic condition rather than one that produced high death rates. Combined with an increasing moralism regarding the disease, the chronic nature of the pox influenced reporting and makes it difficult to obtain reliable numbers.

The Pox soon arrived in England and contemporary accounts noted the presence of the "French pocks" in Shrewsbury at the end of the 1490s and Alice Dymock in Yarmouth may have suffered from it in 1500. The Aberdeen city government took measures by 1497 to control the spread of the "disease of Naples" in the city. The Pox continued to spread and James IV took strong measures to stop its spread in Edinburgh.[26] After that, the disease seemed to disappear from public notice for a time.

Syphilis may have affected England in much the same way as it did the rest of the continent in the years before 1530.[27] Obtaining reliable numbers for England is even more challenging than for the continent for this period. After describing an outbreak of the Sweat (1508), Bernard André goes on to say it was "followed by a far more detestable malady, to be abhorred as much as leprosy, a wasting pox which still vexes many eminent men."[28] This isn't much to go on although André's comment indicates the Pox was present in England. Unlike on the continent, early sixteenth-century English medical commentators often chose to ignore the disease but this was changing by mid-century. The surgeon William Clowes indicates in his work dealing with *morbus gallicus* (first published in 1579) that over a five-year period he and three other surgeons or physicians cured some one thousand sufferers of the French disease at St. Bartholomew's Hospital in London. He goes on to indicate that over a period of nine or ten years every other patient seeking treatment "had the pockes."[29] Clowes's estimates of the incidence of syphilis may be overstated, but the disease did produce large numbers of victims. Surgeons often received gratuities rather than billing their patients and over a 12-month period in 1547–48 the St. Bartholomew's surgeons received gratuities for healing some 87 patients. Twenty-one of these patients are recorded as suffering from syphilis or about a quarter of the number.[30] This sample may not reflect the total patient load at St. Bartholomew's Hospital and does not take into account the elite treated by private physicians. It is suggestive that syphilis had become a major public health problem in England by the mid-sixteenth century.

During the last half of the sixteenth century, numerous English commentators on syphilis stepped forward. Medical men were paying increased attention to syphilis just as it had become a less deadly medical problem. As early as 1533, Thomas Paynel provided a translation of Ulrich von Hutten's treatise on the French disease but it was not until 1547 that Andrew Boorde took independent notice of the disease which he called the "French pockes" and advocated mercury as a cure.[31] The English commentators were surgeons, as well as physicians, who wrote in English in order to reach a wider audience than Latin tracts were likely to reach.

The physician Andrew Boorde was one of the first English commentators to notice the pox in a meaningful way. His *Breviary of Health* was an encyclopedic treatment of the diseases facing England in the sixteenth century and Boorde intended it for a literate audience, not just medical practitioners as he wrote in English. He calls the disease the great pox or the French pox although he indicates that when he was young people called it the Spanish pox. After describing the symptoms of the disease, Boorde advocates an ointment made of mercury sublimate, turpentine, burnt aloe, and butter to be applied to the pustules.[32] There was nothing original about Boorde's work, but by writing in English, he reached a wider audience. Some modern commentators might argue that sixteenth-century observers were unable to distinguish between syphilis and other venereal diseases such as gonorrhea and yet Boorde made a distinction between what he called a "burning disease" (most likely gonorrhea) and the Pox. Boorde further indicated that a woman's "secret member" could be troubled by a variety of diseases such as burning, ulcers, scabies, and the pox. This is not to say that various venereal diseases were not confused in the sixteenth century, but that at least one commentator was aware that there were different sorts of venereal diseases that required different treatments. Boorde's description of the pox and its treatment is devoid of moral condemnation of its victims, he simply described the disease as he did others and provided a treatment for its sufferers.

As Winfried Schleiner has pointed out, the English commentators on syphilis tended to be more moralistic than their continental counterparts, blaming the sinful nature of the victims for their misfortunes although as Boorde's *Breviary of Health* indicates this was not always the case.[33] The incidence of many diseases in the Middle Ages was sometimes seen as resulting from a need for moral reform and the plague engendered this response on occasion. Critics directed their moralism at society as a whole for plague outbreaks rather than individuals. Leprosy, on the other hand, often carried with it a moral condemnation of the victim for a variety of reasons including the mistaken argument for sexual transmission.

Even though a syphilis diagnosis did not carry moral stigma with it in the early years, it gradually came to take on a moral stigma that came close, at times, to indicating that the victims got what they deserved because of their individual moral failings. In 1497, the Emperor Maximilian issued an edict labeling the new disease a plague sent by God as a punishment for blasphemy.[34] His edict was more a call for general moral reform than a pronouncement that blamed individuals for their sins. The Reformation often led commentators to take a more individually moralist approach to society and syphilis seemed to fit this pattern as the Puritanism of several English writers affected how they treated the disease and its victims. Already in the early years of the sixteenth century, efforts were made to curtail prostitution and the Crown closed down the brothels owned by the Bishops of Winchester in 1506 although only briefly.[35] This was not the first time that the Southwark stews had been closed. In 1417, the London Common Council ordered them closed because they harbored women and men of ill repute although they were soon reopened.[36] Both closures seem to have been motivated more by fear of disorder than health issues. Unlike Maximilian's edict, this moralism was directed at sexual impropriety almost exclusively. The coupling of the Pox and moral reform grew stronger as time passed. In 1546, Henry VIII ordered that the London stews that "engender such corruption among the people as tendeth to the intolerable annoyance of the commonwealth, and where not only the youth is provoked, enticed, and allowed to execute the fleshly lusts, but also, by such assemblies of evil-disposed persons haunted and accustomed, is daily devised and conspired how to spoil and rob the true laboring and well-disposed men."[37] This proclamation added the fear of sexual impropriety to an overall unease about social disorder that considers brothels and alehouses as places that hatched forces of social decay that needed to be controlled. Writing in 1567, Thomas Harmon captured these fears in his *Caveat for Common Cursetors*. He described several categories of male and female "vagabonds" who posed a threat to society. His bawdy baskets were women who traded "their lyues in lewed loathsome lechery," and his "Doxes be broken and spoyled of their maydenhead by the vpright men {men at the top of the criminal trade}, and they they haue their name of Doxes, and not afore. And afterward she is common and indifferent for any that wyll vse her."[38] Poverty could lead to an increase in prostitution and poverty appeared to be on the increase in the late sixteenth century and with it a fear of vagrants and the unruly poor. Sixteenth-century commentators, such as Thomas Harmon, were alarmed by vagabonds, but Paul Slack warns that we must be careful to avoid over-emphasizing the problem.[39] Many late sixteenth-century English commentators came to see syphilis as a moral evil brought on by sexual libertinism and related to social disorder and, therefore, something to be punished appropriately. The inclusion of syphilis in medical tracts enabled writers to display their moral and, in some cases, misogynist outrage at what they may have seen as the moral decline of English society.

Three writers stand out in their commentaries on the new disease. William Bullein, Philip Barrough, and William Clowes the elder all prepared treatises in English dealing with diseases, and their treatment with syphilis was one of many ailments dealt with by the writers. All three followed a well-worn path that drew on continental authors in describing the origins of the disease and its treatment. They noted both mercury and guaiacum as treatment options although they also indicated other possible treatments as well. They also largely disdained to discuss preventative measures for doing so might make it easier for malefactors to engage in the pleasures of the flesh. These commentators tended to regard sufferers as evil people who had brought on their own medical problems by their sinful nature. Unlike some of their continental counterparts, English commentators did little to connect the pox with established medical doctrines such as contagion theory. They quickly got to work by describing the diseases and various cures in plainspoken detail. This lack of a theoretical approach probably came, in part, from their intended audience who were less likely to be concerned with theory and more concerned with practice. Even if university-trained physicians looked down on them, the treatises of the three, especially Clowes's, enjoyed a wide readership.

William Bullein was a physician to the gentry in the mid-fifteenth century and the author of several works dealing with medicine.[40] Unlike most sixteenth-century physicians, Bullein wrote in English as he intended to reach a wide audience. His *Bulwarke of Defence against all Sicknesse*, first published in 1562 with another edition in 1579, is composed of five works joined together. Bullein describes a dietary remedy for the pox but has scant hope for it.[41] Most of what he has to say about syphilis is found in the first book of the *Bulwarke* entitled the "Book of Simples," in which Bullein describes various herbal and chemical cures as well as the diseases that they can be used to treat. He describes both the guaiacum and mercury as cures for syphilis although he favors the former, calling guaiacum the "holy wodde or wodde of life." Bullein provides an extensive discussion of its preparation in baths and ointments, noting that March and April are the best months to treat the pox with a guaiacum decoction. His discussion of both treatments follows the conventional approach for compounding and administering the cures. He warns that quicksilver can be misused and is a perilous cure to undertake.[42] Nothing really very new here. Fracastoro and others had described the disease and its treatments earlier so Bullein contributed little save writing in English for a wider audience. What is new is his tone. Bullein does not discuss any preventative measures and even indicates a reluctance to treat those who have acquired the disease through their own fault, i.e. those who "haue liued in most shamles lust and lechery, among painted stinkyng harlots, for which offence, they be smitten with the plague, called the French Pockes."[43] He is kinder to those who have acquired the disease through no fault of their own but comes close to saying that those men who acquired the disease through consorting with prostitutes needed to be punished for their sinful ways. Like other sixteenth-century authors, Bullien focuses entirely on men dealing with women only as agents who convey the disease. He displayed his attitude toward women in an aside during his discussion of syphilis in which he condemns women who use fairy charms and "danable witches" who he considered more harmful to the realm than quatrain fevers, pestilence, or the pox, indicating they should be burned.[44]

Writing about syphilis had become a cottage industry in the latter part of the sixteenth century. Philip Barrough dealt extensively with syphilis in his treatise *The Method of Physick Containing the Causes, Signes, and Cures of Inward Diseases in Man's Body* first published in 1590.[45] The sixth book of the work deals with the cures of the disease called *Morbus Gallicus* in 24 pages. Barrough's favored remedy is guaiacum although he indicates that quicksilver may be a remedy of last resort when all others have failed.[46] There is less of blaming the victim with Barrough than had been the case with Bullein. Not surprisingly given the threat that Spain posed to England when Barrough composed his work there is a distinct anti-Spanish tone to the work. He indicates that the Spanish acquired the disease from the Indians instead of the gold they had intended to gain in America. Moreover, he somehow blames the emperor Charles V for spreading the disease to Italy for his soldiers "were much given to venery," labeling him "a man of great power, and delighted much in shedding of blood, sparing neither man, woman, nor child."[47] Earlier commentators had noted the New World origin of the disease, but more in passing and generally went on to note that guaiacum came from the New World. While the various names such as French disease, Neapolitan disease, or Polish disease might indicate its origin, they did not imply a moral condemnation. Barrough, however, connected the disease with Spain, even though he conventionally called it *Morbus Gallicus*, further contributing to the Black Legend. It was almost as if the disease had become another weapon in the war of words between England and Spain.

After describing the origins of the pox, Barrough gets to work detailing its symptoms. He provides specific examples, often in graphic detail, as well as what he calls "the infection of the natural spirits, which are the immediat instruments of the faculty sustaining and giuing liunelines to the whole body by whole infection."[48] Once he has described the symptoms of the disease, Barrough proceeds to list cures. In keeping with humor theory, he advocates bloodletting as one possible cure although he does warn that this remedy might make the disease worse.[49] Once he has dispensed with older remedies, Barrough turns to guaiacum, providing an extensive discussion of the preparation of the decoction people should use in treating the disease.[50] Although his favored treatment was guaiacum, Barrough grudgingly admitted that quicksilver could be used in some cases as well as other compounds. Overall, there is little of explicitly blaming the victim in Barrough's work. However, his misogyny is apparent as he blames women, especially prostitutes for transmitting the disease. As he puts it: "There be devilish women desirous to be handled and dealt withal, who will beautifie themselves, to inflame mens hearts to lust towards them; abandon these your company, and thrust them out of the dores and house."[51] Barrough follows conventional medical remedies with his prescriptions. He is aware of the sexual transmission of the disease, but unlike Bullein he is content to blame only the female partner rather than the general sinfulness of the sexual act although that may be implicit in his work.

The barber-surgeon William Clowes the Elder served on the staff of St. Bartholomew's Hospital in London and published his first treatise *A Short and profitable Treatise Touching on the Cure of the Disease now Called Morbus Gallicus* in 1579. He published an updated version in 1585 and an expanded and corrected version, retitled as *A Brief and Necessary Treatise, Touching the Cure of the Disease now usually Called Lues Venerea by Unctions and Other Approved Ways of Curing* in 1596. Interestingly he abandoned the term *Morbus Gallicus* in the title for what was coming to be the more accepted term *Lues Venera* with the 1596 edition although he often returned to the older term in the text. Clowes was aware of his outsider status as a surgeon and took pains to defend publishing English rather than Latin in the 1596 edition.[52] In many ways, the barber-surgeons had taken on the cure of syphilis as physicians often tried to avoid it so Clowes was at the center of dealing with the disease.

Clowes' approach was conventional. He described the disease in terms used by most earlier commentators and provided a variety of cures often taken from continental authorities. He takes his readers through a comprehensive list of cures but the two most important cures are guaiacum and mercury. Clowes maintained "that quicksilver is most profitable for the cure of Lues Venerea."[53] He follows up this admonition with various quicksilver compounds and means of application, but these remedies had already appeared in the works of continental writers. In that sense, Clowes does not advance his readers' knowledge of the disease or its treatment. Like William Bullein, Clowes has scant sympathy for the victims of *Lues Venera*. His opening letter to his readers makes his view clear: "*Lues Venerea*, the pestilent infection of filthie lust: a sickness verie loathsome, odious, trouble-some, and dangerous. A notable testimonie of the just wrath of God against that filthie sinne, which at this daie not only infecteth Naples, Spaine, and France, but increaseth yet daily, spreading it self through Englande."[54] Clowes uses syphilis as the vehicle to couple social and moral disorder as he calls for a better-ordered society. He accepts the idea of divine punishment for the disease, jumps over astrological causes, and indicates: "the causes whereof I see none so great as the licencious and beastly disorder of a great number of rogues, and vagabonds, the filthy lyse of many leude and idle persons, both men and women, about the Citie of London."[55] Clowes made the connection in the 1579 edition of lewd people and alehouses, which he indicated harbored them.[56] Clowes was not alone in seeing alehouses as centers of disorder such as prostitution, as many authorities required alehouse keepers to forbid prostitution on their premises.[57] Actions such as closing alehouses would lead to the moral reformation necessary to ward off the disease. Clowes expressed attitudes common among many Puritan reformers of the last third of the sixteenth century. He also displayed a class bias; he no longer was concerned with aristocratic victims of the disease, but instead with controlling vagabonds and others on the bottom rungs of society. In the taverns of the day, male victims of low moral status encountered the women who gave them the "loathsome, odious, and troublesome," disease. No Christian charity for them, but instead harsh and necessary reform of their conduct for he hardly considers victims of the disease worthy of treatment.

Like both Bullein and Barrough, Clowes saw women as the agents of trans-mission of the pox. "The sickness is said first to be ingendered by the unlaw-ful copulation and accompanying with uncleane women, or common harlots," although he admits there could be other means of transmission such as touching infected clothing or from wet nurses to infants.[58] Male victims might deserve the disease they acquired because of their immoral conduct in Clowes' estimation, but it was women who infected them in one way or another as men evidently could not infect women in Clowes' view. Ironically, all three medical men were writing during the reign of Elizabeth I.

Clowes' approach to syphilis illustrates how the disease had become a social disease. In Bruce Boehrer's view, the developing approach to the disease reflected what Clowes perceived as a need to protect the existing social structure that felt itself under threat.[59] Such an approach marginalized sufferers as evil livers. As Qualtiere and Slights argue, this approach enabled non-sufferers to feel a sense of superiority both for their own rectitude in avoiding the disease and as a recommendation of sexual restraint as a means of combating it.[60] There is much to recommend this marginalization argument, but even intense Puritans such as Clowes had to be aware that members of the nobility were also victims of the disease so that medical men had to treat at least some of its victims with care. Moreover, many of the social problems that England was encountering in the late sixteenth century were nothing new and the response was not uniquely Puritan. As Margaret Spufford has pointed out, late sixteenth-century England had much in common with late thirteenth-century England in terms of how some contemporaries saw an unruly lower class that required moral correction through social control. The desire to exercise social control was not uniquely Puritan and it was coming to be expressed in a variety of ways by the turn of the seventeenth century [61] What is more helpful is to regard it as a call for moral reform, but one couched within the existing deference for the aristocracy. As Frédérique Fouassier puts it, Clowes' treatise was both typical and untypical of Renaissance medical literature.[62]

The English commentators on the Great Pox added little to existing knowledge of the disease or its treatment. Syphilis was well understood by the time Fracastoro wrote his *Contagion* in 1546. Medical practitioners understood the treatment options and relied on their favorite. By about 1530, the disease had evolved away from its more virulent form to a chronic form that disfigured, incapacitated, and ultimately killed its victims if they lived long enough. Large numbers of people continued to be affected so syphilis was a public health threat but one different than that presented by the immediacy of the plague or even the English Sweat. The fear generated by its symptoms coupled with the means of transmission continued to drive many commentators such as Clowes, Bullein, and Barrough in the latter part of the century. It had also truly become a social phenomenon in the latter part of the century as discussion of syphilis became a way for Englishmen to point up the Spanish and moral threats to English society arising from the disorderly masses. Although the threats might come from the outside, their cause was internal—the need for moral regeneration that was being expressed by a variety of Puritan writers in the last years of the sixteenth century. With that emphasis, we have come a long way from the cosmopolitanism and devotion to helping to cure the sick of a Girolamo Fracastoro.

The impact of the pox

Syphilis, the French disease, produced a much more long-lasting impact than the English Sweat, lasting well into the twentieth-first century. Its direct demographic impact, especially after the early years was probably less than that of the Sweat for syphilis rapidly became a chronic disease of epidemic proportions, but not an epidemic disease that killed large numbers of people in a short time. Lost production generated by a chronic disease is always hard to track and syphilis is no exception. We might expect that the disease had negative impacts on individual activity, especially in its later stages, but death came more slowly to its victims than in the early sixteenth century.

Syphilis had an impact on the literary world in the short run that exceeded that of the plague. It became a vehicle for mocking aspects of society and social behavior and a means for encouraging moral reform. For example, Shakespeare draws together a depiction of misogyny and moral and physical corruption in *Timon of Athens* (1607–08) with an almost classical depiction of the secondary and tertiary stages of syphilis.[63] This impact extended well into the seventeenth century as writers and playwrights used syphilis to advance their arguments about a variety of social issues. In the hands of some playwrights, syphilis almost became a means of generating humor as much as generating fear. Moral reformers used the disease to illustrate the wages of sin in an n often gruesome fashion so syphilis had an almost bifurcated impact. By the nineteenth century in the hands of writers, such as Charles Baudelaire or Gustave Flaubert, syphilis even came to stand for a free-thinking rejection of conventional morality.

Like other new diseases, especially those with horrifying symptoms, syphilis generated fear in society. Once the death rate declined, the immediacy of this fear may have declined, but chronic syphilis continued to generate a measure of fear in Western society well into the twentieth century. Part of the fear generated by syphilis came from its nature as a venereal disease. By the end of the sixteenth century, it had come to replace leprosy as a great moral evil afflicting society. Syphilis held pride of place as a leading example of the punishment for sin well into the twentieth century when the ability to affect a cure through penicillin and the advent of AIDS led to its replacement. Because of the links of syphilis to prostitution, reformers became increasingly repressive in the treatment of prostitutes, especially those with syphilis. Even more than leprosy, syphilis became the means for reformers to focus on the punishment of sexual license and call for reform through casting sin as a public health threat. Syphilis, like the Sweat and the plague, was a genuine public health threat in the sixteenth century. It went beyond them in becoming a means of illustrating the moral threat facing society and this gave it a lasting impact that the other two diseases did not possess once epidemics ceased to be commonplace.

New challenges to the medical status quo

Syphilis and the English Sweat both posed challenges to the longstanding Galenic and Arabic approaches to medicine that the onset of the plague in the fourteenth century had started to raise.[64] Initially, commentators treated them as new diseases although gradually over time some commentators incorporated them into the Galenic corpus. Both diseases displayed frightening symptoms and the Sweat and syphilis, at first, produced high mortality rates. In neither case did either of the diseases rival the plague in being able to decimate the population by ten percent in one epidemic as the plague was still able to do in the sixteenth century. *Sudor Anglicus* was an epidemic disease with five definable outbreaks. Syphilis seems to have reached nearly epidemic proportions in some communities and among some strata of society in the sixteenth century, but it cannot be labeled an epidemic disease because of its chronic nature

Numerous authors took on syphilis from educated laymen such as von Hutten to empirics, to surgeons such as Clowes to physicians such as Gabriele Fallopius, Fracastoro, or Bullein. While many early writers such as Grünpeck wrote in Latin, the trend seemed to be toward writing in the vernacular. Fracastoro, of course, wrote in Latin but he was coming to be the exception. English medical men wrote their treatises on syphilis in English even though, like Clowes, they might be defensive about doing so. One reason that medical men wrote in English was to combat the increasingly large number of empirics who they referred to as quacks. The remedies provided by empirics were often more deadly than those that came from the medical elite, but at times they had their successes. The medical establishment produced very little new medical knowledge from its encounter with the Pox unless the moralistic approach of some of the English practitioners is noted. As Harold Cook has pointed out, the seventeenth century became the century of self-proclaimed healers who were more than willing to take on the medical elite.[65]

The encounter with the Pox led some medical practitioners to question the Galenic consensus, but others tried to force the disease into the existing structure. Some surgeons and empirics experimented with chemical cures such as mercury and guaiacum and physicians followed suit in order to remain competitive in the medical marketplace. In some circles, the Pox reintroduced and strengthened the relationship between moralism and disease that reappeared with some commentators on HIV/AIDS in the twentieth century. At least in England, the Pox further contributed to the fear of social disorder arising from below even if the fear was overstated. Syphilis did not produce anything like the demographic disaster and its impact that came from the plague. It worked around the edges of society to lead to questioning of the medical consensus and giving moral reformers ammunition to urge social control.

The sixteenth century was an exciting but also a troubling time as various thinkers challenged old outlooks at every turn. The religious movement known as the Reformation had a major impact on society, but so too did humanism, the discovery of the New World, and the printing press. It is perhaps not unsurprising that medical concepts and practices also found challenges. Nor is it surprising that people would reconsider aspects of the social order. The challenges came from many quarters, but the role of new diseases was an important one in helping to push medical and even social thinking in new directions.

Notes

1 Coverage of the disease from its first appearance up through the present day can be found in Claude Quétel, *The History of Syphilis*, Judith Braddock and Brian Pike, trans. (Baltimore: Johns Hopkins University Press, 1990).
2 Jon Arrizabalaga, John Henderson, and Roger French, *The Great Pox: The French Disease in the Renaissance* (New Haven: Yale University Press, 1997). The historicist approach to the disease is enunciated even more forcefully in Roger French and John

Arrizabalaga, "Coping with the French Disease: University Practitioners' Strategies and Tactics in the Transition from the Fifteenth to the Sixteenth Century," in Roger French, Jon Arrizabalaga, Andrew Cunningham, Luis García-Ballester, eds., *Medicine from the Black Death to the French Disease* (Aldershot: Ashgate, 1998), 248–87. Mary Healy, *Fictions of Disease in Early Modern England* (Basingstoke: Palgrave, 2001), 252. Healy and this work follow Margaret Pelling in arguing that denying a role for biology ignores the ability to understand continuity and change in nature that can contribute a good deal to our understanding of disease and help avoid the danger of becoming anthropocentric. Margaret Pelling, *The Common Lot* (London: Longman, 1998), 7.

3 Robert J. Knell, "Syphilis in Renaissance Europe: Rapid Evolution of an Introduced Sexually Transmitted Disease?" *Proceedings of the Royal Society of London, Biology Letters*, 271 (2004), S174–S176.

4 Alfred W. Crosby, Jr., "The Early History of Syphilis: A Reappraisal," *American Antropologist*, 71 (1969), 218–27. Anthropologists have provided further support for the Columbian origin of syphilis through examining various archaeological sites in the New and Old Worlds as well as the documentary evidence. See, for example: Brenda J. Baker, George J. Armelagos, Marshall Joseph Becker, Don Brothwell, Alan G. Morris, et al., "The Origins and Antiquity of Syphilis: Paleopathological Dianosis and Interpretation," *Current Anthropology*, 29 (1988), 703–37, Kristen N. Harper, Molly K. Zuckerman, Megan L. Harper, John D. Kingston, and George J. Armelagos, "The Origin and Antiquity of Syphilis Revisited: An Appraisal of Old World Pre-Columbian Evidence for Treponemal Infection," *Yearbook of Physical Anthropology*, 54 (2011), 99–133.

5 Bruce M. Rothschild, "History of Syphilis," *Clinical Infectious Diseases*, 40 (2005), 1454–63.

6 Simon Mays, Gillian Crane-Kramer, Alex Bayliss, "Two Probable Cases of Treponemal Disease of Medieval Date from England," *American Journal of Physical Anthropology*, 120 (2003), 133–43; Tanya E. von Hunnius, Charlotte A. Roberts, Anthea Boylston, and Shelley R. Saunders, "Histological Identification of Syphilis in Pre-Columbian Engand," *American Journal of Physical Anthropology*, 129 (2006), 559–66; S. Mays, S. Vincent, and J. Meadows, "A Possible Case of Treponemal Disease from England Dating to the 11th–12th Century AD," *International Journal of Osteoarchaeology*, 22 (2012), 366–72.

7 Baker, et al., "Origin and Antiquity of Syphilis," and Harper et al, "Origin and Antiquity of Syphilis Revisited," provide good summaries of the debate.

8 Proponents of the social construction of disease approach Jon Arrizabalaga, John Henderson, and Roger French are unwilling to adopt the term syphilis because contemporaries rarely used it. Their highly useful book deals with the impact of the disease on the continent, but does not address England. *The Great Pox* (New Haven: Yale University Press, 1997). As indicated earlier, this approach also leads to difficulties in understanding the impact of a disease.

9 C. Meyer, C. Jung, T. Kohl, A. Poenicke, A. Poppe, K.W. Alt, "Syphilis 2001—A Palaeopathalogical Reappraisal," *Homo–Journal of Comparative Human Biology*, 53 (2002), 39–58; Kristen N. Harper, Paolo S. Ocampo, Bret M. Steiner, Robert W. George, Michael S. Silverman, et al., "On the Origin of the Treponematoses: A Phylogenetic Approach," *PLOS Neglected Tropical Diseases*, 2 (2008), e148.

10 Reynold H. Boyd, "Origin of Gonorrhoea and Non-Specific Urethritis," *British Journal of Venereal Disease*, 31 (1955), 246–48. Danielle Jacquart and Claude Thomasset, *Sexuality and Medicine in the Middle Ages* (Princeton: Princeton University Press, 1985), 179–80.

11 Andrew Boorde, *The Breuiarie of Health Wherein Doth Follow, Remedies for all Maner of Sicknesses & Diseases the which may be in Man or Woman.* (London: Thomas Este, 1598), c19, 82, 376.

12 W.G. Emmison, *Elizabethan Life: Morals and the Church Courts* (Chelmsford: Essex Record Office, 1973), 31–36.

13 A good synopsis of Grünpeck's views can be found in Paul A. Russell, "Syphilis, God's Scourge or Nature's Vengeance," *Archiv für Reformationsgeschichte*, 80 (1989), 286–306 and Darin Hayton, "Joseph Grünpeck's Astrological Explanation of the French Disease," in Kevin Siena, ed., *Sins of the Flesh* (Toronto: Centre for Reformation and Renaissance Studies, 2005), 81–106.

14 In addition to Hayton's and Russell's essays, Jon Arrizabalaga provides an analysis of the early response to the disease although he goes beyond the astrological explanation of Grünpeck. "Medical Responses to the 'French Disease' in Europe at the Turn of the Sixteenth Century," in Siena, *Sins of the Flesh*, 33–55.

15 Ana Foa, "The New and the Old: The Spread of Syphilis (1494–1530)," in Edward Muir and Guido Ruggiero eds, M.S. Gallucci, M.M. Gallucci, and C.C. Gallucci, trans., *Sex and Gender in Historical Perspective* (Baltimore: Johns Hopkins University Press, 1990), 26–45; William Eamon, "Cannibalism and Contagion: Framing Syphilis in Counter-Reformation Italy," *Early Science and Medicine*, 3 (1998), 1–31.

16 Samuel K. Cohn, Jr., *Epidemics* (Oxford: Oxford University Press, 2018), 95–126.

17 Carole Rawcliffe, *Leprosy in Medieval England* (Woodbridge: Boydell Press, 2006), 252–3.

18 J.G. O'Shea, "'Two Minutes with Venus, Two Years with Mercury'—Mercury as an Antisyphilitic Chemotherapeutic Agent," *Journal of the Royal Society of Medicine*, 83 (1990), 392–95. See also, John Parascandola, "From Mercury to Miracle Drugs: Syphilis Therapy over the Centuries," *Pharmacy in History*, 51 (2009), 14–23.

19 Ulrich von Hutten, *De Morbo Gallico: A Treatise of the French Disease*, Thomas Paynel, trans. (London: John Clarke, [1533] 1730), c. 8.

20 The reception of Fracastoro's theory of contagion and its lasting impact are detailed in Vivian Nutton, "The Reception of Fracastoro's Theory of Contagion: The Seed that Fell among Thorns," *Osiris*, 2d ser, 6 (1990), 196–234. Further discussion of contagion theory and the changing approach to disease will follow in the next chapter.

21 Fracastoro, *Contagion*, 134–41.

22 Fracastoro, *Contagion*, 142–57.

23 Arrizabalaga, Henderson, and French provide an excellent summation of how the new disease fit into theories of contagion at mid-century and what impact changes of thinking had on medical thought. *Great Pox*, 234–51.

24 Fracastoro, *Contagion*, 268–9.

25 Fracastoro, *Contagion*, 277–93.

26 Carole Rawcliffe, *Urban Bodies* (Woodbridge: Boydell Press, 2013), 113.

27 Johannes Fabricius provides the best overall coverage of syphilis and its impact in late sixteenth-century England. *Syphilis in Shakespeare's England* (London: Jessica Kingsley Publishers, 2008). An account of the impact of syphilis and the plague on literature during the period (although it goes beyond narrow treatment of the diseases on writers such as Shakespeare) is Margaret Healy, *Fictions of Disease in Early Modern England*.

28 Bernard André, *Annales Henrici VII.* James Gairdner, ed. (Rolls Series, 10, 1858), 126. André may misdate the syphilis outbreak.

29 William Clowes, *A Brief and Necessary Treatise, Touching the Cure of the Disease Now Usually Called Lues Venerea.* (London: Edmund Bollifant, 1596), 149–50. Clowes used the term *Morbus Gallicus* in 1579 and 1585 editions.

30 Margaret Pelling, "Appearance and Reality: Barbersurgeons, the Body and Venereal Disease in Early Modern London," in A.L. Beier and R. Finlay, eds., *The Making of the Metropolis, London 1500–1700* (London: 1986), 82–112.

31 Andrew Boorde, *The Breuiarie of Health Wherein Doth Follow, Remedies for all Maner of Sicknesses & Diseases the which may be in Man or Woman.* (London: Thomas Este, 1598), c 74, 80–81.

32 Boorde, *Breuiare of Health*, c 217, 237.

33 Winfried Schleiner, "Moral Attitudes toward Syphilis and Its Prevention in the Renaissance," *Bulletin of the History of Medicine*, 68 (1994), 390–7. See also, Schleiner, *Medical Ethics in the Renaissance* (Washington DC: Georgetown Univesity Presss, 1995), especially 162–202.

34 Russell, "Syphilis, God's Scourge or Nature's Vengeance." 292. Although first published more than 90 years ago, Owsei Temkin's "On the History of 'Morality and Syphilis,'" in Owsei Temkin, *The Double Face of Janus* (Baltimore: Johns Hopkins University Press, 1977), 472–84 is still worth reading.
35 A.H. Thomas and I.D. Thornley, eds., *The Great Chronicle of London* (Gloucester: Alan Sutton, 1983 [1938]), 331.
36 Riley, *Memorials of London*, 647.
37 Paul L. Hughes and James F. Larkin, eds., *Tudor Royal Proclamations*, 3 vols. (New Haven: Yale University Press, 1964–1969), 1: 365.
38 F.J. Furnivall, *The Rogues and Vagabons of Shakespeare's Youth* (London: Chatto and Windus, 1907), 65, 73. Johannes Fabricius places Harmon's Caveat and John Awdeley's *Fraternitye of Vacabondes* (1561) into the context of vagrancy in Elizabethan England. *Syphilis in Shakespeare's England*, 88–93.
39 Paul Slack, *Poverty and Policy in Tudor and Stuart England* (New York: Longman, 1988), 91–112.
40 For biographical detail concerning Bullein, see William S. Mitchell, "William Bullein, Elizabethan Physician and Author," *Medical History*, 3 (1959), 188–200.
41 William Bullein, *Bulwarke of Defence against All Sicknesse* (London: Thomas Marshe, 1579), "Book of Compounds," fol 43.
42 Bullein, *Bulwarke of Defence*, "Booke of Simples," fol 57–59, 70.
43 Bullein, *Bulwarke of Defence*, "Booke of Simples," fol 57.
44 Bullein, *Bulwarke of Defence*, "Booke of Simples," fol. 56.
45 A brief biographical treatment of Barrough is Gerald Shklar, "Philip Barrough, Elizabethan Physician with the First English Book on Medicine," *Journal of the History of Dentistry*, 52 (2004), 55–9.
46 Philip Barrough, *The Method of Physick Containing the Causes, Signes, and Cures of Inward Diseases in Man's Body.* (London: Richard Field, 1596), 361–85.
47 Barrough, *Method of Physick*, 361. It appears that Barrough confused the Emperor Charles V with King Charles VII of France whose army is often credited with bringing the pox to Naples in 1493–94.
48 Barrough, *Method of Physick*, 363.
49 Barrough, *Method of Physick*, 367.
50 Barrough, *Method of Physick*, 368–74. Like Bullein, Barrough also considers that spring is the best time for treatment (p 372).
51 Barrough, *Method of Physick*, p. 374.
52 William Clowes, *A Brief and Necessary Treatise, Touching the Cure of the Disease Now Usually Called Lues Venerea, by Unctions and Other Approved Waies of Curing* (London: Edmund Bollisant, 1596), 221. Aspects of Clowes' career are discussed in Celeste Chamberland, "Between the Hall and the Market: William Clowes and Surgical Self-Fashioning in Elizabethan London," *Sixteenth Century Journal*, 41 (2010), 69–89.
53 Clowes, *Brief and Necessary Treatise*, 169.
54 Clowes, *Brief and Necessary Treatise*, 149.
55 Clowes, *Brief and Necessary Treatise*, 149.
56 William Clowes, *A Short and Profitable Treatise Touching the Cure of the disease called (Morbus Gallicus) by Unctions* (London: John Day, 1579; New York: Da Capo Press, 1972), sig Aii^r.
57 Fabricus, *Syphilis in Shakespeare's England*, 96–103.
58 Clowes, *Brief and Necessary Treatise*, pp. 150–51.
59 Bruce Thomas Boehrer, "Early Modern Syphilis," *Journal of the History of Sexuality*, 1 (1990), 200.
60 Louis F. Qualtiere and William W.E. Slights, "Contagion and Blame in Early Modern Europe: The Case of the French Pox," *Literature and Medicine*, 22 (2003), 12–13.
61 Margaret Spufford, "Puritanism and Social Control?" in Anthony Fletcher and John Stevenson, eds., *Order and Disorder in Early Modern England* (Cambridge: Cambridge University Press, 1981), 41–57.

62 Frédérique Fouassier, "William Clowes's Treatise on Syphilis (1579): A Trebly Eccentric Work,' in Sophie Aymes-Stokes and Laurent Mellet, eds., *In and Out: Eccentricity in Britain* (Newcastle Upon Tyne: Cambridge Scholars Publishing, 2012), 80.
63 William Shakespeare, *Timon of Athens*, 4, 3: 153–66. In Harold F. Brooks, Harold Jenkins, Brian Morris, and Richard Proudfoot, *The Arden Edition of the Works of William Shakespeare* (London: Methuen, 1951–82). Margaret Healy, *Fictions of Disease in Early Modern England*, and Johannes Fabricus, *Syphilis in Shakespeare's England* provide other telling examples.
64 Arrizabalaga, Henderson, and French highlight the role of the Great Pox in raising questions about Galenism as it evolved over the course of the sixteenth century. *Great Pox*, 252–77.
65 Harold J. Cook, *The Decline of the Old Medical Regime in Stuart London* (Ithaca: Cornell University Press, 1986). Margaret Pelling, *Medical Conflicts in Early Modern London* (Oxford: Clarendon Press, 2003).

9
A NEW ERA FOR EPIDEMIC DISEASE

Syphilis and the English Sweat, in addition to plague, continued to create medical problems for English society from the late fifteenth century onward. Three other infectious diseases that produced large death tolls on occasion also began to have an impact in the sixteenth century. Influenza, typhus, and smallpox are all diseases that have posed major public health threats in the past and influenza continues to do so.

None of the three diseases was new in the sixteenth century, but people noticed their presence for a variety of reasons. Most people did not see agues or fevers resulting from diseases such as influenza as more than unpleasant episodes even though fevers of various sorts claimed victims every year. There were a few epidemics that might have led people to question this assumption but in 1918–1919 the situation changed and over 50 million people died worldwide in an influenza pandemic. From the sixteenth century through the mid-twentieth century, small and large typhus outbreaks broke out, sometimes killing a few hundred people, and sometimes killing several thousand. Smallpox is an old disease but in the seventeenth and eighteenth centuries something changed and it became a major killer in Europe. Along with other European diseases such as measles, smallpox produced a demographic catastrophe in the New World helping to produce a population decline of up to ninety percent in some cases. Questions arise whether these three diseases were present in the Middle Ages and if they were present why they did not have more of an impact. Addressing these questions helps lead to further insights into how environmental and social factors play a role in spreading infectious diseases. Exploring these questions, when taken together with discussion of other diseases, will help to understand why diseases emerge or re-emerge today.

DOI: 10.4324/9781003215219-10

The changing world of the sixteenth century

By the beginning of the sixteenth century, temperatures in northern Europe were edging downward as the Little Ice Age had begun. Average temperatures varied year to year, but the trend was toward colder winters and cooler summers than had been the case in the fourteenth century and earlier. There were still some warm years during the sixteenth century, but the first decade of the seventeenth century and particularly the last decade of the century would be distinctly colder than most years during the medieval period. As noted earlier, colder and wetter (or drier) conditions had an impact on the growing season and food production. Decreased food production could lead to malnutrition making some people likely to fall victim to disease. Famine remained a threat in some areas and emerged at certain times such as late in the sixteenth century. Colder or wetter conditions might lead more people to remain indoors in close proximity to others during the winter increasing the chances of infection for some diseases. The Little Ice Age made it easier to spread certain diseases, but climatic conditions did not necessarily lead to increased outbreaks.

The population of England and the rest of Europe was growing in the sixteenth century although it did not reach pre–Black Death numbers until the end of the century. As Wrigley and Schofield put it, the sixteenth century, especially the period lasting from 1565 to 1584, saw the end of the medieval disease regime with its widespread epidemic mortality.[1] Diseases, such as syphilis and the English Sweat, helped to retard population growth but did not have the impact of the plague. A somewhat better standard of living also played a role as improved food supply helped lead to a healthier population. England was essentially at peace domestically during the century after the turmoil of the War of the Roses in the fifteenth century. This too could have led to a decline in the death rate and an improvement in the birth rate.

An increasing population is generally a good thing, at least until the size of the population begins to outstrip food supply which was not the case in the sixteenth century save for a few famine years. Increasing population, however, can make it easier to spread diseases such as influenza, typhus, and smallpox, particularly when people are crowded together. As the number of people increased in the countryside, some set off for the towns of England to try their fortunes. Economic circumstances forced many town dwellers to live near to each other often in poor living conditions, making them ready candidates for an epidemic. Indeed, until the nineteenth-century English urban populations grew by in-migration, not by natural growth, as cities remained unhealthy places.

One final component of the disease–human relationship that came into play more strongly in the sixteenth century than before was a growing inter-relationship with the rest of the world. There had always been some contact between England and Asia during the Middle Ages and this overland trade enabled diseases such as plague to spread along trade routes. The discovery of the New World in the late fifteenth century opened up a new ecological world to Europe (and to the

Americas as well). The discovery of the New World operated in the background for the English disease universe of the sixteenth century, and it does not seem to have played a role with the English disease outlook at least as regards, influenza, typhus, and possibly smallpox.

Environmental factors played a role with other diseases and they were at work with the three diseases under consideration here. The overall disease burden of society had an impact on the seriousness of smallpox, typhus, and influenza infections. A person with a weakened immune system, from a disease such as tuberculosis, was more susceptible to death from a viral infection such as influenza than was a healthy person.

Influenza, an old disease that remains a threat today

The viral disease influenza may be one of the oldest diseases to infect humans. The symptoms of influenza are those of many diseases so that identifying it from descriptions in the past is difficult. As anyone who has suffered through a bout of the flu knows, the most common symptoms are high fever, sore throat, runny nose, coughing, joint pain, and headaches. A person with a mild case of the flu is likely to note these symptoms and go on with life until they pass within a week. When the symptoms become more severe, the victim may be forced to bed for a few days and even experience a secondary pneumonia infection that can be fatal. In 1427, the St. Albans chronicler indicated that "in the beginning of October, a certain rheumy infirmity which is called '*mure*' invaded the whole people, and so infected the aged along with the younger that it conducted a great number to the grave."[2] Was this influenza—maybe. Influenza often infects the very young and the aged so this is plausible. A rheumy infirmity could be a description of the flu, but with nothing more to go on, it is difficult to say this was an outbreak of influenza. Because the symptoms of influenza are so non-specific, chroniclers were not likely to note its presence unless a large number of deaths resulted.

Influenza remains a major health threat today and some public health officials indicate that it has the potential to pose a major threat to society. The disease mutates rapidly in small ways (antigenic drift), making it difficult to achieve successful prevention. Antigenic shift in which the virus mutates in a major way, as occurred with the variant that caused the 1918–19 influenza pandemic, also occurs regularly. Birds and hogs are hosts for the influenza virus. Once a strain mutates so that it can infect humans, the virus is transmitted through human-to-human contact and viral discharge. In most outbreaks today, small children and especially the elderly are victims although there have been some notable exceptions such as the 1918–19 pandemic when people in the prime of life were the most commonly affected. The ease in spreading the disease coupled with its almost continual mutation makes the flu a formidable enemy although yearly vaccinations and better palliative care decrease its impact today. Nonetheless, during most flu seasons, which typically run from mid-autumn to spring, between three and five million people will become ill with the flu and between 290,000 and 650,000 people worldwide may die in any one year.

Influenza is caused by an orthomyxovirus. Type A, B, and C Influenza viruses exist and researchers discovered Type D in 2016 although it has not infected humans as yet. Influenza Type A, which has birds as its natural host, infects humans and other mammals such as hogs. Influenza Type B almost exclusively infects humans, but people usually acquire a degree of immunity at an early age. This early immunity combined with a limited host range generally keeps influenza B from being a major health threat. Influenza Type C can infect humans, hogs, dogs and cats, but is not common and usually causes mild infections in children.

Type A influenza virus has been responsible for human epidemics and the influenza A genome consists of eight separate pieces of single-stranded RNA which function as distinct genes. The reassortment of the genetic material can occur readily and has produced several recombinations. Two of the viral genes code for surface glycoproteins, hemagglutinin (H) and neuraminidase (N). The human immunological defense system develops antibodies to defend against these antigens. Over time, a wide variety of subtypes of influenza Type A have emerged with sixteen H and nine N subtypes although not all have been linked to epidemics in humans. At this point, it is not possible to discern the level of mutation in the past, but it is safe to assume that it occurred. Some of these different serotypes can be quite deadly. Researchers identify H1N1 as the cause of the Spanish Flu of 1918–19, which killed more than 50 million people worldwide, as well as the Swine Flu outbreak of 2009. The H2N2 serotype caused the Asian Flu of 1957, while the Hong Kong Flu of 1968 was caused by the H3N2 serotype. More recently, the continued spread of the highly pathogenic H5N1 serotype has raised concern about another major pandemic.[3] Type A Influenza virus is highly adaptable and moves readily from bird hosts to mammals, including humans and often back again, often mutating along the way. The unstable gene combinations found in birds become stable viruses once the virus switches to these secondary hosts. This situation was less important in the past save that each influenza epidemic was likely to have a slightly different impact than the one before it. This continually changing environment makes it difficult to develop a fully successful preventative vaccine today.[4] Influenza has the potential to be a major disease threat today, but was this the case in the past?

Because influenza spreads via human contact and nasal discharge, a large concentrated population is necessary for the disease to pose a major health threat. With an R_0 between three and four, influenza spreads readily through an at-risk population although not everyone who comes in contact with an infected person contracts the disease. Influenza may be an old disease but it would not be until the growth of towns that it became a major health threat. Scholars have considered it among the many possible causes for the Plague of Athens, but this is unlikely. Charles Creighton indicated what he considered influenza with a fever in 1173 with "an evil and unheard of cough," but it is difficult to call this influenza with any certainty.[5] Most likely, the first documented influenza epidemic occurred in 1510, as four medical scientists acknowledged in their commemoration of its 500th anniversary.[6] In late July and August, people throughout Europe were afflicted with an oppressive cough, fever, and a sensation of constriction of the heart and lungs. The disease reputedly first arrived in Italy along trade routes from Asia and quickly spread throughout the continent reaching northern Europe by September and October and ultimately the New World as well. The disease burned out quickly and seemed to cause few deaths, mostly among children.[7] While the 1510 episode was likely influenza, there is consensus that the better-documented pandemic originating in Asia Minor and North Africa in early summer 1580 and reaching England in August, September, and October was influenza.[8] England also appears to have suffered an influenza epidemic in 1557–58. The author of Wriothesley's chronicle indicated that during the summer of 1557 "divers strange and new sicknesses, taking men and women in their heads; as strange agues and fevers, whereof many died."[9] Thereafter, influenza became common with periodic pandemics that affected all of Europe, culminating in the worldwide pandemic of 1918–1919.

Influenza had become one of the "new" diseases of the sixteenth century, largely because of changing environmental circumstances rather than emergence. Today, Asia is often the region in which influenza periodically evolves into a new deadly serotype that then affects the rest of the world. David Patterson maintains that the influenza epidemics of the eighteenth century got their start in Russia and then moved in an East to West direction.[10] The disease occurred at regular intervals throughout the eighteenth and nineteenth centuries reaching pandemic proportions on occasion. What troubled people in the sixteenth century was that influenza claimed victims from all classes, unlike the plague that had come to be a disease largely of the poor by the sixteenth century. The author of the continuation of Fabyn's Chronicle took pains to note in his entry for 1558: "In the beginning of this mayor's year died many of the wealthiest men all England through of a strange fever."[11] Although this is not a good description of influenza, it does indicate the surprise that the well-to-do died during the epidemic.

It seems that the usual pattern of children, the elderly, and those people with already compromised immune systems should have been the victims of medieval outbreaks and sixteenth-century outbreaks even though epidemics claimed victims of all ages. The sixteenth-century chroniclers either ignored child deaths in favor of noting adult victims or the pattern of the disease was different than modern outbreaks, leading to the question—was this influenza? A complication of influenza is secondary infection with pneumonia, a bacterial disease. Pneumonia existed throughout the Middle Ages and was usually called ague as were several other fevers including malaria. It can be deadly at any time to people with weakened immune systems. A combination of an influenza infection followed by pneumonia can be especially devastating. Secondary infection with pneumonia may have been responsible for many of the deaths during the 1918–19 influenza pandemic as well as the 1957 and 1968 pandemics.[12]

Influenza probably was part of the disease regime in premodern England but contemporaries considered it to be one among many fevers that caused problems for people and they tended to see fevers as simply part of life. There seems to have been no outbreaks severe enough to label as epidemics save in 1557–59.[13] The lack of population density and access to new strains (most likely from Asia) contributed to this situation. It is also possible that the influenza serotypes present in medieval Europe were not as virulent as later strains such as H1N1. When influenza infections occurred in combination with other diseases, influenza could have helped to increase the overall mortality rate, especially among children and the elderly. These views changed as the disease became more common and by the eighteenth century, doctors readily identified influenza in part because there were twelve epidemics in addition to yearly cases.[14]

Typhus, killer of prisoners and soldiers

Like influenza, typhus is probably an old disease, but it did not become a major health problem until the early modern era. It is usually a product of crowded conditions and poor sanitary conditions and famine, which make people more susceptible to the disease. Writing in the 1930s, before the development of antibiotic therapy, the bacteriologist Hans Zinsser devoted a book to the disease and its impact indicating that it was one of the major scourges of humankind. Today, typhus receives little notice, except as a possible biological weapon, although there continue to be cases in Africa and parts of Asia such as Afghanistan. Although there is no commercially available vaccine, today typhus is readily treated with the antibiotic doxycycline.

Epidemic typhus is caused by *Rickettsia prowazekii,* a gram–negative bacteria that is transmitted by an arthropod, in this case, the human body louse. Lice feces rather than lice bites serve to transmit *R. prowazekii* and the lice themselves die of the disease. There are two other varieties of typhus, murine typhus and scrub typhus, but only epidemic typhus poses a major health threat. Howard Ricketts first identified the relationship between epidemic typhus and Rocky Mountain spotted fever in 1910, and in 1914, Stanislaus von Prowazek discovered that lice feces rather than their bites transmit the disease. Both men fell victim to the disease, Ricketts in 1910 and Prowazek in 1914. *Rickettsia prowazekii* is one of several infectious diseases such as trench fever and relapsing fever that are lice-transmitted.[15] Long thought to be confined to only humans, it is now known that flying squirrels in the United States can also carry *Rickettsia prowazekii.*[16] After an incubation period of ten to fourteen days, symptoms of typhus begin to manifest themselves. Early symptoms include severe headache, sudden fever, and a rash on the trunk and limbs, and malaise. These symptoms can be the symptoms of several other diseases such as typhoid fever. Later symptoms are the development of a high fever with a temperature of 105°F, chills, and nervous system involvement that can include delirium, seizures, and coma as well as the rash turning a dark color. Some victims also experience severe coughing fits and pneumonia. Severe cases may lead to the rupturing of cells that line the small blood vessels and hemorrhages and blood clots. Untreated the disease may last up to three weeks but full recovery can take up to three months. In the pre-antibiotic era, a typhus outbreak could produce a case fatality rate of upwards of sixty percent. Surviving the disease produces some measure of immunity although it may wane over time.[17] However, the victims remain infected with *R. prowasekii* and under conditions of stress a milder relapsing form of the disease, Brill-Zinsser disease, can emerge.[18]

The presence of human lice can almost be taken for granted in most past societies. Lice serve as the vector for transmitting typhus and once someone in a household became infected, it was almost inevitable that everyone else in the household became infected. Removing the louse vector, either by sanitation improvements or insecticides, makes typhus a preventable disease today, but eliminating it would have been difficult in the past. It seems that people tried to remove lice from their environment, not through an understanding of infectious disease, but to ward off the itching that bites produced, but this was a challenging endeavor.

Historians have often listed typhus as the causative agent for several major epidemics in the past. As always, the indeterminacies of symptoms described by contemporaries and the overlap between the symptoms of typhus and several other infectious diseases makes this a challenging process. There is some likelihood that typhus may have been at least partially responsible for the Plague of Athens in the fifth century B.C.E. although there are other candidates as well, most notably smallpox.[19] When Spanish troops laid siege to the city of Moorish of Baza in 1489 as part of the Reconquistia, Spanish soldiers are described as developing fevers, red spots on their backs, arms, and chests, as well as delirium. One estimate indicates that Spanish battle deaths in the campaign may have numbered 3,000, but deaths from disease, most likely typhus, were as high as 17,000.[20] Outbreaks that were most likely typhus occurred throughout the sixteenth century in Europe, but also in Mexico as Europeans transported the disease across the Atlantic. Typhus was a major player in increasing the death rate during the Thirty Years War and the English Civil War in the seventeenth century and it nearly wiped out the French Grand Army on the retreat from Moscow during the invasion of Russia 1812. Typhus continued to play a role in World War I, the Communist Revolution in Russia, World War II, and most recently in the Burundi civil war in Africa in 1997.[21]

Typhus had become common enough in Europe by the mid-sixteenth century that the Italian physician Girolamo Fracastoro included sections dealing with it and its cure in his comprehensive work *Contagion*, published in 1546.[22] Fracastoro referred to typhus as lenticulae fevers and indicated that the disease first appeared in Italy in 1505 and 1528. While he tried to place the disease within the confines of humor theory, he indicated the disease was contagious and people contracted it by touching afflicted parties. Fracastoro described the fever and rash-like symptoms of the disease and indicated that in serious cases it led to death. His primary weapons against typhus were dietary remedies including the use of fruit juices such as lemon or orange juice or pomegranate wine. He warned against blood-letting and the use of purgatives so at least his remedies were unlikely to inflict further harm on the patient and may have had a palliative effect.

Typhus affected England in the fifteenth century, but first under a different name: gaol (jail) fever. English (and all other European) jails were notoriously unhealthy places in the premodern era and beyond. Prisoners were crowded together with little sanitation or food, often in clothing that might be falling apart. Already in the fourteenth century some notables such as William Walworth and Dick Wittington, Lord Mayors of London, tried to ameliorate conditions with financial contributions to buy food for the prisoners.[23] According to John Stow's account of 1603, sixty-four prisoners in Newgate prison and the jailors of Newgate and Ludgate prisons died in an epidemic of what was probably gaol fever in 1419.[24] Henry V had ordered Ludgate debtors' prison closed in early 1419, but the Crown had to reverse itself and reopen Ludgate prison admitting that some of the prisoners who died in Newgate would still have been alive if they had remained at Ludgate.[25] The unhealthy conditions remained common so that a long stay in jail could be nearly a death sentence even in the best of times.

During Lent in 1522, an assize was held at the castle of Cambridge and jail-ors brought dirty, unwashed, and stinking prisoners into court from the local prison. During the session, many of the spectators as well as the justices and notables such as Sir John Cut and Sir Giles Arlington became ill. The chronicler Edward Hall indicated that the odor of the prisoners or the general filthy conditions may have led to the sickness. Although he presented no symptoms, the circumstances incline toward an outbreak of typhus caused by the lice-infected prisoners.[26] Hall says nothing about whether the prisoners were ill as his concern was only for those he considered the better sort, but a suspicion exists that many of the prisoners died. Following a series of trials at Oxford assizes in July 1577, some three hundred people who had been present in the court during the trials died in less than a month before the outbreak ceased from what was likely jail fever. Sir Robert Bell, Lord Chief Baron of the Exchequer who presided at the assizes, other notables, as well as some students at Merton College, Oxford were all among the victims.[27] Body lice were no respecters of social status and were as likely to burrow into a judge's robes as the rags of an accused prisoner. The Black Assize of Exeter in 1586 also led to wholesale deaths among those present in the courtroom, prisoners, jurists, and spectators. In this case, witnesses blamed some Portuguese prisoners who had been crowded together in a cell that was essentially a hole as the source of outbreak.[28] Prisoners, like soldiers, were often crowded together so that the lice vector made it quite easy to spread the disease. It is somewhat surprising that there were no major typhus epidemics in London in the sixteenth century although reporters may have subsumed them under fever deaths or combined them with plague. Perhaps some improvements in diet, as well as cleanliness and some efforts at quarantine, helped to prevent a typhus outbreak like those that visited German cities during the chaos of the Thirty Years War.

The addition of typhus to the English burden of disease seems to have been spotty in the sixteenth century. The outbreaks noted above illustrate the short time span of only a few days and the limited geographic area of typhus outbreaks. Because England avoided anything like the destruction of the Thirty Years War, it was spared a major typhus epidemic although the Black Assizes each led to a few hundred deaths. There were some outbreaks of typhus during the English Civil War in the mid-seventeenth century when the crowded conditions of army camps led to typhus outbreaks. Environment conditions in the seventeenth century combined with concentrations of people in often unhealthy locales made it possible for a typhus outbreak to turn into an epidemic as occurred in 1643 in Bristol, and among the Parliamentary troops in Berkshire and Oxfordshire and an epidemic in Tiverton that lasted from August until November 1644.[29] Jail conditions did not improve in the eighteenth century and numerous outbreaks of gaol fever occurred that led to local epidemics and generated a good deal of fear.[30] Social prejudice—the poor were coming to be seen as sinful—helps explain how people viewed gaol fever. Just as syphilis took on a prejudicial air by the late sixteenth century, gaol fever followed suit. People blamed prisoners for somehow transmitting the disease to their "betters" even if they did not understand the concept of vector-borne disease. Following miasma theory, contemporaries believed that the "bad" air emanating from prisoners would have been enough to infect a whole courtroom.

The origins of typhus are shrouded by time. Zinsser indicated that typhus may have come to Europe from Africa or Asia, basing his argument on the identification of the disease in Spain in 1489 with its contacts with Africa and Asia.[31] The disease may have been present in the ancient world, but observers came to identify it as a specific disease in the late fifteenth century. Thereafter it continued to play a role, but with antibiotic therapy, typhus lost much of its terror by the latter half of the twentieth century. Many of the symptoms of typhus and typhoid fever are the same and the two diseases were often confused until the nineteenth century. Even had typhus been present in medieval Europe the lack of large concentrations of people in poor sanitary conditions would have made it difficult for a few typhus cases to develop into a full-blown epidemic. The changing environment of the sixteenth century with the growth of urban areas, larger armies, and continued poverty helped to make it possible for a disease such as typhus to turn into an epidemic threat. The expansion of Europe to the New World also made it possible for typhus to cross the ocean in the sixteenth century.

Like influenza, typhus seemed to be a product of the changing conditions in European society. Typhus was not a major contributor to the mortality rate of premodern England, but its presence had become a worrisome entry and could cause a brief spike in the death rate in a community. England avoided a major typhus epidemic primarily because the overall environment was not conducive to it. In many ways, typhus was a subsistence crisis disease as poverty made it possible for the disease to take hold. The poor were generally the ones who died but as outbreaks such as the Oxford and Exeter Black Assizes indicate, typhus was no respecter of social standing. A disease that quite possibly had existed for some time and had even become endemic could become epidemic as happened in central Europe during the Thirty Years War. Typhus could also have been a genuinely new disease of the fifteenth century, but this is not a completely convincing explanation. Until it became commonplace, observers most likely had treated typhus as simply one of many fevers sickening people. Fear created part of typhus's impact and helped observers to take notice. It did not respect social class and by the sixteenth century, many observers had come to regard epidemics as something that primarily killed the poor. The suddenness by which an outbreak started and stopped must have also induced fear because of the unexpected nature of the outbreak.

Smallpox, old or new killer?

Smallpox is almost a forgotten disease today. The last case in the wild occurred in Somalia in 1977 and the World Health Organization declared smallpox eradicated in 1980. Some commentators continue to be concerned with the possibility of the use of smallpox as a biological weapon, but otherwise, the public ignores the disease today. The current disregard for smallpox has not always been the case. It has been a major agent of disease in the past and some commentators have linked it to such major epidemics in the past such as the Plague of Athens in the fifth century B.C.E. and the Plague of the Antonines in the late second century C.E. Aside from the very real high death rates, there is still much that we do not know about the disease although some researchers continue to expand our horizons concerning the origins and historical development of the disease.

Smallpox is caused by the *variola* virus of the *Poxviridae* family and the *orthopoxvirus* genus. The disease exists in two forms, *Variola* major which has posed major health threats in the past, and *variola* minor which is a much less virulent form of the disease. *Variola* major has only one host and disease reservoir—humans—which made the eradication of the disease possible. *Variola* is related to other *orthopoxviruses* such as monkeypox and may have evolved from one of these in the distant past.

The usual means of transmission of smallpox virus is face-to-face contact through inhaling infected droplets although contact with the scabs from a person who has had an active case may of tuberculosis also causes infections. One characteristic that makes smallpox so dangerous is its R_0 of between 3.5 and 6, making it likely that the disease will spread readily through a population that has no immunity. Once the disease enters the body, it develops slowly and victims may not know they have the disease for some time. About the ninth day after infection, symptoms begin to appear and include fever, with a temperature of 101–102° F, chills, headache, backache, and possibly convulsions or delirium. During this stage, which usually lasts three to four days, some victims may also experience terrifying nightmares. Victims begin to develop a reddish flushing of the skin.[32] At the end of the prodrome, the person may even feel somewhat better and the fever subsides. At this point, the characteristic rash begins to develop starting on the face and spreading over the whole body (including the inside of the mouth in some cases). Over the next several days, the patient suffers intensely as the rash turns to pimples, then blisters, and finally large pustules. The pustules are not as large as those produced by syphilis, hence the name smallpox that people used to differentiate between it and the Great Pox. Gradually, the pustules scab over, and the person is often horribly scarred or in some cases loses the sight of one or both eyes. Throughout the period, the victim is contagious. Victims may die at any point in the progression of the disease and some die even as the symptoms begin to subside by day eighteen from secondary bacterial infections. The mortality rate for smallpox is twenty-five to thirty percent with some strains such as malignant confluent smallpox producing death rates closer to seventy percent.[33] Not all victims suffer through all of these symptoms. Some people have such a mild case that they exhibit only fever and possibly a mild rash. In victims of fulminating or hemorrhagic smallpox, the disease attacks the heart, lungs, liver, and intestines. No rash develops and the patient may remain conscious. In extreme cases, the person dies within 24 hours and almost no victim of hemorrhagic smallpox survives longer than four days as hemorrhagic smallpox has a mortality rate of nearly one hundred percent. A full-scale smallpox epidemic must have been horrifying for its victims and for those who had to confront the disease. One senior physician with extensive experience in treating tropical diseases is reported to have walked out of a smallpox ward in Bangladesh during the last stages of smallpox's existence and said: "I don't think I can ever walk through a ward like that. It is unimaginable."[34] The only bright spot is that surviving smallpox infection conveys lifetime immunity. Variola minor produces only mild symptoms and has a mortality rate of one to two percent. Generally, the two do not coexist in the same place at the same time.

Scholars continue to debate the origins of smallpox. It may have first appeared with the development of agricultural settlements 10,000 years ago.[35] Like measles, which also has only a human host, smallpox usually requires a population of 200,000 to 250,000 to sustain an outbreak. One view is that the disease existed in ancient Egypt. The mummy of Ramses V, who died of an acute illness in 1157 B.C.E., has facial lesions that are often characteristic of smallpox victims although other exanthematic diseases may also cause them. Although the mummy is well preserved, no DNA is available so a concrete diagnosis is not possible. Donald Hopkins, who had extensive experience in treating the disease, and who partially examined Ramses' mummy in 1979 indicates the high likelihood of smallpox as the cause of Ramses' death.[36] Some other diseases, most notably measles, can also cause lesions. Moreover, there is no mention of a disease with smallpox-like symptoms in the Old Testament.[37] This is not conclusive evidence for the absence of smallpox, but it is a warning that it may not have been present in the ancient world or if so led to only scattered cases. Although there continues to be some disagreement, the *variola* virus seems to have first surfaced in India or China and then spread to North Africa. Smallpox appears to have been present in parts of Africa, India, and China by the third century BCE although there seems to be little evidence of its spread to Europe.[38] Scholars no longer consider small-pox to have been responsible for the Plague of Athens in the mid-fifth century BCE.[39] There is some consensus that smallpox may have been responsible for the Plague of the Antonines that spread across the Mediterranean world from 165 to 190 C.E. The Greek physician Galen, who was an astute and fulsome observer, provided a description of the symptoms that seem to match those of smallpox but until paleopathology can provide more evidence, the smallpox diagnosis must remain uncertain.[40]

There were few towns large enough to sustain a smallpox epidemic for an extended period in the early Middle Ages although it is possible that some cases developed from time to time. Gregory of Tours describes a disease that spread across northern Europe and southern France in 580–81 CE that seems to dis-play the typical smallpox symptoms. He describes victims with fever and bodies covered with what he calls painful vesicles, that produced extreme pain as they began to break open and discharge pus.[41] Gregory reports that the disease afflicted the families of Chilperic and Guntram, two Merovingian kings, although they took different lessons from the disease. Upon the death of his son, Chilperic realized the transience of life and stopped taxing his subjects. Guntram's wife blamed her physicians for her condition and urged the king to kill them upon her death, which he did.[42] A clear description of the disease comes from the Arabic physician Rhazes in the tenth century, a description that Avicenna echoed and amplified in the eleventh century.[43] Hopkins contends that the disease continued to be active in Europe throughout the Middle Ages although he is forced to admit that there is little evidence of the disease in the fourteenth and fifteenth centuries, possibly because smallpox deaths were masked by the large number of deaths from the plague.[44]

It is more likely that smallpox was a relatively benign disease in late medieval Europe even if a more virulent form had been present in the second century with the Plague of the Antonines. That changed in the sixteenth century and during the seventeenth and eighteenth centuries, a smallpox pandemic affected Europe and the Americas. Writing more than a century ago, Charles Creighton noted the debate concerning the antiquity of smallpox and went so far as to con-clude that the disease was not present in Europe from the tenth to the sixteenth century.[45] Creighton's interpretations are not without flaws, but Carmichael and Silverstein have shown convincingly that although smallpox may have existed in a benign form during the Middle Ages it did not become a virulent killer until the sixteenth century.[46] It may have existed as a relatively benign childhood disease and contracting smallpox as a child provided immunity to adults and if enough people in an area had the disease as children, herd immunity helped protect other adults who were susceptible to the disease.

Carmichael and Silverstein's evidence is textual in nature, but paleopathology also plays a role in understanding smallpox. Paleopathologists have discovered a mummy in Siberia that dates from the late seventeenth to the early eighteenth century that gives some evidence of the presence of smallpox DNA.[47] A child mummy, dating from between 1643 and 1665 from Vilnius, Lithuania has provided a clear DNA sample that enabled researchers to indicate that all later strains of smallpox derived from the smallpox virus present in the later seventeenth century.[48] The authors indicate that using a relaxed molecular clock approach the common ancestor for the strain dates from 1530 to 1654, an observation that aligns with Carmichael and Silverstein's argument that virulent smallpox developed in the sixteenth century.[49] The presence of smallpox of the same virulence as that of the later smallpox pandemics in the late sixteenth century does not rule out that the disease could have existed earlier in a virulent form, but it does raise reservations about the continued presence of a virulent form of the disease during the Middle Ages.

It appears that there was a virulent version of smallpox present in sixteenth-century Europe which occasionally killed or scarred its victims although it was not common. The Italian physician Fracastoro, who was usually very thorough in describing the diseases of the day in *Contagion*, provided only a cursory treatment of poxes and measles (*De variolis et morbillis*) indicating that they did not merit extensive treatment because they usually affected children and did little harm.[50] Writing in 1541, the Englishman Sir Thomas Elyot mentioned measles and smallpox as diseases of children but did not elaborate on something that he appears to have considered a routine disease.[51] Arguing from a lack of information is always a bit tricky, but smallpox seems to have only begun to enter into the consciousness of English observers as a major threat in the sixteenth century. Shakespeare noted every other disease of the day in his plays, but there is no mention of smallpox.[52] Philip Barrough and William Bullein also neglected to mention the disease in works that they intended to be comprehensive treatments of the diseases present in the late sixteenth century.[53] Smallpox epidemics were beginning to break out on the continent in the latter half of the sixteenth century, but they still appear to have been limited in their geographic coverage.[54] Smallpox was present in England and recognized as a potentially deadly disease even if commentators did not devote extensive attention to it. On the tenth of October 1562, Queen Elizabeth I became ill with what her doctors first thought to be a bad cold, but her physicians soon diagnosed it as smallpox much to the consternation of her courtiers who were concerned with a possible succession crisis. Elizabeth survived and suffered some minor scarring. Two other ladies of the court were also stricken with the disease and they too survived although at the cost of considerable scarring.[55] While Elizabeth's illness alarmed members of the court for political reasons, there does not seem to have been the fear-laden response that characterized the court of Henry VIII when the English Sweat broke out. It may have been that people considered smallpox to be potentially deadly on an individual level but did not consider it a highly contagious disease that led people to flee as they did the Sweat.

That situation changed in the seventeenth century as smallpox became endemic, producing a large number of deaths. One estimate is that smallpox killed 400,000 people a year across Europe and had caused more than one-third of all the blindness by the end of the century.[56] We are fortunate that dating from 1629 (with omission from 1636 to 1646) the London Bills of Mortality provide a comprehensive listing of the cause of death of Londoners. The first spike in the number of smallpox deaths occurs in 1632 when smallpox deaths made up 5.6% of the total, up from a background figure of one percent. Thereafter, the figure hovered around five percent spiking upward to greater than eight percent of total deaths in 1649, 1652, 1655, 1664, and 1674.[57] Even so, John Graunt initially lumped smallpox with swine pox, measles, and worms without convulsion and indicated that approximately half of the victims were children younger than six.[58] Smallpox had become a major, if not the major, cause of death for Londoners. Elsewhere in England, the picture is not so clear. One analysis indicates that overall smallpox remained a relatively rare disease in England in the seventeenth century, although not the eighteenth century. Moreover, it appears to have been more of a childhood disease in northern England in the seventeenth century.[59] This situation is a bit surprising as northern England was sparsely settled in the seventeenth century making it difficult to spread the disease. London fits the expected pattern of a disease based on human transmission. This argument can be further evidence that smallpox was re-emerging in a newly virulent form in England in the early modern era, a disease that gathered strength over time. During the eighteenth century, the number of smallpox cases continued to rise in spite of efforts at prevention.

There is another side to the impact of virulent smallpox in the sixteenth- and seventeenth-century world—America. European diseases such as smallpox and measles had a devastating impact on the native population of the Americas. Because these people had never been exposed to European diseases, they had no immunity, making any infection likely to produce a high mortality rate. The disruptions caused by epidemic disease were likely to produce additional deaths through an inability to care for the sick and even starvation or malnutrition. Alfred Crosby has labeled such a situation a virgin soil epidemic and other scholars have used the term to explain the impact of Europeans on the Americas. Smallpox was not a particularly virulent disease in Europe in the fifteenth and early sixteenth centuries when Europeans first began to visit the Americas. The disease appears to have been much deadlier in America than Europe however, producing a large-scale population decline that may have exceeded eighty percent in places.

Scholars have advanced variety of factors to explain the higher morbidity and mortality rate among the Native American population. Much of the debate has concentrated on smallpox although other diseases, especially measles, also played a role in the population decline as the natives faced a new disease cocktail as they encountered Europeans.[60] One biological point to note is that most Native Americans had type O blood. Diseases such as smallpox and measles can more easily affect a homogeneous population than a heterogeneous population. Francis Black has argued that the lack of heterogeneity was a major contributor to the lack of resistance that native population displayed when confronting European diseases.[61] Nonetheless, biology alone does not explain why smallpox was so lethal in the New World. One explanation is that the Africans imported into the New World carried a more virulent form of *variola* major than was then present in Europe. While attractive, the timing for this scenario is not quite accurate as the native population began to experience serious illness long before large numbers of Africans arrived in the New World. Smallpox did not become endemic in the Americas until 1800 so each new epidemic required outside infection.

In addition to biology, other factors have influenced how smallpox affected the Native American population. Large cities in areas of central and South America made it possible to sustain a smallpox (and measles) epidemic for some time. Elsewhere, communities that lived in close proximity to each other helped to spread the disease. There is also some evidence that young infants ran a much higher risk of dying from smallpox than infants in Europe because Amerindian women possessed no antibodies to ward off smallpox.[62]

When cultural and biological factors are combined, they are still somewhat lacking in their explanation of the impact of smallpox. Even if the impact of smallpox as a completely new disease is overlaid on these factors, a troubling point remains—smallpox in Europe in the fifteenth century was not a markedly lethal disease and many of the factors that may have increased lethality in the New World were also present in the Old World. One important limiting factor for smallpox epidemics in Europe was that the disease infected many children who carried their immunity into adulthood helping provide herd immunity to the community. Smallpox truly was a virgin soil epidemic in America, but one that continued to kill long beyond the first generation of contact.

Childhood infection and later variolation (the inoculation of a person with scabs from another smallpox infection) as a protective measure helped to somewhat diminish the impact of smallpox in eighteenth-century Europe although it remained a fearsome presence. America was another matter as the Native American population continued to fall victim to the disease in large numbers. So too, the colonial population. An outbreak in Boston in the summer of 1721 became a full-scale epidemic although a few residents such as the leading clergyman Cotton Mather backed physicians who were willing to variolate people. Mather had his son Samuel inoculated with live *variola* scabs and although he became quite ill, he survived.[63]

Smallpox was not done with America in 1721. Starting in 1775 in New England and finally concluding in the Pacific Northwest and on the Great Plains in 1782 an epidemic swept across the continent infecting everyone in its path. The Mandan and the Hidatsas on the northern plains had never encountered the disease before and suffered greatly so much so that they no longer remained a power in the Dakotas.[64] Although the deaths caused by smallpox in seventeenth- and eighteenth-century Europe were staggering, they were magnified ten-fold or more in the Americas among both the Native American population but also the European colonists who encountered the disease for the first time.

One interesting albeit challenging explanation is that variola major evolved in a more virulent direction in the New World. A corollary would be that the more virulent disease was then exported back to Europe and became the virulent strain that would cause a pandemic in the seventeenth and especially the eighteenth century. At this point, this explanation is speculative but helps to illustrate the continuing difficulty in explaining why smallpox became a virulent killer in early modern Europe.

Carmichael and Silverstein explore several possible explanations for why smallpox became a major health issue in the seventeenth century. An obvious explanation is that the virus was endemic in the fifteenth and sixteenth centuries and mutated into a more virulent strain at some point in the seventeenth century. Biological evidence confirms that the strain of smallpox present in Europe in the eighteenth and nineteenth centuries dates from the seventeenth century.[65] If this was the case, a double mutation is implied as the disease seemed to be more virulent in the late ancient world and so had to mutate in a less virulent direction at some point. Although, as noted above, there are some explanations about why smallpox had such a negative impact on the Native American population dating from the fifteenth century, this complicates the mutation from less to more virulent strain explanation. Carmichael and Silverstone suggest that slaves transported a more virulent strain present in Africa to the New World, but admit that the more virulent strain did not seem to return to Europe. They also indicate that the Spanish may have transmitted a virulent strain from a Variola hotspot in Europe to America. They finally contend that the genetic makeup of the Native American population may have made the disease so deadly.[66] Sixteenth-century smallpox could be deadly, but it seems to have been so on an individual basis. The biological evidence that indicates the presence of a new strain in the seventeenth century helps to explain its virulence. The growth of population centers also made it easier to spread the disease so it was easier for a more virulent strain to take hold.

By the end of the sixteenth century, smallpox had come to pose a major public health problem in Europe, one that intensified by the eighteenth century. Smallpox was not a new disease in the sixteenth century; it was re-emerging disease. The combination of its changing genetic makeup and changing population patterns helped to make a disease with a newly intensified impact. Often a smallpox epidemic seems to have materialized and burned through a town but did not become a nationwide phenomenon. Smallpox in America did reach pandemic proportions on several occasions. Moreover, as Davenport et.al. indicate, the disease did not seem to have wide coverage in England during the seventeenth century.[67] By the end of the seventeenth century, some medical practitioners had turned to variolation, the injection of live smallpox virus into the skin, which produced a mild form of the disease and conferred immunity. Unfortunately, the result at times was a full-blown case of smallpox and the patient died. In the late eighteenth century, Edward Jenner developed the technique of vaccination with cowpox that conferred immunity to smallpox at much less risk. Once society accepted vaccination in the nineteenth century, authorities banned variolation because of the potential danger it posed.

New epidemic diseases for a new era

A relatively static number of epidemic diseases affected England during the Middle Ages. The impact of plague the new disease of the seventh and four-teenth centuries, was devastating helping to indicate how a novel disease could have a large impact on society. During the seventeenth century, observers were often perplexed as some existing diseases such as leprosy no longer seemed to be much of a problem and other "new" diseases appeared.[68] Smallpox, typhus, and influenza did not have a major impact on English population during the Middle Ages. That began to change in the sixteenth and seventeenth centuries as they, and syphilis and *Sudor Anglicus*, the two "new" diseases of the fifteenth and six-teenth centuries, began to affect English health and society. Unlike syphilis or the English Sweat, influenza, typhus, and smallpox may not have been entirely new diseases in the sixteenth century; today researchers would classify them as re-emerging diseases.

The growth of the English (and European) population in the sixteenth cen-tury and particularly the growth of towns helped to create the environment in which crowd diseases such as smallpox, influenza, and typhus flourished. Human-to-human contact transmitted the first two diseases so groupings of larger numbers of people in one place made it possible to sustain a smallpox or influenza epidemic. Typhus is a disease of poverty and poverty was ever-present in early modern England. Its vector, the louse does not have a high mobility range so crowding in urban areas, especially in times of dearth, made it easy to spread the disease and create an epidemic.

Influenza, smallpox, and earlier *Sudor Anglicus* and syphilis could and did claim victims from all classes of society, even monarchs. That aspect made these diseases more frightening to the upper levels of society than plague that by the sixteenth century claimed most of its victims from the peasantry and urban poor. When typhus infected aristocratic victims, people took notice as they con-sidered this abnormal, but otherwise, people did not see it as a major health threat. Increasing mobility in the early modern world also made it possible to spread disease more readily and so influenza, smallpox, and typhus easily spread throughout a country, across Europe, and even to the New World.

Like the English Sweat and syphilis, smallpox posed a challenge to the exist-ing Greco-Arabic structure of medicine grounded in the humor theory. The fevers of influenza and typhus were not entirely new and fevers of one sort or another had always been part of society. It was easier for medical men to place diseases with symptoms similar to existing diseases into a recognizable frame-work than when they confronted what were clearly new diseases such as syphilis and the Sweat. Nonetheless, the pervasiveness of an increased burden of epidemic disease helped to cause some observers to turn to new approaches to explanation in the sixteenth century. Ironically, the impact of Renaissance humanism with its emphasis on recovering Greek texts that scholars regarded as authoritative occurred at the same time as new diseases were emerging. A physician such as John Caius who was committed to ancient learning faced continued explanatory challenges when diseases did not fit Galenic explanations.

First, the plague and then syphilis forced some observers to question aspects of the miasma theory. Human contact appeared to spread both diseases and many authorities, even if not doctors tried to react accordingly. Writing in the mid-sixteenth century, Fracastoro provided a full development of contagion theory, indicating that contagion occurred by contact, by what he called fomes (particles), and from a distance.[69] With contagion theory, the path was started that led to identifying diseases as specific entities, not just a process. Others adopted contagion theory to one degree or another, at times combining it with the miasma theory. Overall, the Galenic theory of the humors continued to dominate. Once people no longer perceived the plague as a major threat, many medical practitioners turned away from contagionism although it would return in the eighteenth century.[70]

In many ways, the sixteenth and seventeenth centuries were a period of transition for English society. The realm of epidemic disease was no different, in how the new or re-emerging diseases affected society, and how society and intellectuals reacted to them. However, after the last plague outbreak of 1665, no other major outbreaks of epidemic disease that had the demographic and fear-generating impacts of earlier disease attacked the country. Smallpox and its scarring aftermath killed and created fear among all as it struck all segments of society, but it did not cause a ten percent decline in population as some late medieval plague outbreaks did. The new epidemic diseases were deadly but they were also new in how they spread and the impact they had on society.

Notes

1 E.A. Wrigley and R.S. Schofield, *The Population History of England, 1541–1871* (Cambridge: Cambridge University Press, 1989), 178–79.
2 H.T. Riley, ed., *Annales monasterii S. Albani, a Johanne Amundesham, monacho, ut videtur, conscripti, A.D. 1421–1440*, 2 vols. (Rolls Series, 1870–71), 1: 19.
3 J.K. Taubenberger and D.M. Morens, "Pandemic Influenza—Including a Risk Assessment of H5N1," *Revue scientifique et technique*, 28 (2009), 187–202. Michael T. Osterholm and Mark Olshaker, *Deadliest Enemy* (New York: Little Brown, 2017).
4 David M. Morens and Jeffrey K. Taubenberger, "Historical Thoughts on Influenza Viral Ecosystems, or Behold a Pale Horse, Dead Dogs, Failing Fowl, and Sick Swine," *Influenza and Other Respiratory Viruses*, 4 (2010), 327–37.
5 Creighton, *Epidemics*, 1: 398.
6 David M. Morens, Jeffrey K. Taubenberger, Gregory K. Folkers, and Anthony S. Fauci, "Pandemic Influenza's 500th Anniversary," *Clinical Infectious Diseases* 51 (2010), 1442–44. David M. Morens, Michael North, and Jeffrey K. Taubenberger assess the descriptive evidence for the 1510 pandemic in "The Art of Medicine: Eyewitness Accounts of the 1510 Influenza Pandemic in Europe," *The Lancet*, 376 (2010), 1894–95. A good brief discussion of early influenza pandemics is K. David Patterson,

Pandemic Influenza 1700–1900 (Totowa: Rowman and Littlefield, 1986). As Patterson's title indicates, he does not consider influenza to have been a threat until the eighteenth century.

7 Morens, Taubenberger, Folkers, Fauci, "Pandemic Influenza," 1442.
8 Gerald F. Pyle and K. David Patterson, "Influenza Diffusion in European History: Patterns and Paradigms," *Ecology of Disease*, 2 (1984), 176–77. W.I.B. Beveridge, "The Chronicle of Influenza," *History and Philosophy of the Life Sciences*, 13 (1991), 233–34. Morens, Taubenberger, Folkers, Fauci, "Pandemic Influenza," 1443. Patrick R. Saunders-Hastings and Daniel Krewski, "Reviewing the History of Pandemic Influenza: Understanding Patterns of Emergence and Transmission," *Pathogens*, 5 (2016), 66. An expanded description of what seems to have been influenza in Berwick in 1580 is J. Stevenson, ed., *The Correspondence of Robert Bowes* (Surtees Society, 14, 1842), 84–85.
9 Charles Wriothesley, *A Chronicle of England during the Reigns of the Tudors, from A.D. 1485 to 1559*, W.D. Hamilton, ed. (Camden Society, N.S., 11, 1875), 139. Slack, *Impact of Plague*, 71. Creighton, *Epidemics*, 401–04.
10 Patterson, *Pandemic Influenza*, 13–28. Also, see Gerald F. Pyle and K. David Patterson, "Influenza Diffusion in European History, 173–84.
11 Robert Fabyn, *The New Chronicles of England and France,* Henry Ellis, ed. (London: F.C. and J. Rivington, 1811), 719.
12 David M. Morens, Jeffrey K. Taubenberger, and Anthony S. Fauci, "Predominant Role of Bacterial Pneumonia as a Cause of Death in Pandemic Influenza: Implications for Pandemic Influenza Preparedness," *Journal of Infectious Diseases* 198 (2008), 962–70. There are several good accounts of the 1918–19 pandemic and Laura Spinney's *Pale Rider* (New York: Public Affairs, 2017) is an excellent recent one.
13 Slack, *Impact of Plague*, 70–71, 127–28.
14 Margaret DeLacy, "The Conceptualization of Influenza in Eighteenth Century Britain: Specificity and Contagion," *BHM*, 67 (1993), 75.
15 S. Badiaga and P. Borouqui, "Human Louse-Transmitted Infectious Diseases," *Clinical Microbiology and Infection* 18 (2012), 332–7.
16 Yassina Bechah, Christian Capo, Jean-Louis Mege, Didier Raoult, "Epidemic Typhus," *Lancet: Infectious Diseases*, 8 (2008), 417–26.
17 Didier Raoult, Theodore Woodward, and J. Stephen Dumler, "The History of Epidemic Typhus," *Infectious Disease Clinics of North America*, 18 (2004), 127–40. Irwin W. Sherman, *The Power of Plagues* (Washington, DC: ASM Press, 2006), 121–22.
18 Emmanouil Angelakis, Yassina Bechah, and Didier Raoult, "The History of Epidemic Typhus," in Michel Drancourt and Didier Raoult, eds., *Paleomicrobiology of Humans* (Washington, DC: ASM Press, 2016), 81–92.
19 The debate concerning the causative agent for the Plague of Athens is extensive focusing on a variety of diseases. A recent entry that takes both textual and epidemiological evidence into account argues for typhus as the most probably candidate. Robert J. Littman, "The Plague of Athens: Epidemiology and Paleopathology," *Mount Sinai Journal of Medicine*, 76 (2009), 456–67.
20 Hans Zinsser, *Rats, Lice, and History* (New York: Little Brown, 1934), 242–44. Typhus may possibly be identified in Spain as early as 1083, but the identification in 1489 is more certain. Raoult, Woodward, Dumler, "History of Typhus," 132.
21 Raoult, Woodward, Dumler, "History of Typhus," 131–36. D. Raoult, J.B. Ndihokubwayo, H. Tissot-Dupont, et al., "Outbreak of Epidemic Typhus Associated with Trench Fever in Burundi," *Lancet* 352 (1998), 353–8.
22 Fracastoro, Contagion, 100–111, 223–37.
23 Creighton, *Epidemics*, 374.
24 John Stow, *A Survey of London*, C.L. Kingsford, ed., 2 vols. (Cambridge: Cambridge University Press, 2015 [1908]), 1: 36–37.
25 Riley, *Memorials of London*, 673–74, 677.

26 Edward Hall, *Hall's Chronicle; Containing the History of England, during the Reign of Henry the Fourth and the Succeeding Monarchs, to the End of the Reign of Henry the Eighth*, Henry Ellis, ed. (London: J. Johnson, F.C. and J. Rivington, 1809), 632.
27 Creighton, *Epidemics*, 1: 376–83.
28 Creighton, *Epidemics*, 1: 383–6.
29 Slack, *Impact of Plague*, 123. Creighton, *Epidemics*, 1: 547–62. The plague visited Bristol two years later producing greater mortality.
30 Kevin Siena, *Rotten Bodies* (New Haven: Yale University Press, 2019).
31 Zinsser, *Rats, Lice and History*, 242–44. Raoult, Woodward, and Dumler indicate the origins of the disease are still unclear although they hold out the hope of using recently developed molecular tools on human remains. "History of Epidemic Typhus," 137.
32 During the early stages of a smallpox infection, it may be confused with measles or chicken pox. The three diseases take different paths thereafter so it is easy to differentiate between them. A severe measles infection may produce scarring as does smallpox. Burke A. Cunha, "Smallpox and Measles: Historical Aspects and Clinical Differentiation," *Infectious Disease Clinics of North America*, 18 (2004), 79–100.
33 C.W. Dixon, *Smallpox* (London: J & A Churchill, 1962), 7. Dixon's work still provides the most extensive discussion of the symptoms and progression of the various forms of smallpox (5–56).
34 D.A. Henderson, *Smallpox—the Death of a Disease* (Amherst, NY: Prometheus Books, 2009), 32. Dr. Henderson led the World Health Organization program to eradicate smallpox.
35 For examples of contrasting views concerning the origins of the variola virus see Sergei Shchelkunov, "How Long Ago Did Smallpox Emerge? *Archives of Virology*, 154 (2009), 1865–71. and Igor V. Babkin and Irina N. Babkina, "The Origin of the Variola Virus," *Viruses*, 7 (2015), 1100–12. Useful discussions of the origins of smallpox and its impact in the ancient and early medieval world are: Dixon, *Smallpox* (187–215), Henderson, *Smallpox* (31–43), Donald R. Hopkins, *Smallpox in History* (Chicago: University of Chicago Press, 1983, 2002), 1–75.
36 Hopkins, *Smallpox*, 14–15. The paleopathology of the disease is discussed in Catherine Thèves, Eric Crubézy, and Philippe Biagini, "History of Smallpox and its Spread in Human Populations," in Drancourt and Raoult, eds., *Paleomicrobiology of Humans*, 161–72.
37 Abbas M. Behbehani, "The Smallpox Story: Life and Death of an Old Disease," *Microbiological Reviews*, 47 (1983), 456. Michael B.A. Oldstone provides a good summary of the early history of the disease that assumes its ancient origin in a virulent form. *Viruses, Plagues, and History*, 2d.ed. (Oxford: Oxford University Press, 2020), 37–69.
38 Hopkins, *Smallpox*, 16–18. Babkin and Babkina, "Origin of the Variola Virus," 1100–12.
39 Littman, "Plague of Athens." 8.
40 Henderson, *Smallpox*, 38; Hopkins, *Smallpox*, 22–3. Kyle Harper provides an extensive discussion of the likelihood of smallpox as the causative agent for the Antonine Plague although he concedes that the diagnosis is uncertain with molecular identification. *The Fate of Rome* (Princeton: Princeton University Press, 2017), 102–111. Harper (p. 106) accepts the conclusion that what Galen may have described was hemorrhagic smallpox. R.J. Littman and M.L. Littman, "Galen and the Antonine Plague," *American Journal of Philology*, 94 (1973), 243–55.
41 Gregory of Tours, *The History of the Franks*, Lewis Thorpe, trans. (Hardmondsworth: Press, 1977), 91–92.
42 Gregory of Tours, *History of the Franks*, 298.
43 Ann G. Carmichael and Arthur M. Silverstein, "Smallpox in Europe before the Seventeenth Century: Virulent Killer or Benign Disease?" *Journal of the History of Medicine and Allied Sciences*, 42 (1987), 151–2. Rhazes made a distinction between

smallpox and measles in his treatise. Richard Mead, *A Discourse on the Small-Pox and Measles, to which is Annexed, a Treatise on the Same Disease by the Celebrated Arabian Physician Abukeker Rhazes*, 3rd ed. (Edinburgh: A. Donaldson and J. Reid, 1763), 62–66, 68–69. Writing in the eighteenth century, Mead indicated that much of what Rhazes said was still correct (5).

44 Hopkins, *Smallpox*, 26–29.

45 Creighton, *History of Epidemics in Britain*, 1: 440.

46 Carmichael and Silverstein, "Smallpox in Europe," 147–67. They focus on the late Middle Ages and do not address the possibility of a virulent form of smallpox in the second century.

47 Philippe Biagini, Catherine Thèves, Patricia Balaresque, et al. "Variola Virus in a 300-Year-Old Siberian Mummy," *New England Journal of Medicine*, 367 (2012), 2057–9. Catherine Thèves, Philippe Biagini, Eric Crubézy, "The Rediscovery of Smallpox," *Clinical Microbiology and Infection*, 20 (2014), 210–18. Both of these articles sound the call for more paleopathalogical work to firmly establish the origins of smallpox.

48 Ana T. Duggan, Maria F. Perdomo, Dario Piombino-Mascali, et al., "17th Century Variola Virus Reveals the Recent History of Smallpox," *Current Biology*, 26 (2016), 1–6. Molecular-clock analyses were used to reveal the timescale of the sample.

49 Duggan, et al., "17th Century Variola Virus," 3.

50 Francastoro, *De contagione*, 72–5, 206–09.

51 Thomas Elyot, *The Castel of Helth* (Miami: HardPress, reprint, first ed. 1541), fol. R1.b

52 Carmichael and Silverstein, "Smallpox in Europe," 158.

53 William Bullein, *Bulleins Bulwarke of Defence against all sicknesse, soarenesse, and woundes that doe dayly assaulte mankinde* (London, 1579; Ebbo Editions reprint), Philip Barrough, *The Method of physick containing the causes, signes, and cures of inward diseases in mans body from the head to the foot* (London, 1596; Ebbo Editions reprint).

54 Carmichael and Silverstein, "Smallpox in Europe before the Seventeenth Century," 158–60.

55 Hopkins, *Smallpox*, 1–3. J.E. Neale, *Queen Elizabeth I* (Garden City: Doubleday, 1934), 121.

56 Behbehani, "Smallpox Story," 458.

57 Carmichael and Silverstein, "Smallpox in Europe," 160.

58 John Graunt, *Natural and Political Observations Made upon the Bills of Mortality* (Baltimore: Johns Hopkins University Press, 1938 {1662}), 15.

59 Romola Jane Davenport, Max Satchell, L.M.W. Shaw-Taylor, "The Geography of Smallpox in England before Vaccination: A Conundrum Resolved." *Social Science and Medicine*, 206 (2018), 75–85.

60 A good discussion of the continuing impact of imported disease from the first contacts in the Caribbean through the impact of the Puritans in New England in the first half of the seventeenth century is Noble David Cook, *Born to Die* (Cambridge: Cambridge University Press, 1998). Other works that place the impact of European diseases in a wider context are: Alfred W. Crosby, *Ecological Imperialism*, 2d.ed. (Cambridge: Cambridge University Press, 2004) and Suzanne Austin Alchon, *A Pest in the Land* (Albuquerque: University of New Mexico Press, 2003).

61 Francis L. Black, "An Explanation of High Death Rates among New World Peoples when in Contact with Old World Diseases," *Perspectives in Biology and Medicine*, 34 (1994), 292–307. Black developed his argument to explain the impact of measles and care must be used when extrapolating to smallpox.

62 James C. Riley, "Smallpox and American Indians Revisited." *JHM*, 65 (2010), 472–4. Riley's article (445–77) is a good summary of questions concerned with the impact of smallpox on the American population.

63 A good account of the 1721 epidemic that examines the reasoning behind supporting and opposing variolation is Stephen Coss, *The Fever of 1721* (New York: Simon & Schuster, 2016).

64 The best account of the 1775–82 smallpox outbreak in America is Elzabeth A. Fenn, *Pox Americana* (New York: Hill and Wang, 2001).
65 Duggan, et al., "17th Century Variola Virus," 1–6.
66 Carmichael and Silverstone, "Smallpox in Europe," 162–67.
67 Davenport, et al., "Geography of Smallpox in England," 75–85.
68 The changing disease mix of the seventeenth century and the medical response to it is examined in Lloyd G. Stevenson, "'New Diseases' in the Seventeenth Century," *BHM*, 39 (1965), 1–21.
69 Fracastoro, *Contagion*, 3–37.
70 Margaret DeLacy, "Nosology, Mortality, and Disease Theory in the Eighteenth Century," *JHM*, 54 (1999), 261–84. DeLacy, *The Germ of an Idea* (New York: Palgrave, 2016).

10

DISEASE AND ITS IMPACT AT THE BEGINNING OF A NEW ERA

At the turn of the seventeenth century, the people of England continued to face challenges to health posed by everyday diseases such as diarrhea, pneumonia, malaria, and tuberculosis. The impact of leprosy had been in decline for some time. The plague was an old and deadly companion long before 1600, and it still produced a large number of deaths on occasion. However, other diseases afflicted society, most notably the English Sweat, syphilis, typhus, influenza, and smallpox. In essence, the English disease burden had increased from the Late Middle Ages onward.

England has been used as a case study in order to examine the impact of various diseases. For the most part, it is possible to generalize across Europe for the impact of the various diseases. There were minor variations of course. The English Sweat was almost exclusively an English problem. Malaria continued to be a major health problem in some parts of southern Europe, such as Rome, well into the nineteenth century. The moralistic response to syphilis by some English medical men was not always repeated elsewhere in Europe. There are also many similarities such as the theoretical response to disease or the decline and slow regrowth of population following the Black Death.

In spite of the large number of deaths arising from continued plague, epidemics as well as other diseases, the population of England grew in the sixteenth century, surpassing the pre-plague level. The growth of population affected society in a variety of ways including increased migration to urban areas that continued to be unhealthy. The population increase came largely from the impact of increased fertility as disease outbreaks drove population size downward in some areas and child mortality rates remained high. Plague outbreaks in the sixteenth century did not cause the death high toll of the Black Death in the fourteenth century and even though other epidemic diseases might cause a decline in one region, they did not have the impact of the plague. Syphilis, tuberculosis, malaria, and diarrheal disease continued to be threats, but they killed individuals, not large groups of people at any one time.

DOI: 10.4324/9781003215219-11

Many works dealing with the impact of disease on society devote most of their attention to the social, economic, and sometimes intellectual impact of disease. As earlier chapters indicate, the impacts of diseases have varied. Some have provided a basis for seeing how moralism colored people's perspective on a particular disease. Some provide insights into the class structure of society. The impact of the Second Plague Pandemic demonstrated how pandemic disease could so disrupt existing structures that major changes ensued. In explaining these impacts, some historians have tended to see disease as a cultural phenomenon, one in which the disease is socially constructed.

Contemporaries named diseases, often applying several different names. As Charles Rosenberg has indicated, a disease does not exist as a social phenomenon until it is named but this isn't the total picture.[1] People in premodern England took note of diseases such as plague or the Sweat when they killed large numbers of people in a short time. They also took note of diseases when they infected the social elite. Typhus probably was present in England before the sixteenth century, but the aristocratic victims of the Black Assizes caused observers to take note of the fever and incidentally to blame the poor for Gaol Fever. The large number of victims in the 1485 English Sweat epidemic caused Thomas Forrestier to take note. He and later observers also focused on the Sweat because of the social status of the victims as when it infected the court of Henry VIII. Dysentery had been a "background" disease throughout the Middle Ages, noted only when it claimed an influential victim. People acknowledged chronic diseases such as tuberculosis and malaria, but little more than that as observers simply accepted that they were part of life. The plague was first noted because of its horrendous mortality rate. By the sixteenth century, it came to be something that some observers blamed the poor for transmitting to their "betters." When leprosy first appeared, it had a large footprint that even included the social elite. Gradually, some commentators tended to marginalize victims as morally suspect individually. Syphilis first appeared in Europe in the early sixteenth century and claimed a large number of victims many from the political and intellectual elite so it received widespread coverage. In England, Puritanism gave another twist to how the disease as medical authors such as Bullein and Clowes considered its victims to be moral degenerates. So yes, there was clearly a cultural aspect to disease in the premodern world.

There is also a biological reality of a disease such as syphilis, whether it was called the French Disease, the Neapolitan Disease, or the Great Pox as the causative agent and the progression of the disease was the same no matter what the name. Understanding the biology of disease enables us to understand how a disease progressed through society, how it claimed its victims, and often why existing remedies failed to cure it. Examining the evolution of smallpox, using paleopathology has helped to understand why it was not the threat in the Middle Ages that it became in the seventeenth and eighteenth centuries. Understanding how plague spread in waves helps us to grasp why it was such a deadly enemy. An awareness of the environmental background for disease, such as climate change, helps in understanding why diseases such as the plague became health threats at certain times and how they spread. This latter relationship of climate and the environment and disease is a complicated one, but one worth exploring further. People defined how they perceived diseases and how they treated diseases as in essence a social construction. The biology remained the same no matter the name and understanding it enhances our understanding.

Addressing the biology of disease furthers our understanding of how the various diseases affected society. Keeping the SIR (susceptible, infected, recovered) and SIRS (susceptible, infected, recovered, susceptible) models in mind as we consider measles, plague, and the Sweat helps to understand why they affected society in the way they did. Once people recovered from measles (the R term), they were immune and the epidemic died down until a new group of susceptibles arose. Plague conferred limited immunity and surviving an attack of the Sweat seemed to confer no immunity so the susceptible group continued to be replaced with new susceptibles (the second S). This situation helps to explain why plague epidemics seemed to come in waves. On the other hand, the replenishment of susceptibles only adds more to the mystery of the Sweat. One possible explanation might be a long incubation period so that most of the second-stage susceptibles were not exposed to active cases. Understanding the mutation of smallpox would enhance our knowledge of a disease that seemed to go from deadly to a childhood malady, to deadly. Paleopathology has helped in providing clear identification of some past diseases through the use of aDNA studies. Unfortunately, we do not have reliable records concerning the prevalence of diseases such as plague, typhus, or smallpox so it is generally not possible to construct mathematical models of the spread of the diseases. Being able to do so would help in understanding how diseases spread and who fell victim to them. When blended with historical understanding, biology can further enhance our understanding of disease in the past.

One set of questions is unanswered by biology and historical evidence rarely provides answers. Although I have occasionally noted the impact of a particular disease on an individual, evidence concerning individuals has usually not been present. History is about individuals as well as society and I have rarely been able to do justice to the emotional pain that various diseases produced.

Changes in medicine, but not always in the health of society

An obvious question is what impact did medicine and science have in reducing the impact of disease? In many ways, medicine did not have a large impact on the reduction of deaths from infectious disease until the nineteenth century. The microbial revolution in the latter third of the century led to better diagnosis and treatment of several diseases such as Yellow Fever, cholera, and malaria. Even the agent for plague, *Yersinia pestis*, was identified in the 1890s through the work of Alexander Yersin in dealing with the Third Plague Pandemic.

All of these advances were a long way off in 1600. Intellectual medicine had not remained static and changes were beginning to be hinted at by the sixteenth century. Some became more significant in the seventeenth century through the impact of the Scientific Revolution. As Roger French notes, already by the 1630s, some doctors were calling aspects of the medicine of Hippocrates and Galen into question and were showing the error in some Galenic suppositions.[2] The theoretical approach of Greco-Roman medicine rooted in Aristotelian natural philosophy continued to dominate physicians' thinking, but already in the sixteenth century, there were those such as Vesalius who advocated a more empirical approach to diagnosis. Other aspects of medicine that went back to the Romans, such as the miasma theory of disease, continued to be influential until the early twentieth century. Sparked in part by efforts to deal with the plague and syphilis, contagionism, enunciated by Fracastoro in mid-century, also came to be used to explain how some diseases spread especially by public officials.

The development of medical education in the Middle Ages starting with medical schools at Salerno and Padua helped to regularize the study of medicine based on the study of particular texts, many of which were assumed to have come from Galen or Hippocrates even though some were often Latin translations of Arabic writers such as Avicenna. University medical education was text-based, not empirical although a few anatomical demonstrations were creeping in and were becoming more common by the sixteenth century. If anything, the "back to the texts" approach of Renaissance humanism that emphasized a return to original Greek texts, as John Caius did with his edition of one of Galen's works, helped to lock in the authority of old texts even when they might be in error.

Part of the changes in medical knowledge that helped to challenge Aristotelian natural philosophy that was the basis of Galenic thought came from the confrontation with "new" diseases. Galen and his Arabic successors, such as Avicenna or Rhazes, described the symptoms of many diseases and noted their treatments. It was thus possible to study the progression of a disease in an individual and prescribe an individual remedy for it consistent with returning the humors to balance. "New" diseases such as plague, syphilis, or the English Sweat were outside this body of knowledge. They affected many people at once with almost all of the same symptoms. Confronting new diseases forced learned physicians to consider how the disease affected a population and so began the transition to regarding diseases as specific entities with similar symptoms, prognosis, and treatment. By the nineteenth century, this approach had evolved into the ontological view of disease that would be reinforced with the discovery of germs as the causative agents of disease. Even if many aspects of medical theory remained the same, people's perception of disease began to change in the Late Middle Ages.

While the perception of disease was changing, treatment for infectious diseases continued to be rooted in the humor theory of disease with miasmas often seen as causative factors that helped to throw the humors out of balance. Medical men also came to use contagion to explain how some diseases spread from one person to another as Fracastoro did with his treatise.[3] Surgical treatment improved in the late Middle Ages, sparked in part by improved anatomical knowledge arising from dissections and military surgery. Dissection was less helpful in revealing truths about infectious diseases so physicians were left with observation and trying to fit the "new" diseases into older theoretical approaches which was proving to be an increasingly uneasy fit. Until physicians better understood the causative agents for infectious diseases, their success in dealing with infectious diseases would be limited. "New" epidemic diseases helped to bring about a gradual medical revolution not completed until the nineteenth century, but they did not bring about better contemporary treatment of infectious disease.

The medical establishment of physicians and surgeons were not the only prac-titioners to confront infectious disease. Most people did not consult the aris-tocrats of the medical profession but used the services of village practitioners, midwives, cunning folk, quacks, or whatever they were called. At least many of the remedies of some of the non-elite practitioners were less harmful than the bloodletting, purging, or some drug treatments advocated by physicians to return the humors to balance. Village practitioners might not cure, but they may have been less likely to kill their patients than even well-intentioned physicians. From the fourteenth century onward, people could consult a variety of writings concerning medicine and become their own physicians. Most of the works by English authors before the seventeenth century were derivative of continental authors. Initially, most of these authors wrote in Latin, regarded as the language of learned medicine, but a large number of specialized and general works dealing with health appeared in English in the sixteenth century. The physician John Caius apologized for writing in English in his *Boke or Counseil against the Disease Commonly Called the Sweate or Sweatying Disease*, published in 1552, but more works were being written in English such as Thomas Moulton's *This is the Myrour or Glasse of Helth* published in 1531 or the physician William Bullein's compre-hensive *Bulwarke or Defence against All Sicknesse, Soarenesse, and Woundes that Doe Dayly Assault Mankinde*, published in 1579.

The health of the public also came to be the purview of municipal and royal authorities in the late Middle Ages. Governmental officials often adopted an approach based on contagion theory although they might blend it with miasma theory. Local officials were advised by physicians, but their actions tended to be directed to the health of the community, not one individual. Trying to combat the miasmas that they saw as causing the plague, may not have prevented the plague, but they helped in dealing with diarrheal diseases. Improved sanitation may have even helped destroy the habitat for fleas or lice although this is harder to trace. Quarantining plague victims did help to limit the spread of the disease. It was not until the nineteenth century and what the medical researcher Charles-Edward Winslow called "the great sanitary awakening" that filth came under full-scale attack.[4] Quarantine had become a way of life in some fifteenth-century Italian cities, but the practice was slower to catch on in England although some responses to the English Sweat were essentially those of exiling the afflicted per-son from society or withdrawing from society as King Henry VIII did in response to the Sweat. Governments, however, did nothing to deal with the overcrowding that led to the spread of many diseases that were transmitted human-to-human or by vectors such as fleas and lice.

The impact of epidemic disease on society

Everyday diseases such as diarrhea or tuberculosis posed a health problem for English society before and well beyond 1600 and people accepted them as almost a way of life, but they generally did not produce immediate impacts on society. When the number of leprosy cases reached almost epidemic numbers in the twelfth and thirteenth century, it affected social relations and led to the building of leprosaria to treat and isolate lepers, but did not lead to major disruptions to economic or political life. Epidemic diseases were another matter. Widespread coverage in time and space as well as large numbers of the dead gave epidemics the power to disrupt the everyday functioning of society in ways that everyday diseases did not.

COVID-19 has disrupted at least some aspects of life in many countries such as causing a drastic temporary decline in the tourist industry, job losses, substantial loss of life, and suffering for many people across the globe. Some of the changes arising from the COVID-19 pandemic will revert back, but others will become permanent. It is hard to predict what sort of disruptions will arise from a pandemic, but they often change life in many ways for many people.

Commentators often see the First and, especially the Second Plague Pandemics as the standard by which to test the impact of other pandemic disease outbreaks. Although we are learning more about the impact of the First Plague Pandemic, much remains unknown shrouded in a lack of records or in suspect and possibly exaggerated contemporary accounts. It appeared to cause at least temporary disruption in the Byzantine Empire although its impact in England is less certain. The Second Plague Pandemic that started in 1347 and continued until the early eighteenth century in Western Europe, and especially the Black Death of 1347–51 and subsequent fourteenth-century outbreaks provides a classic example of pandemic disease as a disrupter. The loss of life was astounding with more than fifty percent of the European population dying in the fourteenth century outbreaks and with subsequent outbreaks capable of producing a ten percent mortality rate in the total population in any one country. Europe's population had generally returned to pre-plague levels by 1600, but it took more than two hundred years to do this in most countries. Other diseases supplemented the mortality of the plague further helping to hold down population numbers. By comparison, the case mortality rate (deaths of people infected with the disease) of COVID-19 has generally been less than two percent with variations in different places.

Earlier chapters detailed the impacts of various diseases on premodern English society. As might be expected, plague had the largest impact, causing population decline, labor shortages, food shortages, and wage increases as well as affecting religion, art, architecture and building, literature, and the overall mentalité of the people. Reaction to the plague and other epidemics also illustrates human resilience to major misfortune as people got on with their lives somehow. One impact of plague on the mentalité of people across Europe was the fear that the disease produced. In some cases, it led to a search for scapegoats to blame for the disease, in others (much harder to document) it may have produced almost an incapacity to act for fear that the end was near.

Some historians argue that the economic and social disruption arising from the Second Plague Pandemic helped to produce first the Little Divergence and then the Great Divergence, a series of changes that catapulted Europe's economy ahead of the rest of the world. Others have argued for almost no impact, but the proponents of the large impact thesis seem to be carrying the day. The consensus seems to be that plague served as a disrupter of society in many ways.

The period of the "Little Divergence," (1300–1600) is not just about demographic, wage, or productivity changes, it is also about changing outlooks in society. Some of these changes came from the discovery of the New World and subsequent colonization efforts, some came from the printing press and how it helped to make knowledge more accessible, and some came from war and religious and political change. The deaths caused by epidemic disease influenced this changing outlook. The social impact of the "new" diseases, such as how people perceived sick people or how society coped with the diseases is also important. It is too strong to say that a modern outlook appeared overnight, but gradually how people viewed their own societies, what knowledge they considered valid knowledge, and how they viewed the future all were changing. Medical knowledge and theories of disease might be slow to change, but confronting disease, especially epidemics did force at least some people to further develop a questioning outlook that affected various aspects of society.

Plague was not the only disease to affect the outlook of society. Leprosy affected one aspect of how society viewed the afflicted, as people often considered lepers to be the victims of their own sinful nature. In some cases, lepers seemed to have been feared as if their very presence could produce moral decay. Some observers also came to see syphilis, which first appeared in the 1490s, as a disease of moral decay. While some victims bore their affliction as almost an acknowledgement of their cosmopolitan lifestyle, many commentators, especially late in the sixteenth century indicated that a syphilis infection was indicative of the sinful nature of the individual. A fear of disorder in society originating from the perceived immorality of the lower orders often accompanied this fear of sin. Syphilis like leprosy produced a fear of the disease in society for what moral individuals would want to be infected with a disease that proclaimed their immorality. The large number of syphilis infections, like the once large number of leprosy sufferers, also had other impacts from the need to care for the afflicted, to loss of productivity. Unlike leprosy, but like plague, syphilis was a new disease that had not appeared in the existing medical canon. While it did appear to be almost epidemic in coverage at times, syphilis took time to kill so it did not have the sudden impact of the plague. *Sudor Anglicus*, which first appeared in 1485 and last appeared in 1551, could produce a large number of infections and even a substantial number of deaths in a location in a very short period. Its unexpected appearance and status as a "new" disease contributed to the fear it generated. Like syphilis, but unlike plague by the sixteenth century, the English Sweat was no respecter of social class infecting cardinals as well as the poor. The suddenness of the disease and its sudden disappearance contributed to its impact, as did the status of its victims. In reality, the Sweat produced a low mortality rate as it did not sweep across the country infecting almost every place for months on end as did the plague. The fear it generated was out of proportion to its actual impact, but *Sudor Anglicus* contributed to at least short-term disruption such as the canceling of court sittings and was widely feared at the time.

Aside from the plague, the "new" diseases that appeared before 1600 did not cause major disruption although they did contribute to tensions in society. The newly evolved smallpox came to have a similar impact from the seventeenth century onward and influenza gradually had a growing impact throughout the nineteenth century culminating in the pandemic of 1918–1919 that killed between 50 and 100 million people worldwide.

By their very nature, epidemic and pandemic diseases had an impact on society as they captured the popular imagination, affected the economy and social attitudes, and challenged existing views of medicine in ways that everyday diseases could not. Famines and natural disasters such as large volcanic eruptions might produce at least short-term disruption, but not the wide-ranging impact of epidemic diseases in pre-modern England. One group of economists and historians questions whether the impact of epidemics has been positive or negative, indicating that people took away different lessons from them so it is difficult to see a long-term economic impact.[5] War had the potential to have a major impact as the Thirty Years War certainly did in central Europe in the seventeenth century. The Hundred Years War between England and France stretching from the mid-fourteenth century to the mid-fifteenth century had more of an impact on France than England as most of the conflict was fought there, but overall, the Hundred Years War or the War of the Roses did not have the impact of epidemic disease. War changed over time and by the twentieth-century World War I and World War II served as the ultimate disrupters of society. The limited nature of war before 1600 meant that the impact of war was often fleeting, affecting people in one region, or affecting one social group, but it had not yet become the disrupter it became in the future.

Of the diseases examined here, plague had the greatest impact, an unsurprising result given the large number of deaths it produced. It is fair to ascribe at least some of the causative force for the "Little Divergence" and possibly even the "Great Divergence" to the impact of the Black Death. This impact needs further evaluation when the continuing number of plague outbreaks, often with substantial numbers of deaths is factored into the explanatory process. Economic and political changes are highly visible and it is easy to discern the impact of the plague. Other, diseases, however, also affected the political and economic processes of English society although their impacts are harder to trace they often affected social attitudes and local economies, at least in the short term. Epidemic diseases, in particular, also had other impacts on society. The existing medieval medical paradigm survived into the nineteenth century, but cracks were beginning to appear in its explanatory framework, as medical practitioners were unable to explain fully the "new" epidemic diseases of the premodern world with the existing body of medical knowledge.

Understanding the impact of disease in premodern England is a matter of seeing the big issues such as death rates and political and economic change. It is also a matter of observing and explaining issues that might be less visible such as the increasing impact of moralism, in essence blaming the victim, used in explaining who was infected and why. Another part of the explanatory process involves observing the changing medical framework of society. This observation encompasses medical knowledge and the growth of public health regulation by government when existing medical practice was unable to cope with new diseases such as plague or old diseases such as diarrheal diseases. The impact of disease needs to be seen from the perspective of human reaction to disease, reaction that sometimes helped to alleviate problems and sometimes made them worse. The relationship of the environment, especially climate, in helping to foster an environment for disease to appear and spread or to retard it must also be part of this relationship. Human diseases do not exist in a vacuum; they are influenced by a variety of factors that have been noted in specific chapters.

Premodern England did not enjoy the medical advances of the twentieth century such as advanced diagnostic tools or antibiotics and other drug therapies. People coped the best they could, but challenges to health were all around them. Understanding these challenges helps to give us a better understanding of society in the past. Understanding how people coped with disease, especially "new" diseases, also gives us some insight into our current situation. COVID-19 has had a large impact on the world, as it truly is a pandemic disease. A large number of people have died, even more have been sick for some time. Economic loss has been substantial in counties across the globe. Economic distress has not been evenly shared across societies and some commentators call for changes in order to produce more equitable economies. Some commentators have suggested that the impact of COVID-19 will help to lead to a changing work environment in some industrial countries with more people working from home than in centralized locations. In this case, some glimmer of this change has already been underway, and it will be interesting to see if the pandemic furthers a larger paradigm change. At times, fear and scapegoating, not that different than that generated by some diseases in the premodern world, have been present. A variety of remedies have been advanced, some such as vaccines have been successful, others less so, and others downright dangerous. Scientific knowledge and the scientific method have helped in coping with COVID-19 in ways that people in the premodern world could not imagine. Unfortunately, junk science continues to be present and is more accessible than in the premodern world. Perhaps there is more that we can learn from disease and its impact on the premodern world than we would like to admit.

Notes

1 Charles Rosenberg, *Explaining Epidemics and Other Studies in the History of Medicine* (Cambridge: Cambridge University Press, 1992), 306.

2 Roger French, *Medicine before Science* (Cambridge: Cambridge University Press, 2003), 157.

3 Fracastoro, *Contagion*, 3–69.

4 Charles-Edward Amory Winslow, *The Conquest of Epidemic Disease* (Madison: University of Wisconsin Press, 1980 {1943}), 236–66.

5 Bas van Bavel, Daniel R. Curtis, Jessica Dijkman, Matthew Hannaford, Maïka de Keyzer, Eline van Onacker, Tim Soens, *Disasters and History* (Cambridge: Cambridge University Press, 2020), 147.

GUIDE TO FURTHER READING

What follows is a brief indication of useful works starting with general treatments. For the most part, I've confined myself to books with a few articles where book-length treatments are unavailable. I've also tried to indicate recent works for the most part. The references for each chapter provide more fulsome treatment of the secondary literature. Primary sources of two types make up much of the support for this work. The first are those sources that historians regularly utilize such as contemporary chronicles, authors, and governmental documents. The second is not what historians would call a primary source, but these sources are important to the understanding of the science behind the diseases. These sources are reports from scientists concerning aspects of the various diseases and are indicated in the chapter references.

General sources

Although many of his interpretations are out of date, Creighton provides a well-documented discussion of disease in Britain into the nineteenth century. Rawcliffe provides a useful discussion of medieval health problems from the perspective of public health. Cohn describes the human response to epidemics from the Plague of Athens to Ebola in West Africa in 2014. Although some of the essays in Webster are dated, there are insightful treatments of subjects such as medical practitioners, diet, and Paracelsian medicine. Oldstone and Snowden are good, recent general works. Although his focus is largely on the impact of the Black Death, Campbell provides an important discussion of the relationship between climate and disease in the Late Middle Ages.

Bruce M.S. Campbell, *The Great Transition*. Cambridge: Cambridge University Press, 2016.

Samuel K. Cohn Jr., *Epidemics*. Oxford: Oxford University Press, 2018.
Charles Creighton, *A History of Epidemics in Britain*, 2 vols., 2d ed. London: Frank Cass, reprint 1965, (1894).
Michael B.A. Oldstone, *Viruses, Plagues and History*, 2d ed. New York: Oxford University Press, 2020.
Carole Rawcliffe, *Urban Bodies*. Woodbridge: Boydell Press, 2013.
Frank M. Snowden, *Epidemics and Society*. New Haven: Yale University Press, 2020.
Charles Webster, *Health, Medicine and Mortality in the Sixteenth Century*. Cambridge: Cambridge University Press, 1979.

Medical practice and theory

The treatments in these works tend to be weighted in the direction of intellectual medicine, but Rawcliffe and Wear also provide helpful treatments of non-elite practitioners.

Luke Demaitre, *Medieval Medicine*. Santa Barbara: Praeger, 2013.
Roger French, *Medicine before Science*. Cambridge: Cambridge University Press, 2003.
Mirko D. Grmek, ed., *Western Medical Thought from Antiquity to the Middle Ages*. Cambridge: Harvard University Press, 1998.
Carole Rawcliffe, *Medicine and Society*. Gloucester: Alan Sutton, 1995.
Nancy Siraisi, *Medieval and Early Renaissance Medicine*. Chicago: University of Chicago Press, 1990.
Alan Wear, *Knowledge and Practice in English Medicine, 1550–1680*. Cambridge: Cambridge University Press, 2000.

Diarrheal diseases and public health

Articles, noted in c. 2–3, provide the best sources for these health problems although Rawcliffe's *Urban Bodies* addresses some of them.

Piers D. Mitchell, ed., *Sanitation, Latrines and Intestinal Parasites in Past Populations*. Burlington: Ashgate, 2015.

Leprosy, tuberculosis, measles, malaria

Demaitre addresses Europe as whole while Rawcliffe covers England and Bynum provides an overview of measles. Dobson addresses malaria and environmental factors influencing the incidence of the disease in her wide-ranging study. The articles noted in c. 3 provide coverage for measles, tuberculosis, and malaria.

Helen Bynum, *Spitting Blood*. New York: Oxford University Press, 2012.
Luke Demaitre, *Leprosy in Premodern Medicine*. Baltimore: Johns Hopkins University Press, 2007.
Mary J. Dobson, *Contours of Death and Disease in Early Modern England*. Cambridge: Cambridge University Press, 1997.
Carole Rawcliffe, *Leprosy in Medieval England*. Woodbridge: Boydell Press, 2006.

Plague

There is a large volume of works dealing with aspects of the plague. The scientific literature is noted in Greene's article and book below and in the references for c. 4–6. Her *Pandemic Disease* is a collection of articles that first appeared in *The Medieval Globe* in 2015. Slack's work deals with other diseases, such as influenza, in addition to the plague.

John Aberth, *The Black Death*. New York: Oxford University Press, 2021.
Ole J. Benedictow, *The Complete History of the Black Death*. Woodbridge: Boydell Press, 2021.
Monica H. Green, ed., *Pandemic Disease in the Medieval World*. Arc Humanities Press, 2015.
Monica H. Green, "The Four Black Deaths," *American Historical Review*, 125 (2020), 1601–31.
Lester K. Little, ed., *Plague and the End of Antiquity*. Cambridge: Cambridge University Press, 2007.
Paul Slack, *The Impact of Plague in Tudor and Stuart England*. Cambridge: Cambridge University Press, 1985.

Syphilis and the English Sweat

Quétel provides an overview of syphilis and Fabricius focuses on the sixteenth century, but much of the best work is in articles noted in the references for c. 8. The Sweat is addressed by articles in the references for c. 7.

Johannes Fabricius, *Syphilis in Shakespeare's England*. London: Jessica Kingsley, 1994.
Claude Quétel, *The History of Syphilis*. Judith Braddock and Brian Pike, trans. Baltimore: Johns Hopkins University Press, 1992.

Smallpox, typhus, influenza

Several of the references in c. 9 address smallpox although Hopkins provides an overview and the Carmichael and Silverstein article serves as an introduction to some important questions. Typhus receives little coverage and Zinsser's older work is still the best general work although Snowden provides some coverage. There are many treatments of the 1918–1919 influenza pandemic, but only a few articles and sections in larger works found in the references for c. 9 treat earlier epidemics.

Ann Carmichael and Arthur Silverstein, "Smallpox in Europe before the Seventeenth Century: Virulent Killer or Benign Disease," *JHM*, 42 (1987), 147–168.
Donald R. Hopkins, *The Greatest Killer*, (Baltimore: Johns Hopkins University Press, 1983.
Hans Zinsser, *Rats, Lice and History*. New York: Little Brown, 1934.

INDEX

For Product Safety Concerns and Information please contact our EU
representative GPSR@taylorandfrancis.com
Taylor & Francis Verlag GmbH, Kaufingerstraße 24, 80331 München, Germany

*9 7 8 1 0 3 2 1 0 4 1 3 3 *